A Textbook of
PHARMACOGNOSY

THEORY AND PRACTICALS

(Exactly as per ER 1991)
Thoroughly Revised and Remodelled

For Diploma Course in Pharmacy

Seventeenth Edition

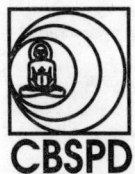

Prof. J.S. Qadry
M.Pharm. (Pb.), D.Sc. (Germany)
MSEI, FGAF (Germany), MASP (USA)

Dean-Director, Shekhawati College of Pharmacy, Dundlod, Rajasthan

Formerly
Professor and Dean, Dubai Pharmacy College, Dubai, UAE
Founder Dean and Vice Chancellor, Hamdard University, New Delhi
Founder Principal, Hamdard College of Pharmacy, University of Delhi
Specialist Advisor, Traditional Medicine, Ministry of Public Health, Kuwait
Head, Deptt. of Pharmacognosy, LM College of Pharmacy,
Gujarat University, Ahmedabad
President, Pharmacy Council of India

CBSPD
CBS Publishers & Distributors Pvt Ltd

New Delhi • Bengaluru • Chennai • Kochi • Kolkata • Lucknow • Mumbai
Hyderabad • Jharkhand • Nagpur • Patna • Pune • Uttarakhand

A Textbook of
PHARMACOGNOSY
THEORY AND PRACTICALS

ISBN: 9787-81-239-2532-5

Copyright © Author

Seventeenth Edition: 2014
Reprint: 2017, 2018, 2019, 2020, 2023, **2024**

Science and technology are constantly changing fields. New research and experience broaden the scope of information and knowledge. The editors have tried their best in giving information available to them while preparing the material for this book. Although all efforts have been made to ensure optimum accuracy of the material, yet it is quite possible some errors might have been left uncorrected. The publisher, the printer and the author will not be held responsible for any inadvertent errors, omissions or inaccuracies.

Published by **Satish Kumar Jain** and produced by **Varun Jain** for

CBS Publishers & Distributors Pvt Ltd
4819/XI Prahlad Street, 24 Ansari Road, Daryaganj, New Delhi 110 002, India.
Ph: 011-23266838, 23289259   Website: www.cbspd.com
                                    e-mail: delhi@cbspd.com

Corporate Office: 204 FIE, Industrial Area, Patparganj, Delhi 110 092
Ph: 011-4934 4934   Fax: 011-4934 4935
                           e-mail: publishing@cbspd.com; publicity@cbspd.com

Branches

- **Bengaluru:** Seema House 2975, 17th Cross, KR Road, Banasankari 2nd Stage, Bengaluru 560 070, Karnataka, India
  Ph: +91-80-26771678/79   Fax: +91-80-26771680   e-mail: bangalore@cbspd.com
- **Chennai:** 7, Subbaraya Street, Shenoy Nagar, Chennai 600 030, Tamil Nadu, India
  Ph: +91-44-26680620, 26681266   Fax: +91-44-42032115   e-mail: chennai@cbspd.com
- **Kochi:** 42/1325, 1326, Power House Road, Opp KSEB, Power House, Ernakulum Kochi 682 018, Kerala, India
  Ph: +91-484-4059061-65,67   Fax: +91-484-4059065   e-mail: kochi@cbspd.com
- **Kolkata:** 147, Hind Ceramics Compound, 1st Floor, Nilgunj Road, Belghoria, Kolkata-700056, West Bengal, India
  Ph: +033-25633055, 033-25633056   e-mail: kolkata@cbspd.com
- **Lucknow:** Basement, Khushnuma Complex, 7 Meerabai Marg (Behind Jawahar Bhawan), Lucknow-226001, UP, India
  Ph: +0522-4000032   e-mail: tiwari.lucknow@cbspd.com
- **Mumbai:** PWD Shed, Gala no 25/26, Ramchandra Bhatt Marg, Next to JJ Hospital Gate no. 2, Opp. Union Bank of India, Noorbaug, Mumbai-400009, Maharashtra, India
  Ph: 022-66661880/89   e-mail: mumbai@cbspd.com

Representatives

• Hyderabad	0-9885175004	• Jharkhand	0-9811541605	• Nagpur	0-8692091830
• Patna	0-9334159340	• Pune	0-9664372571	• Uttarakhand	0-9716462459

Printed at Glorious Printers, Jhilmil Industrial Area, Delhi, India

Preface

During the past decade and a half or so educational institutions in India offering the technical and professional courses have mushroomed without sparing a thought on the resultant imbalance that would ensue in the student-teacher ratio at the teaching level that could also affect the job prospects of the future graduates. With a view to satisfying the legal requirements of PCI and AICTE, the newly established institutions of pharmacy had to appoint different categories of the teaching staff diluting the level of their qualifications and teaching experience, including of those heading the institutions. Needless to mention that the institutions, mostly private, were established by persons not even connected with the field of education let alone pharmacy and allied technical subjects. This new phenomenon impacted the continuity of teachers' learning and the acquisition of professional knowledge and adversely affected professional excellence. The situation led to serious calls for maintaining higher standards for teachers for the benefit of students that required to develop their skills in professional assessments. With fast development of computer technology and its applications in all branches of knowledge, the students deserve new measures to be adopted in teaching by the teaching faculty in both the theory and its practical application.

This scenario calls for the remedy to drastically overhaul the teaching techniques that do not lie in just changing the curriculum and examination system. What is required is adopting new measures to improve students' performance and new ways of teaching and assessment. In fact there is need to undertake concrete attempt for professional development in order to achieve the suggested teaching reform. This further calls for concerted efforts to enhance professionalism in pedagogy through adopting new approaches to the process of teaching and learning by implementing the newly coined dictum: "teach the teachers".

The suggested new approach could have been initiated by PCI under the aegis of Education Regulation Committee (ERC). I am of the opinion that the authors of books on professional subjects can also streamline courses and their topics in a way that makes the process of learning and teaching the subjects in a serially rational characterization of the curriculum. Keeping this in mind I have now authored all my revised editions in different subjects in a way that topics follow each other serially and scientifically. Owing to the nature of its subject matter this new pedagogic approach in pharmacognosy, as per ER 1991, is being followed in letter and spirit, dealing the theoretical course in a separate section for lectures, while conducting the practical course directly in the laboratory in a separate section.

Talking about the present revised and remodelled edition, I have presented the theoretical and practical parts separately to help the new as well as the experienced teachers, as also the students, to treat the whole course in theory and practical classes separately in an easy-to-grasp mode.

The above mentioned approach has also made the book more comprehensive in that the course content is now tackled in two broad sections. Section One deals with Theoretical Topics under Part I, Part II and Part III, while Section Two deals with Applied Work, under Part IV, Part V and Part VI. Included separately at the end are Appendices and Index.

The subject of pharmacognosy or pharmaceutical biology in the past couple of decades has rapidly undergone drastic expansion in the molecular biology/phytochemistry. Thus even though this book is written for the students of diploma course as per the archaic 1991's ER, I feel there is now need for the students to know more of phytochemistry. Hence separation of theoretical syllabus through section one from the inter-mingling practical syllabus through section two will to some extent help to create interest in phytochemical background for both the teachers and the students.

To the globally well known CBS Publishers & Distributors Pvt. Ltd., in particular to Mr. Satish K. Jain, Chairman & Managing Director and Mr. Vinod K. Jain, Production Director, I am thankful for their highly constructive and active cooperation in printing and finishing of the book.

New Delhi   **J.S. Qadry**

A Textbook of
PHARMACOGNOSY

Other Books by Professor J.S. Qadry

- Pharmacognosy (With 140 Colour Photographs), 16/e
- Organic Pharmaceutical and Medicinal Chemistry
  (in 3 Volumes), 3/e
- Textbook of Inorganic Pharmaceutical and Medicinal
  Chemistry, 11/e
- Biochemistry and Clinical Pathology (Theory and Practical)
  – by Pillai / Qadry

Contents

SECTION 2
Applied Work (Practical Course)

Appendices

SECTION 1

Theoretical Topics

- General Introduction
- Phytochemistry: Chemistry of Plant Constituents or Phytochemicals
- Description of Drugs Under Specific Therapeutic Efficacies

General Introduction

PHARMACOGNOSY, HISTORY AND SCOPE

Pharmacognosy

Pharmacognosy is the study of crude drugs obtained from plants, animals and mineral *kingdoms* and constituents obtained therefrom. Even though the science of pharmacognosy has been practised since the advent of mankind, the term Pharmacognosy was first used by **C.A. Seydler**, a German scientist, in 1815 in his book *Analecta Pharmacognostica*. It is derived from two Latin words *pharmakon*, 'a drug', and *gignosco*, 'to acquire knowledge of'. It means knowledge or science of drugs.

Drugs used in medicine today are either obtained from nature or are of synthetic origin. Natural drugs are obtained from plants, animals or mineral kingdom. Drugs from microorganisms like antibiotics were not known in the earlier times. Synthetic drugs or syntheticals like aspirin, sulpha drugs, some vitamins and some antibiotics are synthesized in laboratories from simple chemicals through various chemical reactions.

Natural drugs obtained from plants and animals are called drugs of biological origin and the active principles, because of which they have their therapeutic use, are produced in the living cells of plants and animals.

Crude drugs are plants or animals or their parts which after collection are subjected only to drying or making them into transverse or longitudinal slices or peeling them in some cases. Most of the crude drugs used in medicine are obtained from plants and only a small number comes from animal and mineral kingdoms. Drugs obtained from plants consist of entire plants, while senna leaves and pods, nux vomica seeds, ginger rhizome and cinchona bark are parts of the plants. Though in a few cases, as in lemon and orange peels and in colchicum corm, drugs are used in fresh condition, most of the drugs are dried after collection. Crude drugs may also be obtained by simple physical processes like drying or extraction with water. Thus aloe is the dried juice of leaves of *Aloe* species, opium is the dried latex from poppy capsules and black catechu is the dried aqueous extract from the wood of *Acacia catechu*. Plant exudates such as gums, resins and balsams, volatile oils and fixed oils are also considered as crude drugs.

Further drugs used by physicians and surgeons or pharmacists, directly or indirectly, like cotton, silk, jute and nylon in surgical dressing or kaolin, diatomite used in filtration of turbid liquid or gums, wax, gelatin, agar used as pharmaceutical auxiliaries of flavouring or sweetening agents or drugs used as vehicles or insecticides are treated in Pharmacognosy.

Drugs obtained from animals are entire animals, as cantharides, glandular products, like thyroid organ or extracts like liver extract. Similarly, fish liver oils, musk, bees wax, certain hormones, enzymes and antitoxins are products obtained from animal sources.

Drugs are organized or unorganized. **Organized drugs** are direct parts of the plants and consist of cellular tissues. **Unorganized drugs**, even though prepared from plants, are not the direct parts of the plants and are prepared by some intermediary physical processes like incision, drying, or extraction with water and do not contain cellular tissue. Thus aloe, opium, catechu, gums, resins and other plant exudates are unorganized drugs.

Drugs from mineral sources are kaolin, chalk, diatomite, the well-known *Makardhwaj* and other *bhasmas* of Ayurveda.

HISTORY OF PHARMACOGNOSY

Diseases are born with man and drugs came into existence since a very early time to remove the pain of diseases and to cure them. Thus, the story and the history of drugs is as old as the mankind.

In the early period, primitive man went in search of food and ate at random plants or parts like tubers, fruits, leaves, etc. If he found that no harmful effects were observed, he considered them as edible materials and used them as food. If he found that by their eating other actions were found, they were considered inedible and according to the actions he used them in treating symptoms or diseases. If it caused diarrhoea, it was used as purgative, if vomiting it was used as an emetic and if it was found poisonous and death was caused, he used it as an arrow poison. The knowledge was empirical and was obtained by trial and error. He used drugs as such or as their infusions and decoctions. The results were passed from one generation to another generation and new knowledge was added in the same way.

In India knowledge of medicinal plants is very old and medicinal properties of plants are described in Rigveda and in Atharvaveda (3500–1500 BC) from which Ayurveda has developed. In Ayurveda, the ancient well-known treatises are Charak Samhita dealing mostly with plants and Sushrut Samhita in which surgery is also mentioned. In Egypt, people were familiar with medicinal properties of plants and animals. They were familiar with human anatomy and knew of enbalming the dead and preserving their bodies as described in Papyrus Ebers (1550 BC), an ancient book found in one of the mummies.

Greek scientists contributed much to the knowledge of natural history. Hippocrates (460–370 BC) is referred to as father of medicine and is remembered for his famous oath which is even now administered to doctors. Aristotle (384–322 BC), a student of Plato was a philosopher and is known for his writing on animal kingdom which is considered authoritative even in twentieth century. Theophrastus (370–287 BC) a student of Aristotle, wrote about plant kingdom. Dioscorides, a physician who lived in the first century AD, described medicinal plants, some of which like belladonna, ergot, opium, colchicum are used even today. Pliny wrote 37 volumes of natural history and Galen (131–200 AD) devised methods of preparation of plant and animal drugs, known as 'galenicals' in his honour.

Pharmacy separated from medicine and materia medica, the science of material medicines, describing collection, preparation and compounding, emerged. As mentioned earlier in 1815 Seydler introduced the name pharmacognosy.

Even up to the beginning of 20th century pharmacognosy was more a descriptive subject akin mainly to botanical science and it consisted of identification of drugs both in entire and powdered conditions and concerned with their history, commerce, collection, preparation and storage.

Period 1934–1960

The development of modern pharmacognosy took place later during the period 1934–1960 by simultaneous application of disciplines like organic chemistry, biochemistry, biosynthesis, pharmacology and modern methods and techniques of analytical chemistry, including paper, thin layer and gas chromatography and spectrophotometry.

The substances from the plants were isolated, their structures elucidated and pharmacological active constituents studied. The development was mainly due to the following four events:

1. Isolation of penicillin in 1928 by William Fleming and large scale production in 1941 by Florey and Chain.
2. Isolation of reserpine from Rauwolfia roots and confirming its hypotensive and tranquilizing properties.

3. Isolation of vinca alkaloids, especially vincristine and vinblastine. Vincristine was found useful in the treatment of leukemia. These alkaloids also have anticancer properties.

4. Steroid hormones like progesterone were isolated by partial synthesis from diosgenin and other steroid saponins by Marker's method. Form progesterone by chemical and microbial reaction cortisone and hydrocortisone are obtained.

Antibiotic age

This period is also antibiotic age, as besides penicillin active antibiotics like streptomycin, chloramphenicol, tetracycline and several hundred antibiotics have been isolated and studied extensively.

Some of the important aspects of the natural products which led to the modern development of drugs and pharmaceuticals are as follows:

Isolation of phytochemicals: Strong acting substances such as glycosides of digitalis and scilla, alkaloids of hyoscyamus and belladonna, ergot, rauwolfia, morphine and other alkaloids of opium were isolated and their clinical uses studied.

Structure activity relationship: Tubocurarine and toxiferine from curare have muscle relaxant properties because of quaternary ammonium groups. The hypotensive and tranquillising actions of reserpine are attributed to the trimethoxybenzoic acid moiety which is considered essential. Mescaline and psilocybin have psychoactive properties. Presence of a lactone ring is essential for the action of cardiac glycosides. Likewise anthraquinone glycosides cannot have their action without satisfying the positions at C_3, C_1, C_8, C_9 and C_{10}.

Drugs obtained by partial synthesis of natural products: Oxytocic activity of methyl ergometrine is more than that of ergometrine. In ergotamine, by 9 : 10 hydrogenation, oxytocic activity is suppressed and spasmolytic activity increases. We have already referred to the preparation of steroid hormones from diosgenin by acetolysis and oxidation and further preparation of cortisone by microbial reactions.

Steroid hormones and their semisynthetic analogues represent a multi-million dollar industry in U.S.A.

Natural products as models for synthesis of new drugs: Morphine is the model of a large group of potent analgesics, cocaine for local anaesthetics, atropine for certain spasmolytics, dicoumarol for anticoagulants and salicin for salicylic acid derivatives. Without model substances from plants a large number of synthetics would have been missed.

Drugs of direct therapeutic uses: Among the natural constituents, which even now cannot be replaced, are important groups of antibiotics, steroids, ergot alkaloids and certain antitumour substances. Further, drugs such as digitoxin, strophanthus glycosides, morphine, atropine and several others are known since long and have survived their later day synthetic analogues.

Biosynthetic pathways: Biosynthetic pathways are of primary and secondary metabolites. Some of the important pathways are Calvin's cycle of photosynthesis, shikimic acid pathway of aromatic compounds, acetate hypothesis for anthracene glycosides and isoprenoid hypothesis for terpenes and steroids via acetate mevalonic acid-isopentyl pyrophosphate and squalene.

Progress from 1960 onwards: During this period only a few active constituents mainly antibiotics, hormones and antitumour drugs were isolated or new possibilities for their production were found. From 6-amino penicillanic acid, which has very little antibiotic action of its own, important broad-spectrum semisynthetic penicillins like ampicillin and amoxicillin were developed.

From ergocryptine, an alkaloid of ergot, bromocryptine has been synthesised. Bromocryptine is a prolactin inhibitor and also has activity in Parkinson's disease and in cancer. By applications of several disciplines, pharmacognosy from a descriptive subject has again developed into an integral and important discipline of pharmaceutical sciences.

Scope of Pharmacognosy

To talk about the scope of pharmacognosy now will mean undermining the importance of this branch of pharmaceutical sciences. Pharmacognosy is really that subject which has been continuously contributing all it could for the development of other fields of pharmaceutical and medical sciences. It has led to the discoveries of modern medicines and treatment of diseases.

Pharmacognosy is, therefore, rightly referred to as the mother of the above-mentioned sciences, though some like to call it mother of all the sciences. If the natural products – plants, animals and minerals – were not studied for their origin, occurrence and phytochemicals, the medical science would not have been what it is today.

Pharmacognosy, as mentioned above, has long given us hundreds of drugs, technical products, pharmaceutical aids and many new medicines from plants, many of which have been serving important prototype for improved medicines. The plant and animal kingdoms will surely continue to yield many more substances of pharmaceutical and medicinal values in times to come for the latest and future aliments.

A new role of pharmacognosy concerns the study of the biochemical pathways, which opens new vistas for formation of secondary constituents that can be utilised as drugs.

Given below are some of the contributions made by the subject of pharmacognosy.

PHYTOCHEMISTRY

Phytochemicals are non-nutritive plant chemicals that contain protective and disease-preventing compounds. They are often lumped together under the term "phytochemicals" – *phyto* from the Greek word for plant, denoting their plant origins. More than 900 different photochemicals have been identified as components of food, and many more phytochemicals continue to be discovered today. It is estimated that there may be more than 100 different phytochemicals in just one serving of vegetables. As early as 1980, the National Cancer Institute Chemoprevention Program of the Division of Cancer Prevention and Control began evaluating phytochemicals for safety, efficacy and applicability for preventing and treating diseases. Researchers have long known that there are phytochemicals present for protection in plants, but it has only been recently that they are being recommended for protection against human disease.

Phytochemicals are not yet classified as nutrients or substances necessary for sustaining life. They have been identified as containing properties for aiding in disease prevention. They are associated with the prevention and/or treatment of amongst others at least four of the leading causes of deaths in the United States and elsewhere – cancer, diabetes, cardiovascular disease and hypertension. They are involved in many processes including ones that help prevent cell damage, prevent cancer cell replication, and decrease cholesterol levels. Some phytochemicals work as antioxidants, while others are enzyme inhibitors. One compound might have an impact via several different mechanisms.

Importance of Phytochemicals

Scientists have long known the importance of plants and the chemicals they produce in overcoming disease. Over 25% of all prescription drugs still use plants as their principal ingredient. Research is now starting to reveal that these compelling compounds protect humans, just like they do plants, by keeping degenerative diseases at lower levels or preventing them completely when used on a regular basis.

Discovery of new medicines from plants – Nutraceutical use versus drug development

Little work was carried out by the pharmaceutical industry during 1950–1980's; however, during the 1980–1990's massive growth has occurred. This has resulted in new developments in the area of combinatorial chemistry, new advances in the analysis and assaying of plant materials and a heightened awareness of the potential plant materials as drug leads by conservationists. New plant drug development programs are traditionally undertaken by either random screening or an ethnobotanical approach, a method based on the historical medicinal/food use of the plant. One reason why there has been resurgence in this area is that conservationists, especially in USA, have argued that by finding new drug leads from the rainforest, the value of the rain forests to society is proven and that this would prevent these areas being cut down for unsustainable timber use. However, tropical forests have produced only 47 major pharmaceutical drugs of worldwide importance. It is estimated that a lot more, say about 300 potential drugs of major importance, may need to be discovered. These new drugs would be worth $147 billion. It is thought that 1,25,000 flowering plant species are of pharmacological relevance in the tropical forests. It takes 50,000 to one million screening tests to discover ONE profitable drug. Even in developed countries there is a huge potential for the development of nutraceuticals and pharmaceuticals from herbal materials. For example, the UK herbal materia medica contains around 300 species, whereas the Chinese herbal materia medica contains around 7000 species. One can imagine what lies in store in the flora-rich India!

Technical Products

Natural products besides being used as drugs and as therapeutic aids are used in a number of other industries as beverages, condiments, spices, in confectioneries and as technical products.

The coffee beans and tea leaves besides being the source of caffeine are used as popular beverages. Ginger and wintergreen oil are used less pharmaceutically but are more used in preparation of soft drinks. Mustard seed and clove are used in spice and in condiment industry. Cinnamon oil and peppermint oil besides being used as carminatives are used as flavouring agents in candies and chewing gum. Colophony resin, turpentine oil, linseed oil, acacia, pectin and numerous other natural products are used widely in other industries and are called technical products.

Pharmaceuticals Aids

Some of the natural products obtained from plants and animals are used as pharmaceutical aids. Thus gums like acacia and tragacanth are used as binding, suspending and emulsifying agents. Guar gum is used as a thickening agent and as a binder and a disintegrating agent in the manufacture of tablets. Sterculia and tragacanth, because of their swelling property are used as bulk laxative drugs. Mucilage-containing drugs like isabgul and linseed are used as demulcents or as soothing agents and as bulk laxatives. Starch is used as a disintegrating agent in the manufacture of tablets and because of its demulcent and absorbent properties used in dusting powders. Sodium alginate is used as an establishing, thickening, emulsifying, defloculating, gelling and filming agent. Carbohydrate-containing drugs like glucose, sucrose and honey are used as sweetening agents and as laxative by osmosis.

Agar is used as a laxative by osmosis. Agar is also used as an emulsifying agent and in culture media in microbiology. Saponins and saponin-containing drugs are used as detergents, emulsifying and frothing agents and as fire extinguishers. Tincture quillaia is used in preparation of coal tar emulsions. Saponins are toxic and their internal use requires great care and in some countries internal use as frothing agents is restricted. Glycyrrhiza is used as sweetening agent for masking the taste of bitter and salty preparations.

Fixed oils and fats are used as emollients and as ointment bases and vehicles for other drugs. Volatile oils are used as flavouring agents.

Gelatin is used in coating of pills and tablets and in preparation of suppositories, as culture media in microbiology and in preparation of artificial blood plasma. Animal fats like lard and suet are used as ointment bases. Beeswax is used as ointment base and thickening agent in ointments. Wool fat and wool alcohols are used as absorbable ointment bases.

Thus, from the above description it can be seen that many of the natural products have applications as pharmaceutical aids.

Animal Products

In the introduction it was stated that the drugs are also obtained from the animal kingdom. Animal kingdom, therefore, needs to be given an equal importance and pharmacognosist has to consider the products obtained from the various classes of animals. They, like plants, are also classified into Phyla, Classes, Orders, Families, Genera and Species.

There is an immense interest in the chemistry of many marine creatures, which form a potential source for products derived from animal sources, although these sources are not as large as those from the plants.

The animal products can be obtained from wild or domesticated animals. These two sources of animals roughly correspond to the vegetable drugs in that the wild animals are required to be hunted, while the domesticated animals are cared and reared like cultivated drugs. For detailed study of animal products, the advanced book on pharmacognosy by the same (senior) author may be consulted.

PHARMACOGNOSY AND INDIGENOUS SYSTEMS OF MEDICINE

Indigenous systems of medicine or traditional systems of medicine have been prevailing in almost all the countries of the world. These systems, as primitive as they could be, have been there ever since the mankind existed. The practitioners of these systems have been utilising natural products, mostly plants and animals, based on the knowledge acquired by them from their forefathers' experience.

India has been playing a leading role in practising the indigenous systems of medicine, which have been treating about 80% of India's population highly successfully. There are three well-known traditional systems of medicine, viz.

Ayurvedic, Unani and Siddha systems of medicine. The fourth system of medicine, which has become quite popular during the last century or so, though originated in Germany by the German physician, Samuel Hahnemann, is **Homeopathy.**

Of the other global traditional systems of medicine a mention must also be made of the significant and well respected Chinese system of medicine, which has been having a long, perhaps longer than Indian systems, history as a traditional system based on use of natural products for preparing traditional Chinese medicaments.

It is no surprise that India, which boasts of its age-old use of natural products, and rightly so, should be the first to take the lead in rationally and scientifically developing its indigenous medicines and its art of healing. The Vaids and Hakims, the physicians as they are called in Ayurveda and Unani medicines respectively, who were only recognizing or identifying the herbal drugs, animal products and minerals through their experience, were the ones who welcomed the subject of pharmacognosy, as it helped them to know the biological and geographical sources, identities, macro- and microscopic characters, chemical constituents and correct uses. The advancement brought about by research in pharmacognosy, phytochemistry and pharmacology plus the fact that 80% of India's (as also world's at large) population depends on herbal medicines, the Ministry of Health, Government of India, started a separate department to look after the interests of Indian systems of medicine. The government decided to amend the Drugs and Cosmetic Act 1948 to an Act of 1964, according to which the medicines/formulations were supposed to show/display on the label of the container all the ingredients. The government of India then took very bold steps to bring the Indian Systems of Medicine (ISM) almost at par with the allopathic system of medicine. It formed a separate Ayurvedic and Unani Drugs Technical Advisory Board (AUDTAB) just like the Drugs Technical Advisory Board (DTAB) for allopathic drugs and cosmetic products. The World Health Organisation (WHO) also started looking after the interests of traditional systems of medicine and it came forward to allocate funds and sponsored the development of ISM and other global traditional systems of medicine elsewhere. Thus, presently WHO recognises the traditional/indigenous systems of medicines as such and also additionally as complementary and alternative medicines (CAM) the new and cosmetically decorated words used for the same. This expression also brought the herbal drugs and traditional remedies closer to the allopathic medicine in some way or the other and gave them the chance to boast to an extent that all over the world, including USA, they (herbal remedies/CAM) are becoming more and more useful day-by-day. Surely, the scientific appraisal of these remedies and their modern way of presentation also justified their widespread use as of today. The USA as usual took immediate opportunity to frame rules and regulations for controlling their manufacture, sale and use. Thus traditional remedies with the support of scientific findings and good manufacturing practices are now prescribed and marketed under the caption as complementary and alternative medicines.

For all the above developments, the lead, in my considered opinion, has come from India, where the Indian government under the aegis of its Ministry of Health had started ISM department and separate councils for research in the concerned indigenous systems of medicine.

There are now Central Council for Research in Ayurvedic Medicines and Siddha Medicines and Central Council for Research in Unani Medicines. These councils and other centres and organisations are allocated liberal grants to fulfil their aims and objectives for conducting thorough research to develop the indigenous systems in a way that their practice for treatment with indigenous drugs and formulations is justified. More details on this subject are beyond the scope of this book.

However, since the subject matter of the chapter refers to and deals with the indigenous systems of medicine, it is considered prudent here to in short dilate upon the important indigenous systems of medicine practised in India.

AYURVEDA OR AYURVEDIC SYSTEM OF MEDICINE

The word Ayurveda can be analysed as **ayur** meaning life and **veda**, which means knowledge. Popularly speaking, Ayurveda can be defined as a medical science which helps the human body to keep fit, while providing cures for disease from indigenous plants, animal products and minerals. Another definition given to Ayurveda is:

Ayurveda literally means "science of life and longevity". It is considered to be one of the traditional systems of medicine of India. Ayurveda is a science in the sense that it is a complete system. It is a qualitative, holistic science of health and longevity, a philosophy and system of healing the whole person, body and mind.

Ayurveda is one of the oldest documented healthcare systems with a consistent theoretical basis and practical clinical application. The Ayurvedic system believes that the body becomes susceptible to a host of diseases mainly due to accumulation of various metabolic wastes and toxins in the body. Hence, treatment is directed towards proper elimination of these wastes and toxins from the body.

According to ancient Indian Philosophy, the universe is composed of five basic elements or Pancha Bhutas: Prithvi (*Earth*), Jala (*Water*), Agni (*Fire*), Vayu (*Air*) and Akash (*Sky*). The Pancha Bhutas are represented in the human body as Doshas, Dhatus and Malas. To be healthy, equilibrium of three doshas, seven dhatus and three malas is essential.

The prime aim of the Ayurveda is to restore the balance of the three **Doshas** and ensure good health. The combination of our Doshas is determined at birth and remains by and large constant throughout the lifetime. When at their natural state of balance, our Doshas provide the strength our bodies need to prevent conditions that may allow disease. When out of balance, the body becomes susceptible to disease. Our Doshas can go out of balance due to toxin accumulation, improper diet, climatic conditions, unhealthy habits and stress. In order to derive any benefit from Ayurvedic medicines, it is of utmost importance that we evaluate our constitution on the basis of these three Doshas. The following passages will describe the basics somewhat in more detail.

Ayurvedic theory is profoundly useful in analyzing individual patient's constitution and understanding variations in disease manifestation.

The Ayurvedic framework can be used to structure working models of the unique state of each patient, and to project a vision or goal for a whole state of health, again unique to each case.

Ayurveda offers specific recommendations to each individual on lifestyle, diet, exercise and yoga, herbal therapy, and even spiritual practices to restore and maintain balance in body and mind. Ayurveda sees a strong connection between the mind and the body, a huge amount of information is available regarding this relationship.

This understanding that we are all unique individuals enables Ayurveda to address not only specific health concerns but also offers explanation as to why one person responds differently than another.

Physiological Perception

As stated above, all matter is thought to be composed of five basic elements (*Panchamahabhutas*) which exhibit the properties of earth (*Prithvi*), water (*Jala*), fire (*Tejas*), wind (*Vayu*) and space (*Akasha*). These elements do not exist in isolated forms, but always in a combination, in which one or more elements dominate. According to Ayurveda, the human body is composed of derivatives of the five basic elements, in the form of **doshas, tissues (*dhatus*)** and waste products (*malas*).

DOSHAS: The most fundamental and characteristic principle of Ayurveda is called "**tridosha**" or the Three Humours. Doshas are the physiological factors of the body. They are to be seen as all pervasive, subtle entities, and are categorized into vata, pitta and kapha. **Vata** regulates movement and is represented by the nervous system. **Pitta** is the principle of biotransformation and is the cause of all metabolic processes in the body. **Kapha** is the principle of cohesion and functions through the body fluids. Together, these three doshas determine the physiologic constitution of an individual.

DHATUS: The tissues are classified into seven categories: plasma, blood cells, muscular tissue, adipose tissue, bony tissue, bone marrow and the reproductive tissue.

MALAS: Three main waste products are urine, faeces and sweat.

For the metabolic processes in the body, there are three main groups of biological factors, probably exhibiting enzymatic functions (agnis). **Jatharagni** is responsible for the digestion and the absorption of nutritious substances. During this process, digestion takes place in three stages: first the digestion of sweet (**madhura**) and salty (**lavana**) nutrients, then the digestion of sour (**amla**) nutrients, and finally the digestion of sharp (**tikta**), bitter (**katu**) and astringent (**kasaya**) nutrients. The respective products of these three stages are sweet, sour and sharp.

PANCHABHUTAGNIS: There are five types of biological factors which are responsible for the processing of the five basic elements into a composition useful to the body.

Dhatvagnis: The third group contains seven types, each for the assimilation of the seven tissues. This assimilation takes place successively. From the absorbed nutritious substance, plasma (rasa) is produced first; from plasma, blood (rakta) is formed, then muscular tissue (mamsa), adipose tissue (meda), bony tissue (asthi), bone marrow (majjan) and the reproductive cells (shukra).

Basics of Ayurveda

Pathological perception – Samprapti, the Disease Process

Under normal conditions the doshas, dhatus and malas correspond to certain standards regarding their quantity, quality and function. However, this situation is not static and due to several endogenous and erogenous factors, the doshas may become unbalanced, resulting in disease. Every disease is related to an imbalance of the doshas. Other coherent factors can be: the disturbance of the biological factors (*agnis*), the formation and accumulation of undigested nutrients (*ama*), obstruction of the body channels (*shrotorodha*) and a disturbed assimilation in the tissues.

Ayurveda gives us a model to look at each individual as a unique makeup of the three doshas (*Prakruti*) and thereby design treatment protocols that specifically address a person's health challenges. When any of the doshas (*Vata, Pitta* or *Kapha*) become unbalanced, Ayurveda will suggest specific lifestyle and nutritional guidelines to assist the individual in reducing or increasing the doshas that have become unbalanced. If toxins in the body are abundant, then a cleansing process known as *Pancha Karma* is recommended to eliminate these unwanted toxins.

Pharmacological Perception

The materia medica of the Ayurveda, composed of the five basic elements, has been categorized according to the derivatives of these elements. They include: taste (*rasa*), potency (*virya*), taste of the digestion product (*vipaka*), properties (*guna*), specific properties (*prabhava*) and action (*karman*).

Taste (*rasa*) is six fold: sweet (*madhura*), sour (*amia*), salty (*lavana*), sharp (*tikta*), bitter (*katu*) and astringent (*kasaya*). Each taste is composed of two of the five elements. The condition of the food substances after digestion is also expressed in terms of taste (*vipaka*). However, it can only be sweet, sour or sharp.

The properties (*guna*) are grouped in 10 pairs, each one complementary to the other: heavy and light, cold and hot, fat and dry, slow and sharp, stable and labile, soft and hard, clear and slimy, smooth and raw, fine and massive, and viscous and liquid.

The potency (*virya*) of a drug is defined as its capability to express its property. Sometimes potency is grouped in the same way as the property, but for practical reasons, it is usually expressed in terms of hot (*ushna*) and cold (*shita*).

The specific property (*prabhava*) distinguishes two drugs that have the same taste, taste after digestion and potency: This might be due to the composition of the drug or the location in the body where the drug acts.

Finally the action (*karman*) of a drug on the body is expressed in terms of the three doshas. A drug can increase or decrease the vata dosha, the pitta dosha and the kapha dosha.

The drugs used in Ayurveda are made by several processes from vegetable and mineral raw materials. Mostly plant alkaloids and other phytochemicals are the active ingredients. Obviously, barring some chemical changes, these are mostly natural derivatives.

The Ayurvedic preparations are now-a-days manufactured in modern scientific way and represent all kinds of formulations, like pills, tablets, syrups, pastes, confections, oils, ointments, etc. quite comparable in their presentations with those of allopathic formulations. Of course, Ayurvedic medicines make use of metals like gold, silver, tin, mercury, lead, etc. in the form of *bhasmas* (ashes). In many respects Ayurvedic preparations and their formulations now-a-days closely resemble the Unani medicines/ formulations, both utilizing the natural products. The main difference in both the systems i.e. Ayurvedic and Unani being that Ayurvedic medicines and the system are of purely Indian origin, while the Unani system (see details in the following pages) is said to be Graeco-Arabic system of medicine, which has been enriched by contributions from Greeks, Arabs and Persian philosophers and medical men.

UNANI SYSTEM OF MEDICINE (UNANI TIBB)

The Unani System of Medicine may be described as that system of medicine whose fathers were the ancient Greek physicians. Later on it was adopted by Arabs, who further developed it. Ultimately it reached Europe during the Middle Ages (Fig. 1.1). Muslims called it Unani Medicine because of its origin in Greece, whereas European historians would prefer to call it Arab Medicine.

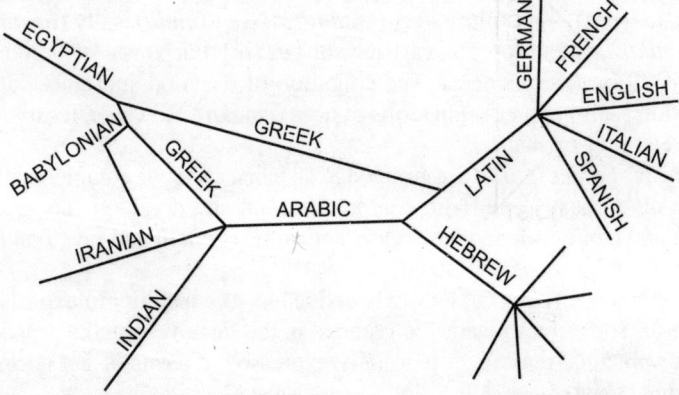

Fig. 1.1. Graphic representation of the course of acquirement of knowledge, showing "that the Arabic tradition was a continuation and revivification not only of Greek science but also of Iranian and Hindu ideas" (George Sarton, 1952).

The disease in the Unani system of medicine varies from person to person. Though disease as a universal phenomenon has common features, yet in Unani medicine it is treated differently according to the different individuals. Unani system of medicine owes much to Greek medicine as well as to Greek medicine philosophy. First it was based on Pythagorean theory of the four proximal qualities: **hot, cold, wet** and **dry elements** (*Arkan*). These qualities are characteristics of the elements *fire, air, water* and *earth*. Conjoined with this is the famous **Hippocratic Humoral Theory**. According to this theory, body has four humors: *blood, phlegm, yellow-bile* and *black-bile*. Each individual has a temperament of his own and these temperaments are four: *sanguine, phlegmatic, choleric* and *melancholic* (*saturnine*). The temperament does not exclude other humors, but only shows the preponderance of any one humor. If blood predominates, the temperament will be sanguine, if phlegm predominates, it will be phlegmatic, if yellow-bile predominates, it will be choleric and lastly, if black-bile predominates, it will be melancholic or saturnine. The humors are given temperaments. Blood is hot and moist, phlegm is cold and moist, yellow-bile is hot and dry, and black-bile is cold and dry.

These bodily humors are surveyed in Fig. 1.2.

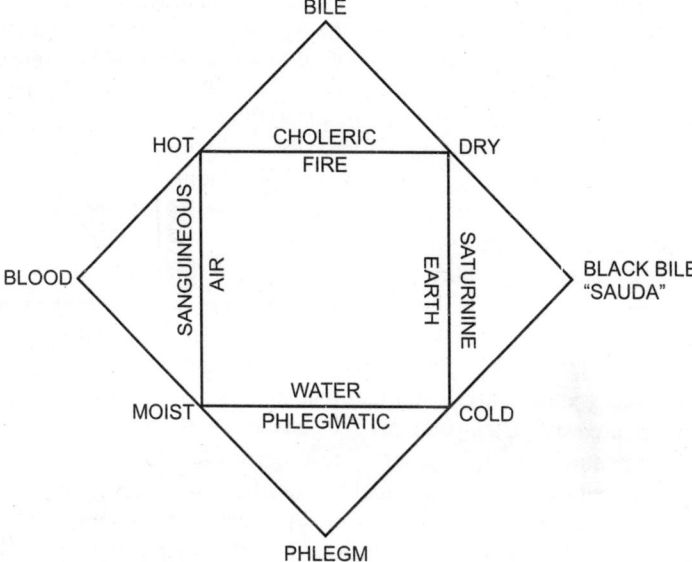

Fig. 1.2. Temperaments, Elements and Qualities representing the view of Graeco-Islamic authorities.

Table 1.1 shows the humors which make up the nature of human body and through which he feels pain and enjoys health.

Table 1.1. Survey of the bodily humors

	Phlegm	**Blood**	**Yellow-bile**	**Black-bile**
Qualities	Cold Moist Salty	Warm Moist Sweet	Warm Dry Bitter	Cold Dry Sour
Seat	Head	Heart	Liver	Spleen
Preponderance in	Winter	Spring	Summer	Autumn

A person enjoys the most perfect health when these humors (elements) are duly proportioned to one another in respect to compounding, power and bulk and when they are perfectly mingled. Pain is felt when one of these elements is in defect or excess, or is isolated in the body without being compounded with all the others. For when an element is isolated and stands by itself, not only must the place which it has left become diseased, but the place where it stands in a flood must become in excess, causing pain and distress. In fact, when more of an element flows out of the body than is necessary to get rid of superfluity, the emptying causes pain. If, on the other hand, it be to an inward part that there takes place an emptying, the shifting and the separation from the other elements, the man certainly must, according to what has been said, suffer from a double pain, one in the place left, and another in the place flooded.

On the basis of humoral theory, for example, abnormal phlegm arising in the head was supposed to be the cause of pneumonia, pleurisy, dropsy, diarrhoea, dysentery, vertigo or sciatica; when phlegm penetrates the blood it is supposed to cause fever or chill.

The "dyscrasia", i.e. the disturbance of the four humors which determined the nature of the disease, was often to be found under unfavourable external influences, such as the seasons of the year, climatic conditions, faulty habits of life and morbid inheritance.

But what is interesting is the fact that in Unani system of medicine even drugs are assigned temperament and that they are to be given according to the temperament of the person. Every person has his own humoral constitution, which indicates a healthy state. If there is any change, his health is disturbed and it is the duty of the physician to restore normalcy. Every individual has within him a power to self-preservation and if the disturbance is not great the state of the health is restored without any medical intervention. One can think the view that the body has within itself a defence mechanism and has the power to restore normalcy within limits is now generally conceded. The Unani system of medicine does not only strive to exploit nature's resources within the organism, but it also aims at helping the organism to attain greater power of resistance after the recovery.

It must, however, be noted that though the scientific and physiological language might strike us as outdated and archaic, we should consider it pragmatically by its results. Let us now leave aside the specific aspects of humoral theory and study carefully the view that every man has his own temperament and that the temperament of every individual requires a specific response from the physician. That drugs also are not just pieces of chemical substances but have different effects with different persons, is a fact which cannot be ignored. What is required is to give expression to the insight of Unani medicine in a different language so as to bring it in tune with the requirements of the present day scientific knowledge.

The Unani system of medicine like any other indigenous system of medicine makes use of drugs belonging to the various sources. A large number of drugs have been used from very early time. The famous Ebers Papyrus believed to have been written about 1500 BC contains collection of prescriptions and formulae covering a wide range of uses. Of these the following drugs have been identified and are still used by the Unani physicians.

Oil, wine, beer, yeast, vinegar, turpentine, figs, castor oil, myrrh, mastic, frankinscense, wormwood, aloes, opium, cumin, peppermint, anise, fennel, saffron, lotus flowers, linseed, juniper berries, henbane, mandragora, poppy, gentian, colchicum, squill, cedar, elder berries, honey, grapes, onion, garlic, acacia and date blossoms.

Among the mineral and metallic substances used by the Egyptians were iron, lead, bitumen, manganese, nitre, vermillion, copper sulphate, white lead, crude sodium carbonate and precious stones were employed in a finely divided condition.

Unani system of medicine uses more than 2,000 drugs in its prescriptions and formulations. A survey of records shows that more than 950 drugs from natural resources have been recognized and are procured and used in routine in most of the Unani Pharmaceutical Manufacturing Concerns. According to the available Unani literature, 186 vegetable drugs are exclusively used in Unani system of medicine. Besides, Unani Tibb claims to use 24 animal drugs and 21 mineral drugs exclusively in its system.

The Unani medicine and compounds, which are purely prepared by using drugs from all kinds of natural resources, comprise of multi-constituent formulations. This means that not only they contain a large number of different drugs but also total constituents (phytochemicals) of the drugs consisting of a formulation.

CLASSIFICATIONS OF DRUGS

VARIOUS SYSTEMS OF CLASSIFICATION OF NATURAL DRUGS

In the study of pharmacognosy drugs are arranged according to the following systems of classification:

1. Alphabetical classification
2. Biological (Taxonomical) classification
3. Morphological classification
4. Chemical classification
5. Pharmacological classification
6. Biochemical classification
7. Geographical classification

1. Alphabetical Classification

The time-tested alphabetical classification is now-a-days considered to be the least disputed way of classification in all walks of life. Pharmacopoeias have always been written on this basic mode of classification. For drugs either Latin names or common vernacular names can be used.

2. Biological (Taxonomical) Classification

In biological (taxonomical) classification, drugs first be classified as plants and animal drugs. At first sight this classification looks appealing; however, many drugs are not entire plants but they are only the parts of the plants, which have been subjected to drying and sometimes peeling and even slicing. Thus, from the drugs, as they occur in commerce, say cinchona bark, it is difficult to identify the plant from which it is obtained. Botanical names' knowledge is, therefore, necessary to classify the drugs in phyla, classes, orders, families, genera and species. In textbooks drugs are arranged under families (N.O.).

3. Morphological Classification

In morphological classification drugs are arranged according to their morphological or external organized or unorganized characters. Thus, all leaves like digitalis, senna and vasaka are grouped under leaf drugs and barks like cinchona, cinnamon and kurchi as bark drugs. Similarly, seeds fruits and subterranean parts are arranged together as organized drugs and laticis, gums, oils, fats, waxes, etc. as unorganized drugs. Dr. T.E. Wallis, a great exponent of this classification, says that if pharmacognosy is to be an independent science, drugs should be classified according to some inherent or intrinsic properties of the drugs. This classification is useful in teaching of practical pharmacognosy. In modem pharmacognosy the importance of this classification is decreasing.

4. Chemical Classification

In chemical classification, as the medicinal action of the drugs is due to active chemical constituents, the drugs are classified according to the chemical nature of their active constituents. Thus alkaloid containing drugs like opium or solanaceous drugs or rauwolfia are arranged under alkaloidal drugs and even according to the chemical nature of alkaloids. Drugs containing cardiac glycosides like digitalis, strophanthus and scilla are grouped together. Similarly drugs containing volatile oils like clove, cardamom and umbelliferous fruits are put together.

5. Pharmacological Classification

Pharmacological classification deals with the grouping of drugs on the basis of pharmacological action of the most important constituent of the drugs on the body or its organs. This classification is also referred to as physiologic or therapeutic classification of drugs. Thus drugs are grouped together as cardiotonic drugs, hypotensive drugs, purgative drugs, anti-diarrhoeal drugs, astringent drugs, anticancer drugs, etc.

6. Biochemical Classification

Recently, biochemical classification which is more natural and takes into account the biogenetic relationship of natural orders is followed. Thus in modem pharmacognosy more importance is given to chemical and biochemical classifications.

7. Geographical Classification

In geographical classification drugs are classified or arranged on the basis of their availability in different parts of the world. Not all the drugs are growing everywhere. Hence this classification is also of some consequence. In fact, in Germany, the renowned pharmacognosist, late Prof. E. Schratz taught pharmacognosy by following this classification under the caption "Wirtsschaftliche Geographie" and supported the geographical, commercial and political roles of drugs.

Natural drugs arranged in important classes are given at the end of the book before the index.

ADULTERATION AND DRUG EVALUATION AND SIGNIFICANCE OF PHARMACOPOEIAL STANDARDS

ADULTERATION

Adulteration literally means an act of making something – material or a product – poorer in quality by adding something seemingly similar of lesser value. In other words, when a drug is made substandard or inferior by mixing it with extraneous (worthless) material or by substituting it with the exhausted drug or by replacing some part/parentage with similar but cheaper material, adulteration is said to have been done. In the worst case an entire lot of a genuine drug material may be replaced by a totally different material with clear and fraudulent intentions. However, it is not always to be taken for granted that adulteration is done intentionally, rather adulteration can take place accidentally with no intention at all on the part of a person who is dealing in adulterated or substandard products, which here are to be considered as natural products, mostly plant drugs, and to a lesser extent animal products. There are many reasons for adulteration.

A. The first and foremost reason being to earn more profits through unfair and foul means. This is the kind of intentional adulteration and the adulterator's intention is clear-cut cheating. Such an act is undertaken when the drug is costly and is in high demand, but is in short supply. Typical example of such a drug is **saffron**.

B. The other kind of adulteration is accidental or unintentional adulteration, which results due to the faulty or unplanned cultivation, careless collection, improper drying after harvesting, unattended transportation and careless storage.

This type of adulteration takes place due to untrained and unskilled workers and by employees with no knowledge and experience in the trade. Some examples of deliberate adulteration are given below.

1. **Mixing of inferior materials:** This kind of material may be a material which is quite akin to the authentic material (drug) i.e. it may be a different species, subspecies, a variety or a chemical race of the same genus as that of the authentic drug. A typical example is that of Indian senna, *Cassia angustifolia*, mixed with other species of *Cassia*, including *auriculata*, *obovata*, the authentic *Anethum graveolens* adulterated by its other species *A. sowa* or its variety, *Ghoda sowa*. Similarly roots of *Rauwolfia serpentina* are considered adulterated with the roots of other species of *Rauwolfia* like, *canescens*, *vomitora* and *hirsuta*.

2. **Substituting exhausted materials:** These are those materials (organized and unorganized) whose active principals are removed, partly or in total, by special methods, e.g. steaming, extracting with water or solvents, followed by special treatment like carefully drying, colouring, etc. to see that the materials retain their original appearance and morphologic characters. Examples of such materials are many like volatile oil containing drugs, like cloves, umbelliferous fruits, cascara, ginger, saffron and others like tea, gentian, jalap, balsams, etc. For details see the description of individual drug.

3. **Substituting similar or closely resembling materials:** In this form of adulteration materials which are somewhat resembling or are similar in kind but have no relation to the authentic materials and are cheaper and easily available are added. In other words, if the drug material is that of a leaf, then leafy material similar to genuine drug is substituted, e.g. leaves of *Ailanthus* are added in place of **belladonna** leaves; leaves of *Phytolacca* and *Scopolia* are added in or substituted for belladonna; leaves of *Xanthium* are added in **stramonium** and **dandelion** in **henbane**, *blown clove* and *stalks* and *mother cloves* allowed in **cloves**; Indian dill is substituted for **European dill**; fixed oil of some seeds/kernels of plants like peach kernel oil is substituted or partly mixed in the **olive oil**; **sterculia** gum is substituted for **tragacanth**. Such examples are plenty and be noted under individual drugs.

4. **Adding useless heavy materials:** This type of adulteration is of worst kind and is done with highly unscrupulous conscience on the part of adulterator. This is done by incorporation in the genuine drug useless material like stones, iron pieces, sand, etc. with a view to increase the weight of the drug to receive more money. In some unorganized drugs, this kind of adulteration is more common. For example **benzoin** is commonly made into lumps putting **colophony**, small-sized stones and sandy/earthy material; **asafoetida** is found to contain small pieces of lime

stone; **opium** because of its dark colour has been found containing lead shots. **Silver-grain cochineal** and **black-grain cochineal** have been found having barium sulphate and manganese dioxide, respectively.

5. **Mixing or overlooking the adventitious material:** In this type of adulteration care is not taken, surely deliberately, to remove the undesirable extra part or portion of the genuine drug material. This is done with a view to increase the volume and weight of the genuine drug. Best examples are the leafy materials like the **solanaceous leaf** drugs, where one finds more sterns than allowed by size. Also **lobelia** shows excessive amount of stem than permitted. In cases of **bark drugs** excessive presence of cork makes the drug adulterated. In **umbelliferous fruits** one finds the pedicels, umbel stalks and thin stem portions. In root drugs many times one finds rhizome portions and older roots.

6. **Adding synthetic products to strengthen the inferior materials:** This is done in products which satisfy to start with organoleptic characters, followed by physical and chemical tests. For example, **citral** is added to the **citrus fruits oil** i.e. **oil of lemon**; benzyl benzoate is added in **balsam of Peru**. Synthetic vanillin is added to unorganized materials. Such type of fortification with synthetic principles is rather more common in nutrition and food products.

7. **Adding or replacing with artificially created materials:** In this kind of serious adulteration some articles resembling the genuine materials (drugs) are artificially or so to say artistically manufactured, so that they simulate the original genuine drugs. A typical and historic example is that of ergot. Portugal's ergot consisted of up to 25% of sclerotium made from flour dough moulded into correct shape and size of ergot sclerotium painted and coloured to resemble the authentic product. Nutmegs have also been similarly simulated from brass-wood pieces to their usual size and shape or by use of mixture of clay and leguminous meal and moulding them in shape, size and colour. Other examples are that of coffee beans and berries. **Beeswax** has also been simulated from paraffin wax which is coloured yellow. Likewise artificial invert sugar has been substituted for honey.

8. **Using powdered waste materials for adulteration of powdered drug materials:** This exercise is done to adulterate a number of powdered drugs like **pepper, liquorice, gentian, nux vomica, cinnamon**. In these powders, powder of olive stone is used. In cinnamon hazelnut, shell powder is added. Some exhausted powdered drugs are used in powders of other drugs. Thus exhausted powdered ginger is added to the **colocynth** and **ginger** powder. There are many examples of this kind of adulteration, which is also very commonly undertaken in other edible materials e.g. in **chilies powder** red sandal's wood powder is added, Powder of neutral materials like almond shells, walnut shells and coconut shells are made use of in mixing these in other genuine drug powders.

EVALUATION OF DRUGS AND NATURAL PRODUCTS

Evaluation means determining identity, purity and quality or activity of the drug. According to Tyler, Brady and Robbers evaluation is expressed as organoleptic (macroscopic and organoleptic), microscopic, physical, chemical and biological evaluation. Both have the same purpose and are expressed differently.

Identity

Morphological Characters

Identity of the drugs if they are in entire condition can be determined by systematic morphological characters, characteristic of each group as leaves, barks, fruits, etc. Thus, seeds of different species of strophanthus, caraway and dill and Alexandrian and Tinnevally senna leaves and pods are distinguished.

Sensory Characters

The sensory characters are colour, smell, taste and consistency. Leaves or herbs like lobelia should be green in colour. If dried in shade they are green in colour but if dried in sunlight they are bleached or pale in colour. Leaves of different species of Mentha as *Mentha piperita*, *M. arvensis* and *M. spicata* can be distinguished by smell. Clove and exhausted clove are distinguished by smell. Cantharides if deteriorated has ammoniacal smell and deteriorated ergot has rancid and ammoniacal smell. Thus, it is possible to distinguish deteriorated drugs by smell. By taste bitter drugs such as gentian, chirata and quassia, sweet drug like glycyrrhiza and pungent drugs like capsicum and ginger can be determined. Consistency, texture and nature of fracture give important information. If leaves are overdried they become brittle and if underdried are flexible. In starchy drugs such as aconite if dried at higher temperature starch gets gelatinised and fracture is horny. Colocynth has loose parenchyma and is compressed easily. Glycyrrhiza is hard and its fracture is fibrous. Fracture of ipecac is brittle, of nux vomica horny and of nutmeg oily.

Microscopic Characters

If drugs are in broken or even in powdered condition they can be identified by microscopic characters. In leaf, in surface preparation types of stomata, trichomes and calcium oxalate crystals, if present, are seen. Similarly in other drugs transverse and longitudinal sections are taken and arrangement of tissues is observed. Bark contains phloem elements and wood contains xylem elements. Aleurone grains are present in seeds only. Some barks such as cinchona contain only phloem fibres, while some such as kurchi contain stone cells, while some such as cascara contain both phloem fibres and stone cells and thus can be identified.

The diagnostic elements such as stomata, trichomes, vessels, fibre stone cells, starch grains, calcium oxalate crystals persist in powdered condition and are used in identification of drugs.

Linear measurements such as diameter of starch grains or length and breadth of fibres and vessels are also useful in identification. Quantitative microscopic constants such as vein islet number, palisade ratio and stomatal index are also important.

Chemical Tests

Group tests such as anthraquinone test or tests of cyanogenetic glycosides or Vitali's test for mydriatic alkaloids, or test of mucilage are used. Sometimes individual tests such as ammonium vanadate and sulphuric acid for strychnine and potassium chlorate and hydrochloric acid emetine are applied. For colophony copper acetate test is used which is used when colophony is met with as an adulterant in other drugs. Iodine test is used for determining Persian and Smyrna tragacanth and sterculia gums. Persian gum contains scattered starch grains. Smyrna contains more starch. Grains and starch is absent in sterculia gum.

Microchemical Tests

Tests are seen on slide as strychnine test. Drugs containing anthraquinone derivatives are microsublimed and colour test and crystals of sublimate are seen. By microprecipitation on slide, as in cinnamon, cinnamic aldehyde is extracted and reacted with dinitrophenylhydrazine. Clove containing eugenol is reacted with sodium hydroxide and observed.

Solubilities

Solubility, especially abnormal behaviours of unorganised drugs towards solvents, is important for identification. Peru balsam is soluble in equal parts of 90 per cent alcohol, but if alcohol is more a turbidity is produced. 5 ml of light petroleum (50°–60°) with 10 ml of castor oil at 15.5° show clear solution. If light petroleum is increased to 15 ml the mixture becomes turbid.

Physical Constants

Physical constants such as specific gravity, refractive index, swelling factor, optical rotation and viscosity are useful in determining the identity, purity and quality. The specific gravity of dill oil containing a higher percentage of dillapiol is more than oil containing less quantity of dillapiol. Paper, thin layer, gas, and now high pressure liquid chromatography give us information not only about the drugs but also about constituents present in the drugs and their quantity. Methods have been developed for quantitative estimation and determining the quality. Thus, in senna sennosides A, B, C and D and aloe-emodin and rhein are seen. Similarly, in belladonna presence of hyoscyamine and hyoscine and absence of apoatropine, a poisonous constituent, is necessary. Constituents of volatile oil can be identified and quantitatively determined by gas chromatography. High pressure liquid chromatography has wide applications including estimation of monoterpene irridoids.

Purity of Product

If foreign organic or inorganic matter is in excess than the pharmacopoeial limits, drug is not according to standard. Organic matter may be innocuous, as parts of the same plant or other plant and is determined by weighing the drug, separating the foreign parts by eye or with a lens and weighing the same. The sample should be representative of entire drug and should be preferably an average of upper, middle and lower parts of the drug from container. Foreign organic matter may be animal, animal excreta, insects or mould and is determined by sedimentation or floatation method. In sedimentation method drug is boiled with chloroform and cooled. Foreign organic matter settles below. It is separated, weighed and identified, if necessary, by seeing under microscope. In floatation method drug is boiled with water, cooled and less dense phase like mineral oil is added. Organic matter is separated in the upper part and identified and determined as above. If the drug is deteriorated much and even if the foreign organic matter is within limits, it should not be used.

Foreign Inorganic Matter

If the drug is not properly prepared, or if coated, total ash of the drug is more. Total of unpeeled drugs is more than those of peeled drug. In case of rhubarb total ash varies within wide limits and so acid-insoluble ash determination is carried out. Total ash is treated with hydrochloric acid and the remaining ash is acid-insoluble ash. In senna leaves acid-insoluble ash determination is important because of possibility of sand being admixed and should be used only if sample passes acid-insoluble ash standard. Trichomes containing drugs as hyoscyamus with glandular trichomes have capacity of retaining clay and in these drugs acid-insoluble ash may be more.

In cases of exhausted drugs such as ginger or tea total ash is not very critical and water-soluble ash determination is also carried out. In Pharmacopoeia, sulphated ash determination is also recommended. If moisture is more than the limit, drug is inferior. Moisture determination is carried out by heating the drug at 100°C till the weight remains constant and by loss of weight moisture is determined. Moisture is determined by adding a solvent immiscible with water like toluene or xylene and distilling the same and collecting the distillate in a measuring cylinder and reading the level of water. Moisture is also determined by Karl-Fischer method.

Purity of the drug is also determined by crude fibre and fluorescence analysis.

Quality or Activity

During collection attention is paid to macroscopical characters. Digitalis stored for many years and not having medicinal activity will by identified as digitalis. Similarly, exhausted or over-fermented gentian containing less percentage of bitter glycosides is identified as gentian. Thus, it is important to determine medicinal activity or quality of the drugs. For determining the activity physical, chemical, biological or microbiological methods are used.

Physical Methods

In mucilage-containing drugs swelling factor, in gums viscosity, in saponin-containing drugs froth number and in anethole-containing drugs congealing point are used for determining the quality. Further soluble extractives of different solvents such as water, alcohol, light petroleum are useful to some extent in determining the activity of the drug. In gentian water-soluble extractive is not less than 33 per cent. In overfermented or exhausted gentian this value is less. Water-soluble extractive is useful in cascara, quassia and glycyrrhiza. In ginger, ipomoea, jalap and buchu leaves, alcohol-soluble extractive is used. In asafoetida, catechu and myrrh, alcohol-insoluble matter should not be more than the standard. In colocynth if light petroleum extract is more it suggests that seeds containing fixed oil are more than the limit. The insoluble matter gives information about adulterants and impurities. Besides the above other physical constants such as specific gravity, optical rotation, refractive index and melting point give information about the activity as well as active constituents like alkaloids, volatile oils, fixed oils, etc.

Chemical Methods

The chemical methods are gravimetric, volumetric, colorimetric, fluorimetric and spectrophotometric. By chemical assay total alkaloids in solanaceous drugs or individual alkaloids, like strychnine in nux vomica, resin in jalap and podophyllum, volatile oil or eugenol in clove, carvone in caraway and dill and allyl isothiocyanate in black mustard are determined. By colorimetric method alkaloids of Solanaceae by Vitali-Morin reagent, ergot alkaloids by p-dimethyl aminobenzaldehyde reagent and vitamin A by antimony trichloride reagent are determined. Quinine in cinchona bark and reserpine in rauwolfia are estimated by fluorimetric method. In anthracene drugs, free and combined anthracene derivatives, lobeline in lobelia and strychnine in nux vomica are determined in visible or UV region. Anthracene derivatives are determined at 510 nm maxima and strychnine at 254 nm maxima in UV.

Biological evaluation

When evaluation is to be done by above methods biological evaluation on living tissue or living organisms is carried out. Cardiac glycosides-containing drugs like digitalis are bioassayed on cat, frog or pigeons. Evaluation of ergot is done on cockscomb or rabbit intestine or rabbit uterus. Saponin is assayed by haemolytic index. Saponins are toxic to lower organisms and are assayed on fish known as fish index and tubifex worms. Anthelmintic drugs like male fern are evaluated on earth worms. Curare and tubocurarine cause relaxation of muscles and evaluation is carried out by rabbit head-drop method. In ophthalmology local anaesthetics are evaluated on eyes of rabbit. According to Claus biological activity is seen under microscope of living transparent organisms Daphnae and thus purgative activity of cascara, cardiotonic activity of digitalis and depressant action of veratrum are seen. For assay of vitamins mice with corresponding avitaminosis are used. Some bacteria like *Staphylococcus aureus* are used for the determination of phenol coefficient and antiseptic value. Certain bacteria are used for antibacterial activity. For bitter drugs like gentian and quassia bitter value, for sweet drugs like glycyrrhiza sweet value, and for pungent drugs like capsicum and ginger pungency value are determined.

Microbiological Assays

Microbiological assays are used for assay of living bacteria, yeast, moulds and some vitamins like B_{12}, riboflavin, nicotinic acid and antibiotics.

SIGNIFICANCE OF PHARMACOPOEIAL STANDARDS

A plant drug or herbal medicine has been defined by WHO (1993) as a plant derived material or preparation with therapeutic or other benefits which contains either raw or processed ingredients from one or more plants.

Active principles of plant drugs exist in a complex environment along with several other inactive, and/or neutral constituents of varied nature and composition. Therefore, a large number of tests and methods are required to determine the identity, strength, quality and purity of these drugs. In addition, the undesirable or harmful substances present in the material need to be evaluated to ensure the safety and efficacy of the material.

Many plant drugs and their preparations (e.g. extracts, tinctures, elixirs, syrups, mixtures, inhalants) are official in pharmacopoeias such as European Pharmacopoeia (EP), British Pharmacopoeia (BP), United States Pharmacopeia/National Formulary (USP/NF) and Indian Pharmacopoeia (IP) and their methods of quality control according to the prescribed standards are well established. Persons engaged in the quality control of plant drugs and their preparations should be well-versed in the use and application of modem instrumental techniques to ensure the accuracy and reliability of their results.

The significance of pharmacopoeial standards is evidenced through the tests and methods employed in the above mentioned pharmacopoeias for the determination of identity, strength, quality and purity of plant drugs and their preparations. In the forthcoming description one can see at a glance to which drug or preparation a certain test or method has been applied for a particular purpose.

Based on above observations of the pharmacopoeial methods, plant drugs may be classified, to a large extent, into the following three groups:

1. For which only the standards of purity (physical and chemical constants) and limits of impurities (specific/non-specific, metallic) are given. Examples: Most of the essential oils and fixed oils.
2. For which standards of identity, purity and limits of impurities are given. Examples: Gums, agar, some fixed oils, ginger, balsams, starch, cellulose, etc.
3. For which standards of identity, strength, purity and limits of impurities are given. Examples: Alginic acid, aloes, belladonna, benzoin, caraway, cascara, digitalis, inulin, ipecac, opium, podophyllum, rauwolfia, resins, senna, some essential oils and fixed oils, etc.

The various tests and methods used to determine the identity, strength, quality and purity of plant drugs and their preparations according to pharmacopoeial specifications (EP, BP, USP, NF and IP and Ayurvedic Pharmacopoeia of India) are as follows:

I. **Identification tests and purity assessment**
   - A. Macroscopic and microscopic examination
   - B. Test for bitterness value
   - C. Chemical identification tests
   - D. Chemical tests for rancidity (oils)
   - E. General physical methods
   - F. Spectrophotometric methods
     - i. Ultraviolet and visible spectrophotometry
     - ii. Infrared spectrophotometry
     - iii. Fluorimetry
   - G. Chromatographic methods
     - i. Thin-layer chromatography
     - ii. Gas-liquid chromatography

II. **Assay methods**
   - A. Chemical methods
   - B. Instrumental methods
   - C. Biological methods
   - D. Microbiological methods

III. **Limit tests**
   - A. Determination of specific impurities/contaminants/adulterants
   - B. Determination of non-specific impurities/contaminants

Further details in connection with tests and methods are beyond the scope of this book. IP and the Ayurvedic Pharmacopoeia of India may be consulted for individual tests and methods.

In this book, however, drugs are described as per the requirement of the syllabus, prescribed by the Pharmacy Council of India (PCI) for the Diploma in Pharmacy Course.

CULTIVATION, COLLECTION AND PREPARATION OF CRUDE DRUGS

This chapter 8, given as Chapter 6 in the syllabus, is again inconsistent in that it does not mention the intended concrete subject matter of the content of the chapter. It mentions partly a repeated version, but a better or somewhat more comprehensive version, of the words used as occurrence and distribution in Chapters 4 and 5 of the syllabus. However, one is left to infer that the chapter should deal with cultivation, as the drugs, Ergot, Opium, Rauwolfia, Digitalis and Senna, given as examples, and for that matter any other drug, cannot be collected and prepared for the market as crude drugs, unless they are first cultivated. Hence, in this Chapter 8 it is deemed necessary to describe cultivation and its importance followed by collection and preparation of crude drugs for the market as exemplified by ergot, opium, rauwolfia, digitalis and senna. Needless to mention here that these five drugs have already been discussed under the pharmacognostic scheme in Chapter 6, and the readers' attention would be drawn to each one of them as and when the need be.

CULTIVATION OF MEDICINAL PLANTS

At present one finds it difficult to have a regular production and adequate supply of the proper and authentic raw material from plant origin. This is obviously due to the fact that the wild growing plants' resources are shrinking, due to not only partly the climatic changes and ruthless collection, but also due to the encroachment of civilization and continued urbanization. Besides, the producers/farmers find it difficult and unprofitable to produce/cultivate, harvest and prepare for market for which processes include controlled drying, garbling, packaging, storage and proper preservation. However, due to the present unlimited popularity of the use of complimentary and alternative medicines (CAM), a large number of drug houses and agencies have come forward to undertake the controlled production for self-utilization and for the market of those plant drugs that form part and parcel of CAM formulations.

In the following paragraphs it is intended to give a brief account of the processes and techniques used for the production of natural drugs.

COLLECTION AND PREPARATION OF DRUGS FOR THE MARKET

As stated above you cannot collect the drugs and prepare them for the market unless they are produced and are there (!). And thus to produce them they are required to be cultivated (or obtained from naturally occurring wild sources). Hence, the chapter will understandably first deal with cultivation, followed by collection and preparation.

Cultivation

Indian subcontinent represents quite different topographic regions and climatic conditions which enables us to produce wide variety of vegetation. The subcontinent, known to be one of the world's twelve biodiversity centres, also encompasses sixteen different agro-climatic zones in which about 45,000 plants species occur. This number represents about 20% of the total global species. It is estimated that of these about 35,000 higher and lower plant species are of medicinal values. Further, Indian forest land affords us about 80% medicinal and aromatic plants which are being collected from the available natural sources. Since they are used in the indigenous systems of medicine and are also exported, an over-exploitation of some important medicinal plant species necessitates their cultivation not only to get their regular supply but also to improve the quality of drugs. Besides, the current and continued popularity of Complementary and Alternative Medicines (CAM) based on plant drugs, the demand for the cultivation of medicinal plants has increased many folds. India is one of the major suppliers of natural products to some developed countries like USA, Germany, France, Switzerland, etc. In view of the fact that the United States of America has taken ultimate interest in the Complementary and Alternative Medicines (CAM) and have gone to the extent of framing under its FDA the rules and regulations and laws to govern the manufacture, sale and intricate utility (with some cautionary notes on the products like "These statements have not been evaluated by the Food and Drugs Administration. This product, e.g. "Osteo Bi-Flex" *www.osteobiflex.com*, is not intended to diagnose, treat, cure or prevent any disease) of such products, the whole world is now coming forward to follow suit. This latest obsession and use of CAM's formulations has further given the fullest justification and further impetus to the indigenous systems of medicine practised in India and elsewhere, like Ayurveda, Unani, Siddha and even Homoeopathy (this system though originated in Germany is now naturalized in India and has claimed its importance as one of the four indigenous systems of medicine), resulting in the use of rich wealth of medicinal plants. The World Health Organization (WHO) has recognized that about 80% of the world's population depends on traditional systems of medicine for its primary health requirements. According to WHO more than 21 plant species are found useful in the traditional systems of medicine. The global market now utilizes herbal plants to the extent of about 85 billion dollars. The Planning Commission of Government of India has established a task force to see that the Indian market should grow from its insignificant 0.5% share to about 15%. Hence, the cultivation of medicinal plants opens a new vista for medicinal plants industry in India. This, in turn, necessitates acquiring technologies and latest techniques for regulated and properly programmed cultivation of medicinal plants. Since CAM has now become popular all over the world, the natural products (medicinal plants, their organs/parts and extracts derived from them) trade is looking to procure them from India for the production of pharmaceuticals, nutraceuticals and cosmeceuticals (aroma therapeutic) preparations.

In the following pages overall information about the general methods of cultivation of the important medicinal plants, discussing especially the ones included in the syllabus i.e. ergot, opium, rauwolfia, digitalis and senna, will be given. A short to moderate account of cultivation has already been given under each of the above drugs. Yet under this chapter additional information, especially concerning the collection (harvesting) and preparation, as expected in the syllabus for information of students, will be given.

Cultivation, in a nutshell, is a well-known activity or process undertaken for growing crops of grains, cereals, vegetables and medicinal plants (all those not obtained from wild plants, and they are now many, more than 90%, as wild locations are now few and far between, having been fully exploited or urbanized). Hence, such drugs which are exclusively procured from cultivated plants need special requirements and treatments in terms of soil, quality of seeds and other forms of vegetative propagations, supply of water for irrigation, including the consideration of extent of rainfall, climatic conditions – proper temperature, humidity, etc. A detailed general account of process of cultivation, including the conditions and requirements thereof, is beyond the scope of the readers of this book.

COLLECTION

The chapter in the syllabus refers, as stated above, to only collection and preparation of drugs, without mentioning cultivation. Collection is actually followed by cultivation. Of course one can argue about collection from wild plants; but how many drugs are now collected from wild sources? Hence, consideration of cultivation and harvesting of drugs has to be a part and parcel of this Chapter 8.

Collection of medicinal plants (drugs) and their parts i.e. representing actual organs comprising of drug e.g. flowers (clove), fruits (coriander, cardamom), leaves (digitalis, senna), roots (belladonna, ipecac), barks (cinchona, cinnamon), woods (quassia), etc. is undertaken at a particular season and by skilled workers (or unskilled natives in case of wild growing plants). Collection (harvesting?) is done by taking into consideration the age of the plant, nature of the active constituents, their quality, composition and quantity at a particular season and even at a particular time of the day.

The mode of harvesting, as mentioned above, though varies with each kind and type of drug, yet the use of mechanical devices (use of machines) is now-a-days preferred due to economic reasons.

There are a large number of agencies in India and abroad which are now engaged in the production of crude drugs. Such agencies, both governmental and private, are located in different regions in India, where the soil and climatic conditions are best suited for the production of medicinal plants and drugs procured from them. Such areas are in and around hilly regions like Nainital (Ranikhet), Dehradun, Darjeeling, J&K State, Kullu and Manali, and some districts in Punjab, Gujarat, Maharashtra, Karnataka, Assam, etc.

DRYING

Drying follows harvesting and is intended to dry the material, as such or after cutting into smaller pieces or separating the parts required, to remove the moisture and ensure proper preservation of the material. It is done to prevent moulding, undesirable action of enzymes and bacteria and changes – chemical and others – taking place in moisture. Drying should take place soon after harvesting as this will stabilize the chemical constituents and reduce the weight due to loss of water. Further, there are many more reasons for quick, proper and controlled drying. Controlled drying operation requires control of temperature, air circulation and duration of drying and the operation also takes into consideration the nature of the material to be dried. The drugs can be dried by use of sun or by artificial heat. Sometimes drying shades are constructed in and around the field to dry the material under shade and in controlled temperature, humidity and air circulation. Artificial drying is more rapid and is desired in tropical countries. In Europe continuous belt dryers are used and generally leaves, herbs and flowers are dried at temperature between 20–40°C and harder tissues containing organs like roots, woods and barks between 30–60°C. Drugs containing volatile oils should be dried immediately and with great care. Hence, the drying operation is determined by experience depending upon the type of plant parts to be dried and the required final appearance of the material.

Sometimes enzymatic action is desirable and is facilitated. In such cases delayed or slow drying at moderate temperature is necessary.

More discussion with intricacies of the drying processes based on conventional artificial heat dryers and machines with examples does not merit consideration here. However, the drugs mentioned as examples in this chapter will be dealt with in detail.

The **preparation of drugs** for the market does not end here i.e. after cultivation, collection (harvesting) and drying. Rather the product, as obtained above, further undergoes other processes like garbling and sorting or selection.

Garbling, which means removal of unwanted material, is the final step in the preparation of drugs for the market.

Selection or **sorting** into grades is sometimes referred to as **"working"**. **"Garbling"** essentially should form the part and parcel of the chapter; as it is concerned with the removal of unwanted extraneous matter like other parts of the same or other plants, stones, dust and other admixed adulterants termed also as **foreign matter**.

"Working" meaning sorting into grades is not essentially included in preparation, as it is intended for grading the same material for consideration other than purifying and garbling the material. It is done from a commercial point of view.

Adulteration: Adulteration is yet another topic which may be considered during the preparation of crude drugs for the market or commerce. The consideration of adulteration here is being made just to introduce the students that the drugs can be said to be adulterated if they are found mixed with another material, intentionally/deliberately or by accidents. Deliberate adulteration is done in cases of drugs which are either costly (like saffron) or are in short or limited supply. This is now very common with those materials which are illegally and secretly sold (like opium, cocaine, Indian hemp, heroin, LSD, etc.). For more details see Chapter 3 on Adulteration and Drug Evaluation.

Evaluation: Another important aspect that the commerce in crude drugs has to bother about is the evaluation of crude drugs. The evaluation involves the authenticity of the drugs, their quality and ultimate purity. For the determination of quality and purity, there are certain standards (numerical values – biological, physical and chemical) laid down in pharmacognosy books, other standard reference books and in pharmacopoeias and formularies. A detailed discussion concerning the determination of adulteration, quality and purity of drugs, as also the factors which affect the quality during collection, drying and storage is given in Chapter 3.

Chapter 6 includes the following five drugs whose cultivation, collection and preparation for the market is to be discussed in the light of foregoing discussion. They are: **Ergot**, **Opium**, **Rauwolfia**, **Digitalis** and **Senna**.

ERGOT

A detailed systematic pharmacognostic account has already been given in the last chapter. However, here a brief outline in respect of its production (cultivation!!) is being given. Appearance or discovery of ergot in olden days was surrounded by mythical consideration. Little did the ancients, aware as they were about "Saint Antony's fire", know how ergot came into being? It is now known that ergot sclerotium is a result of two totally different types of plants, which represent highly diversified species, namely *Claviceps purpurea*, a lower plant of the family Clavicipitaceae and *Secala cereale*, a higher plant of the family Graminae. The sclerotium of *Claviceps purpurea* develops on rye plant, the *Secale cereale*.

Now it can safely be said that ergot is cultivated, as a field is utilized for the cultivation of rye plants. The flowers of rye are utilized for the development of sclerotium of *Claviceps purpurea*. This mode of obtaining or developing ergot from the rye plant flowers is called parasitic. The other mode of producing ergot is saprophytic source. In this case ergot is produced by germinating spores in a nutrient medium in a laboratory (i.e. saprophytic growth), producing hyphae. The hyphae produce mycelium and conidiophores saprophytically in submerged culture. Thus, it can be said that ergot alkaloids on commercial scale can be produced from both parasitic and saprophytic sources and the quality and quantity as also composition of alkaloids produced from these two sources depend upon a number of factors, like the kind of strain used.

The life cycle of ergot fungus, which in nature is parasitic, is quite interesting, through a bit difficult, when one has to understand the different methods of production of alkaloids by both parasitic and saprophytic means. The fields are utilized for growing the rye plants, and now-a-days the flowers of rye are artificially inoculated with cultured conidiophores of *Claviceps purpurea*. Earlier, before the introduction of modern method of inoculation as stated above, the fungus invaded the rye plant fields and the ergot sclerotium used to be harvested/collected with rye grains.

For further details of the production of ergot via its life history, the student is advised to read the pharmacognostic account 011 ergot.

OPIUM (*Papaver somniferum*)

This is a plant which can only be cultivated under an excise license issued by the Excise Department of the State Government concerned. The cultivation of opium is also restricted to about 25,000 hectares in the districts of:

i. Neemach, Mandsur and Ratlam in Madhya Pradesh;
ii. Faizabad, Bara Banki, Bareilly and Saharanpur in Uttar Pradesh; and
iii. Chittoor, Jhalawar and Kota in Rajasthan.

The plantation is undertaken in a well-drained, fertile, clayey loam to rich sandy-loam soils, in moderately cool weather and open sunny locations. The crop is given, in all, about 15 irrigations.

The seedlings are thinned to keep 25–30 cm between two plants, weeding and hoeing are done regularly once a month. The crop is saved from the attack of leaf-minor (*Phyllocnistis* species) by spraying it with 0.2 % Metasystox. The plants flower in about 80 days in U.P. and in about 105 days in M.P. The petals fall in 3–4 days. While the capsules mature in about 10 days for lancing.

The collection of opium and preparation for market is given under opium.

RAUWOLFIA

The plant (*Rauwolfia serpentina*) on an average grows to a height of about one metre. Earlier the drug has been collected from wild plants. Nowadays the drug is systematically cultivated in many favourable locations in India. Another species which is also cultivated successfully is *Rauwolfia canescens*. The cultivation, collection and preparation of the drug i.e. Rauwolfia is discussed under the complete pharmacognostic scheme of the drug.

DIGITALIS

Digitalis has been occupying a very important place in medicinal plants, belonging to the important group of cardenolides.

The species *Digitalis purpurea* has been of common occurrence in England and is naturalized in North America. In Kashmir it is found along with *D. lanata*, which it can be said now occupies rather more important a place than the all time famous *D. purpurea.*

The plant is cultivated and collected very carefully and its preparation for market and storage calls for strict control of processes, than is the case with most of the other crude drugs. Thus, the pharmacopoeias and other treatises mention the storage and its conditions in detail.

The general pharmacognostic description of digitalis under Chapter 6 includes the cultivation, collection, preparation for market and storage conditions and the readers are advised to see the same.

SENNA

There are two products of senna plants, namely senna leaf and senna fruit. The senna plant, *Cassia acutifolia* has been earlier growing wild in Egypt and Sudan, but now-a-days they are also cultivated there, However, the Indian plant *C. angustifolia* is now cultivated in Southern India, especially in Tinnevalley. Most of the commercial supply comes from India. Senna, as a purgative, is highly esteemed and is found in a number of CAM formulations globally.

The cultivation, collection and preparation for market of senna leaf and senna pod are outlined under the pharmacognostic schemes of these drugs and the author does not feel necessary to reproduce the same here.

Chapter

2

Phytochemistry
Chemistry of Plant Constituents or Phytochemicals

According to the syllabus of Pharmacy Council of India, this chapter should deal with "brief outline of occurrence, distribution, outline of isolation, identification tests, therapeutic effects and pharmaceutical applications of alkaloids, terpenoids, glycosides, volatile oils, tannins and resins". The authors note that there is no mention of certain groups or classes of phyto-chemicals, like carbohydrates, fixed oils and proteins and even enzymes in the above named phytochemicals classes by the PCI in its syllabus. This may surely be an oversight either at the time of framing the syllabus or at the time of typing/printing, as these are included in the syllabus under drugs and pharmaceutical aids and necessities belonging to the classes of carbohydrates and fixed oils, fats and waxes and proteins and enzymes. Besides, knowledge of the chemistry of carbohydrates becomes all the more important in the study of phytochemicals, as a large number of phyto-chemicals, e.g., glycosides and glycosidal alkaloids, etc. have carbohydrate compounds associated with them very intimately as an entity in their chemical structures.

Further, the current pharmacognostic syllabus as per the existing E.R. requires the drugs to be discussed under the suitable pharmacognostic scheme according to the therapeutic efficacy (on the physiological and pharmacological bases) (see next chapter). This requirement as also the fact that the students be exposed first to the easier and less complicated phytochemicals, it is considered prudent that the different classes of phyto-chemicals be described starting from easier groups like carbohydrates, proteins, essential oils and fixed oils followed by glycosides, alkaloids, etc.

PHYTOCHEMISTRY

Phytochemistry, literally, is the chemistry of plants or chemical constituents of plants. Phytochemistry, as it is understood in Pharmacy, is the chemistry of natural products used as drugs or of drug plants with emphasis on biochemistry.

The constituents are therapeutically active or inactive. The inactive constituents are structural constituents of cell wall, like cellulose, lignin, suberin, or reserve constituents of the plants like starch, sugars or proteins. The inactive constituents have, however, other pharmaceutical uses. The active constituents are secondary metabolites like alkaloids, glycosides, volatile oils, tannins, etc. They are single substances or usually mixtures of several substances.

The plant, during biosynthesis, produces carbohydrates, fats and proteins and these are called primary products of metabolism as they are utilised by the plant when required. The secondary products of metabolism are formed from primary products, and the plant is not able to utilise them and they are deposited in the cells and so they are called secondary metabolites.

CARBOHYDRATES AND RELATED COMPOUNDS

Carbohydrates

Carbohydrates, as the name suggests, are compounds which are made up of carbon, hydrogen and oxygen elements. The proportion of hydrogen and oxygen elements is usually the same as that in water (H_2O). Carbohydrates are amongst the first or primary products resulting from the process of photosynthesis. They form by far the largest proportion of the plants biomass, being responsible for the structural and skeletal cellulose and other rigid cellular framework. Carbohydrates supply energy and provide important food reserve as starch in plants and as glycogen in animals. They are precursors of biosynthesis of fats and proteins and secondary metabolites and phytoconstituents like alkaloids, glycosides, etc. Mucilages found in certain plant organs including seeds, e.g. psyllium and gums, formed in plants as normal, physiological or abnormal pathological products, e.g. acacia, are similar to carbohydrates in composition and properties, as they are made up of uronic acid and sugar molecules. Carbohydrates find universal application and are of great medicinal, biochemical and pharmaceutical importance and use.

Carbohydrates are classified into two following groups:
1. Sugars or saccharides
2. Polysaccharides

Sugars or Saccharides

Sugars or saccharides may be monosaccharides, disaccharides, trisaccharides and tetrasaccharides.

Monosaccharides are sugars which have three to nine carbon atoms. However, in plants mostly one finds sugars with five or six carbon atoms, being respectively called pentoses, $C_5H_{10}O_5$ and hexoses, $C_6H_{12}O_6$ which are the ones found very commonly accumulated in plants. Chemically simple sugar is either a ketonic or an aldehydic substitution product of polyhydroxy alcohol. The chemical formulae of sugars can be written in a number of ways. It was in 1886 that Kiliani first established the structure of glucose as a straight chain pentahydroxy aldehyde. Glucose, because it has an aldehyde group, is called an aldose or aldo sugar, while fructose with a ketonic group is called a ketose. Based on these facts the terms such as "aldopentose" and "ketohexose" are well understood.

Sugars are termed D-sugars (dextro-sugars), if the remotest secondary alcohol group at the asymmetric carbon atom is to the right and L-sugars (levo-sugars), if it is to the left. D-substances are more common in nature. A pentose example given below will explain this.

Pentose structures

$$
\begin{array}{cc}
\text{CHO} & \text{CHO} \\
\text{H}-\text{C}-\text{OH} & \text{H}-\text{C}-\text{OH} \\
\text{HO}-\text{C}-\text{H} & \text{HO}-\text{C}-\text{H} \\
\text{H}-\text{C}-\text{OH} & \text{HO}-\text{C}-\text{H} \\
\text{CH}_2\text{OH} & \text{CH}_2\text{OH} \\
\text{D-Arabinose} & \text{L-Arabinose}
\end{array}
$$

Optical rotation is also indicated by (-) levo or (+) dextro signs. Soluble sugars represented by straight chains explain their stereochemistry and isomerism. Many of the properties of sugars are better explained by 1 : 5 oxide or amylene oxide or 1 : 4 oxide or butylene oxide structures or according to Haworth they are ring structures. α- and β-sugars are known according to the position of OH and H groups. Sugars are of special interest to phytochemists and pharmacognosists as they occur combined with a wide variety of simple to complicated compounds called glycosides (see chapter on glycosides).

From amongst the monosaccharides, pentoses and hexoses are more familiar and important.

Pentoses

Pentoses contain five carbon atoms with general formula $C_5H_{10}O_5$. Ribose is present in nucleic acids. Arabinose is present in some glycosides and saponins. Arabinose and xylose are obtained from the hydrolysis of pectins, gums and mucilages. Rhamnose is a methyl pentose and is present in anthracene and flavone glycosides and in some gums, mucilages and resins. Thevetose is present in the cardiac glycoside, peruvoside. Desoxyribose is present in DNA (desoxynucleic acid). Digitoxose, digitalose and cymarose are all desoxy sugars and are present in cardiac glycosides (see structures under drugs).

Hexoses

Hexoses contain six carbon atoms and have the general formula $C_6H_{12}O_6$. Glucose and galactose, as they contain aldehyde group, are known as aldohexoses, and fructose, because of the keto group, is known as ketohexose. Hexoses can be represented by straight chain formulae which illustrate the isomerism and stereochemical relationship. However, their biological properties are explained by the ring formula which shows that sugar may exist as five-membered ring (furanose) or six-membered ring (pyranose).

Hexose structures

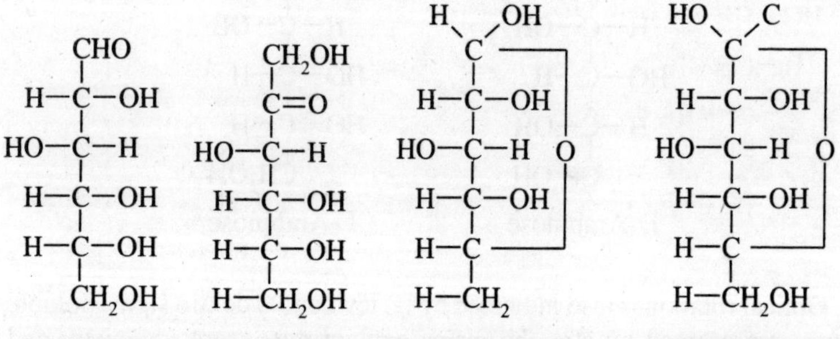

| D-Glucose | D-Fructose | α-D-Glucopyranose | β-D-Glucopyranose |
| (Aldohexose) | (Ketohexose) | (Aldohexose) | (Aldohexose) |

(α- and β-D-glucose, showing pyranose ring and the OH taking part in glycoside formation)

Hexoses are by far the most important monosaccharides found in plants. They are the first detectable sugars synthesized by plants and form the units from which most of the polysaccharides are constructed. There are 16 possible aldohexoses and 8 ketohexoses which, if we consider both the alpha and beta forms, permit 48 isomers. Of these, only 2 are found occurring in the free state in plants: they are levulose (fructose) and dextrose (glucose). Both are found in sweet fruits, honey and invert sugar. When starch is completely hydrolyzed it yields dextrose (D-glucose), while inulin yields fructose upon hydrolysis.

Glucose is an aldohexose, that is, a polyhydroxy alcohol having an aldehydic group while fructose having a ketone group is a ketohexose. These groups explain the reducing properties of the monosaccharides and account for the commonly applied term reducing sugars. The hexoses may be considered as six-membered open chain compounds, five of the carbon atoms each having an attached alcohol group and the sixth the aldehyde or ketone group. Such an aliphatic formula readily illustrates and explains stereoisomerism, but many of the other properties of the hexoses can only be explained on the basis of a ring structure. Thus glucose possesses an amylene-oxide ring. The formulas below have been assigned to glucose.

Similarly, fructose may be represented as a straight chain compound or as a butylene oxide ring. The formulas below have been assigned to it.

Glucose

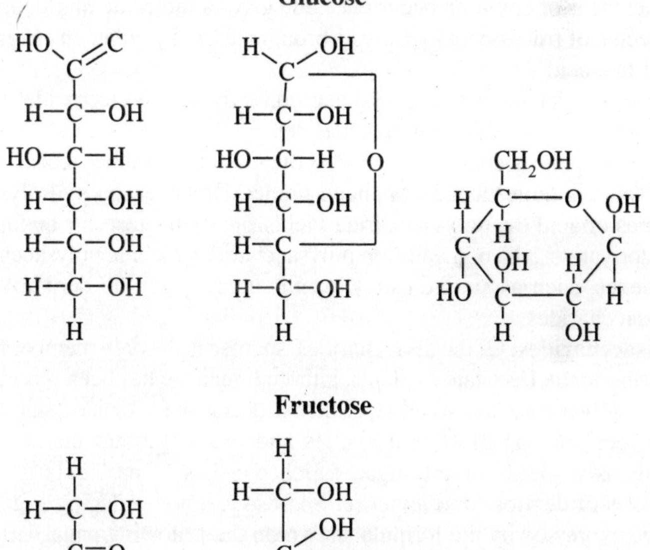

Fructose

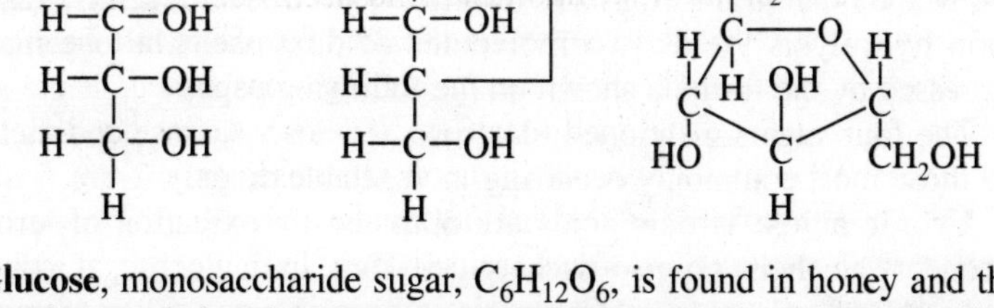

Glucose, monosaccharide sugar, $C_6H_{12}O_6$, is found in honey and the juices of many fruits; the alternate name grape sugar is derived from the presence of glucose in grapes. It is the sugar most often produced by hydrolysis of natural glycosides. Glucose is a normal constituent of the blood of animals (see Sugar Metabolism).

Polysaccharides

Polysaccharides (di-, tri-, tetra-, etc.) are derived by condensation process from sugar phosphate and sugar nucleotides of monosaccharides during the process of photosynthesis. If the resultant polysaccharide is derived from two monosaccharides with the elimination of one water molecule, it is called disaccharide and if it is derived from three and four mono-saccharide molecules, it is called trisaccharide and tetrasaccharide. respectively. These saccharides can also be termed as bioses, trioses and tetroses. Condensation of sucrose in photosynthesis by uridine diphospho-glucose (UDPG) is shown as under:

UDPG + Fructose-6-phosphate → UDPG + Sucrose-6-phosphate →
Sucrose + Pi (α-D-glucopyranoside . β-D-fructofuranoside)

Sucrose is of common occurrence and gives a molecule of glucose and a molecule of fructose on hydrolysis brought about by either an enzyme or by a dilute acid.

Oligosaccharide is an expression used for those polysaccharides which have two to ten units of monosaccharides.

In other polysaccharides in general the number of monosaccharides or sugar units is more than 10 or much higher. However, on hydrolysis by enzymes or acid the polysaccharide yields finally pentoses or hexoses or their derivatives. Also in addition polysaccharides include polysaccharide complexes, such as sulfate esters, uronic acids or amino derivatives of monosaccharides.

Disaccharides: Of the disaccharides, sucrose is the only member found occurring in the free state in plants, although maltose has been reported as occasionally present in the cell sap. Sucrose occurs in fruit juices, sugarcane, sugar beet, the sap of certain maples and in many other plants. Upon hydrolysis it yields invert sugar which consists of molecularly equal quantities of dextrose and levulose. Sucrose is a non-reducing sugar and may be expressed by the formula shown on the following page.

Maltose, while seldom occurring in the free state in nature, is produced in large quantities by the hydrolysis of starch during the germination of barley and other grains (diastatic fermentation). It is a reducing sugar and upon hydrolysis yields two molecules of dextrose. Maltose may be expressed by the formula shown on the following page.

The four sugars mentioned (dextrose, levulose, sucrose and maltose) are those most commonly occurring in vegetable drugs.

Uronic acids: Uronic acids are obtained by oxidation of terminal secondary alcoholic group of saccharides. Thus, from glucose, glucouronic acid and from galactose, galactouronic acid are obtained. Glucouronic acid is present in saponins of glycyrrhiza and quillaia bark, in gums and mucilages. Galactouronic acid is present in gums, mucilages and pectins.

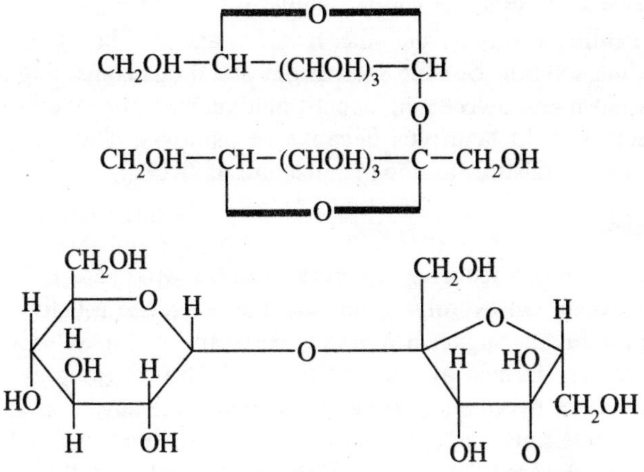

$$CH_2OH-CH-(CHOH)_3-CH$$
$$CH_2OH-CH-(CHOH)_3-C-CH_2OH$$

Sucrose

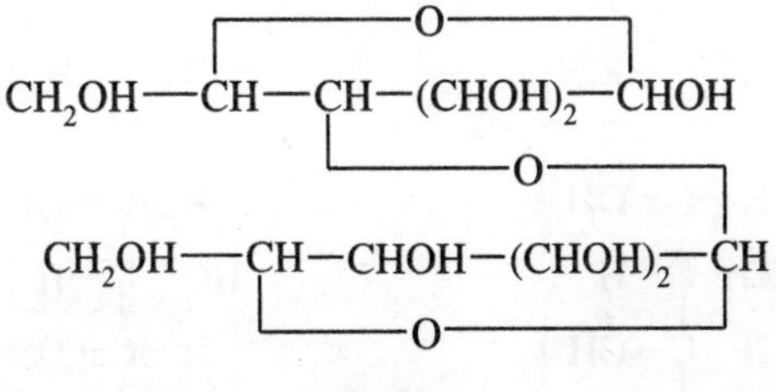

$$CH_2OH-CH-CH-(CHOH)_2-CHOH$$
$$CH_2OH-CH-CHOH-(CHOH)_2-CH$$

Maltose

It is present in tragacanth and sterculia gums and in mucilages of linseed and ishabgul.

Glucosamine is present in chitin. Chitin is a polymer of acetyl-glucosamine and is present in exoskeleton of insects and cell wall of some fungi as ergot.

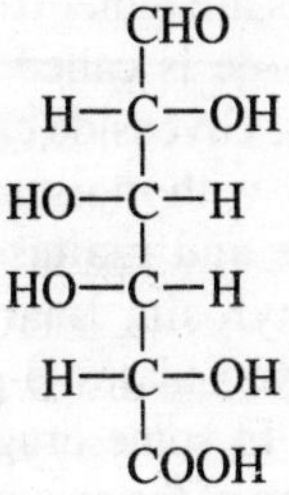

D-galactouronic acid 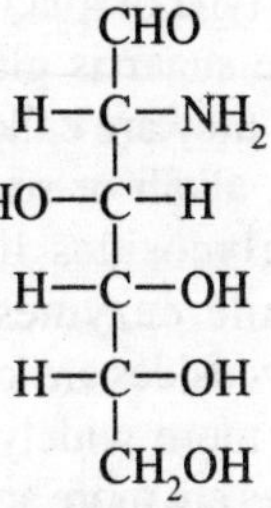   Glucosamine

Sugars are crystalline solids soluble in water, have sweet taste and reduce Fehling's solution and other reducing agents. They give no colour with iodine solution. Soluble saccharides and drugs containing them are used as nutritives, sweetening agents, and vehicles for other medicines. They act as mild laxatives because of osmosis. They are used in fermentation industries for the manufacture of alcohol.

Glycosides

Glycosides are non-reducing organic substances widely distributed in the plant kingdom. On hydrolysis they yield an aglycone usually known as genin and sugar. Sugars are hemiacetals and occur as oxide rings. Glycosides are formed by condensation of hydroxyl group of aglycone and hemiacetal hydroxyl group of sugar. Thus, the sugars in glycosides occur as oxide rings and glycosides may be considered sugar ethers. The simplest glycosides are α-methyl glycoside, and β-methyl glycoside obtained by Emil Fischer by passing dry hydrogen chloride in methyl alcohol.

α-Methyl glycoside   β-Methyl glycoside

By hydrolysis of α-methyl glycosides, α-glucose and methyl alcohol and of β-methyl glycosides, β-glucose and methyl alcohol are obtained. According to the type of glucose glycosides are either α-glycosides or β-glycosides. If the sugar is glucose, glycoside is called glucoside while with other sugars they are called glycosides. Glycoside can be hydrolysed by enzyme, acid, alkali or sometimes only with moisture. The enzymes hydrolysing α-glycosides like invertase and maltase are called α-glycosidases while enzymes emulsin, myrosin, linarase, gentianase hydrolysing β-glycosides are known as β-glycosidases. β-glycosidases and β-glycosides are more widely distributed. In some drugs as in digitalis original glycosides are more active and action of the enzyme is undesirable and steps should be taken to prevent it. In cyanogenetic and isothiocyanate glycosides hydrolysis products are active and action of enzymes is desirable.

Glycosides are classified according to the nature of sugar, according to the chemical nature of aglycone or according to their action. One of the modern classifications is according to the linkage and is mentioned as follows:

A. (1) *O-glycosides:* In these glycosides sugar is combined with phenol or OH group of aglycone.

$$—O\boxed{H + HO}C_6H_{11}O_5 = OC_6H_{11}O_5$$

These glycosides are very common and are met with to a great extent. Cyanogenetic, flavone, cardiac and a number of other glycosides are O-glycosides.

(2) *C-glycosides:* In these glycosides sugar is attached directly to the carbon atom.

$$—C\boxed{H + HO}C_6H_{11}O_6 = C, C_6H_{11}O_5$$

Aloin in aloe and cascarosides of cascara and some flavone glycosides are C-glycosides. These glycosides are resistant to normal hydrolysis and they can be hydrolysed by ferric chloride and hydrochloric acid or sodium metaperiodate i.e. by oxidative hydrolysis.

(3) *S-glycosides:* In this group S of SH group is combined with sugar.

$$—S\boxed{H + HO}C_6H_{11}O_5 = S—C_6H_{11}O_5$$

Isothiocyanate glycosides are S-glycosides.

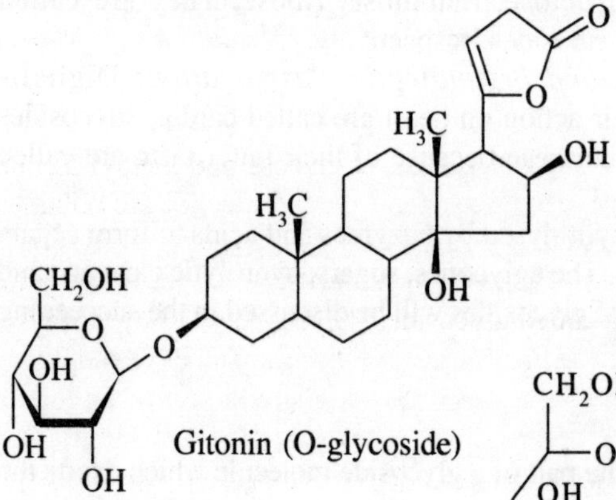

Gitonin (O-glycoside)

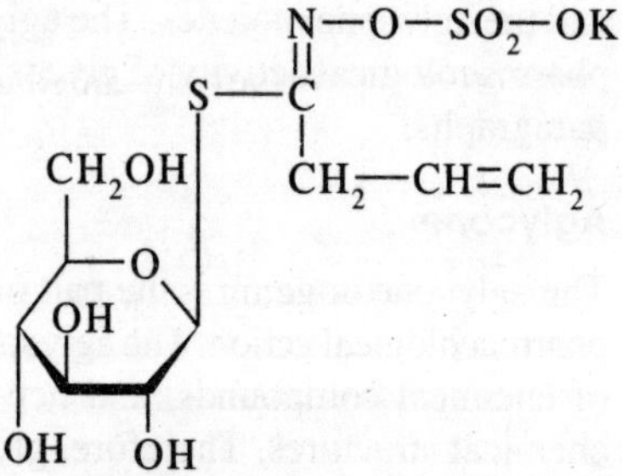

Sinigrin (S-glycoside)

(4) *N-glycosides:* In these glycoside N of the NH (amino group) is combined with sugar.

$$-O \boxed{H + HO} C_6H_{11}O_5 = OC_6H_{11}O_5$$

Nucleosides and some enzymes are N-glycosides.

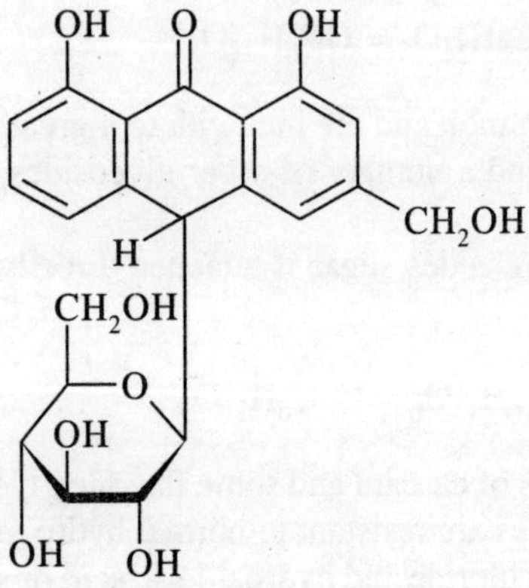

Barbaloin (C-glycoside) 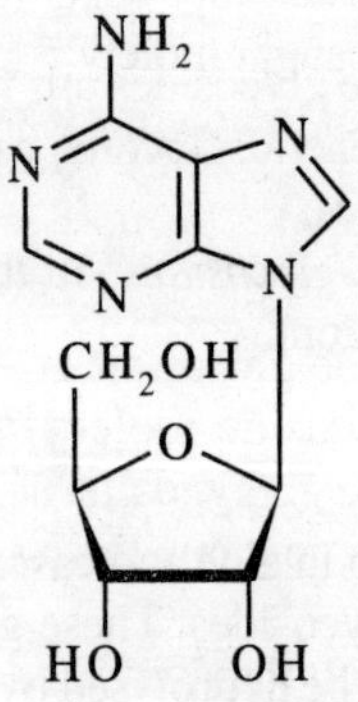   Adenosine (N-glycoside)

B. *Chemical classification:* Glycosides are classified according to the chemical nature of aglycone, as flavone, cyanogenetic, anthracene, alcohol glycosides.

C. *Sugar classification:* They are classified according to the nature of sugar as glycosides of fructose, rhamnose, ribose. They are called fructosides, rhamnosides, ribosides, respectively.

D. *Pharmacological and organoleptic classification:* Digitalis glycosides because of their action on heart are called cardiac glycosides while glycosides of Gentianaceae because of their bitter taste are called bitter glycosides.

These glycosides are hydrolysed by enzymes and acids to form sugars and the aglycone moieties. The aglycones, sugars, hydrolytic cleavage and pharmacological activity of glycosides will be discussed in the succeeding paragraphs.

Aglycone

The aglycone or genin is the part of a glycoside molecule which exerts the pharmacological action. The aglycones occur in a variety of different classes of chemical compounds, and hence the glycosides vary widely in their chemical structures. Therefore, glycosides can be grouped as cyanogenic glycosides (amygdalin), glucosinolates (glucocapparin), lactone or coumarin glycosides (daphnin), iridoid glycosides (swertiamarin, therpagoside), lignan glycosides (arctiun), quinone glycosides (barbaloin), phenolic glycosides (sennoside A), flavonoid glycosides (quercetin), cardiac glycosides (digitoxin), steroidal alkaloid glycosides (solanine), xanthone glycosides (mangiferin), and triterpenoid glycosides or saponins (glycyrrhizin).

SUGARS IN GLYCOSIDES

The glycosides are generally classified on the basis of their sugar moiety. When the sugar moiety is glucose, the glycoside is called a glucoside; if it is fructose, then a fructoside; and, similarly, it is called a rhamnoside, a galactoside, and a riboside when, on hydrolysis, rhamnose, galactose, and ribose, respectively, are liberated. Beside that, two series of stereoisomeric glycosides are possible, based on the configuration at the carbon atom forming the glycosidic linkage, and are known as α and β glycosides.

A glycoside molecule may contain either a single unit of monosaccharide (amygdalin has one unit of glucose) or more than one unit (digitoxin contains three digitoxose units). In other cases, the glycoside may contain two or more different sugar units, for example, rutin has one unit of both rhamnose and glucose, whereas K-strophanthoside possesses one unit of cymarose and two units of glucose.

Generally, in the case where two or more units of sugar are found in a glycoside molecule, the sugars are linked in a chain as a disaccharide, trisaccharide or polysaccharide and this chain is then linked to the aglycone at one particular place. There are cases, however, of glycosides in which two monosaccharides are attached to the aglycone at different positions, such as in sennoside, and cascaroside A and B.

Mostly, the sugar in the glycosides is β-D-glucose. But there are glycoside molecules containing **hexoses** such as mannose, galactose and fructose; **pentoses** such as xylose, arabinose and ribose; and **5-methyl pentoses** such as digitoxose, digitalose and cymarose. In some glycosides, the "sugar" moiety may not be a true sugar but rather a sugar derivative, as, for example, glycyrrhizin, in which the sugar unit is a diglucuronide.

HYDROLYSIS OF GLYCOSIDES

The glycosides are hydrolysed either by acid or alkali, and by enzymes resulting in the cleavage of the glycosidic linkages. However, some of the glycosides are modified or broken down, as in the case of cardioactive steroidal glycosides, which can be opened by strong alkali, resulting in the loss of pharmacological activity. The glycosides in general are hydrolysed energetically by acids, but in many cases artefacts may be formed. Enzyme hydrolysis is specific, for example, emulsin hydrolyses β-glycosides, whereas maltase brings about cleavage of α-glycosides only.

The enzymes frequently occur along with the glycosides in the same plant, and therefore the compounds may be hydrolysed when the two come in contact during extraction and isolation procedures. Therefore, appropriate measures are necessary to inactivate the enzymes. All polysaccharides can be hydrolysed; in some cases, it is also possible to bring about cleavage at a specific monosaccharides linkage in the chain.

PHARMACOLOGICAL ACTION

Many glycosides exert their potent pharmacological activity in milligram doses in human beings. Generally, the pharmacological action of a glycoside is due to its aglycone. Therefore, owing to the variety of aglycone structures, different types of physiological or pharmacological activities are encountered. The clinically useful glycosides, such as digitoxin, digoxin, lanatoside C and ouabain are cardiotonic. Plants containing various glycosides employed medicinally as cathartics are **Aloes**, **Senna**, **Cascara**, and **Rhubarb**; whereas **Glycyrrhiza** and its fluid extract are used as an expectorant.

However, certain glycosides, such as the cyanogenic glycoside amygdalin, exhibit toxicity to man and animals. The sugar part in the glycoside molecule, when administered orally, helps to carry the aglycone to the site of action of a particular organ or tissue where the physiological or pharmacological action is desired.

ANTHRACENOSIDES:
Anthracene/Anthraquinone Glycosides

Chemistry/Phytochemistry

Anthracenosides, as the name suggests, are those glycosides whose basic ring structure is anthracene and the aglycones are anthracene derivatives. These derivatives are popularly referred to as anthraquinones, though we would recommend that they be called Anthracenosides.

According to Tshirch, the famous German pharmacognosist, they are anthraglycosides and their aglycones are anthraquinones, anthranols, anthrones or dimers of anthrones or their derivatives. In the drugs, however, aglycones and sugars of glycosides are found. A large number of these substances are pharmacologically active as cathartics (evacuating bowels) and purgatives. Drugs containing anthracenosides are said to have been used as natural purgative products much before the chemical nature of these active principles was brought to light.

The earliest phytochemical work concerned the isolation of hydrolysed products and not the intact primary glycosides and this was obviously because of the fact that the glycosides are easily hydrolysed.

It was only in early forties when the Swiss scientist Stoll and his co-workers (1941) developed better methods of extraction that not only led to the isolation of sennosides A and B from senna leaflets and pods, but also improved the isolation of primary anthracenosides from other purgative herbal materials. The anthracenosides are mostly found in dicoyledenous plants and some important families amongst them are Polygonaceae, Rhamnaceae, Leguminosae, Rubiaceae, Euphorbiaceae, Verbinaceae, Lythraceae, etc.

Liliaceae is the only family in monocots which contains some of the important anthracenosides. Anthracenosides seem to be absent in Gymnosperms, Pteridophyta and Bryophyta but certain lower plants like fungi and lichens have given evidence of their presence in them.

The stimulant laxatives of plant origin that have been included in the official books i.e. Compendia are *Aloe* species (Aloes), *Cassia* species (senna), *Rhamnus purshiana* (cascara sagrada), *R. frangula* (Frangula), and *Rheum* species (Rhubarb). They will be discussed under individual headings. The anthracene glycosides occur in all the aforementioned genera as derivatives of anthraquinone, anthrone, oxanthrone, anthranol and dianthrone (dimeric) compounds. A list of some representative anthracene glycosides is being given in a table in subsequent text.

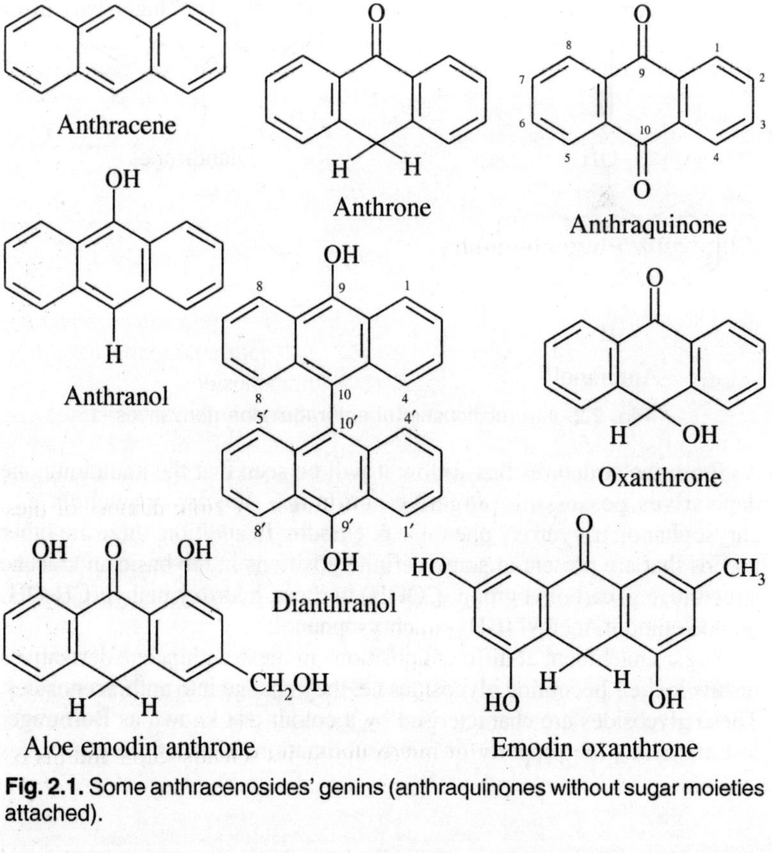

Fig. 2.1. Some anthracenosides' genins (anthraquinones without sugar moieties attached).

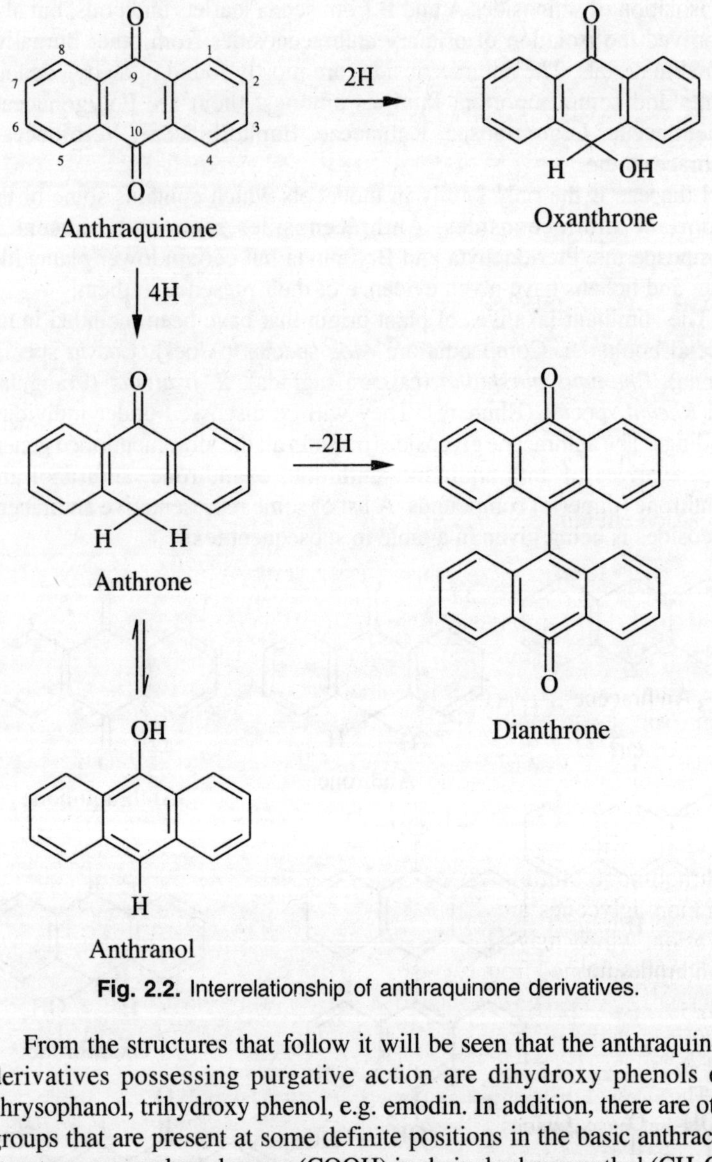

Fig. 2.2. Interrelationship of anthraquinone derivatives.

From the structures that follow it will be seen that the anthraquinone derivatives possessing purgative action are dihydroxy phenols e.g. chrysophanol, trihydroxy phenol, e.g. emodin. In addition, there are other groups that are present at some definite positions in the basic anthracene structure, e.g. carboxyl group (COOH) in rhein, hydroxymethyl (CH_2OH) in aloe emodin, methyl (CH_3) in chrysophanol.

Sugar attachment at different positions in these anthracene derivatives results in their becoming glycosides i.e. they change into anthracenosides. These glycosides are characterised by a colour test known as Borntrager test and show the property of microsublimation. Most of the glycosides

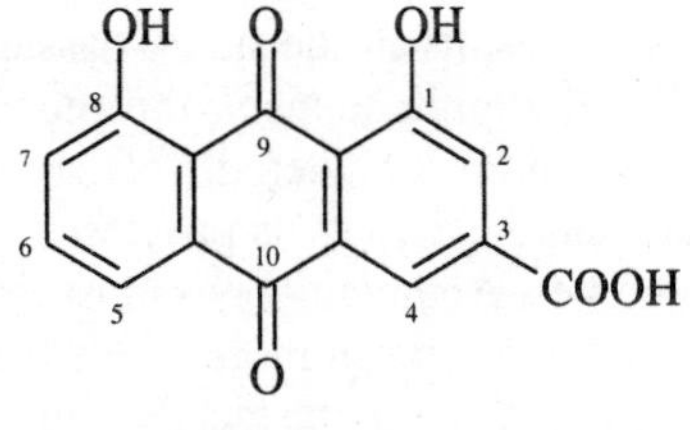

Rhein

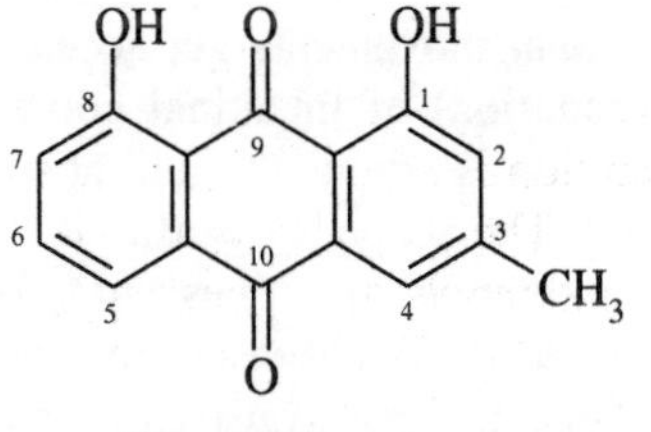

Chrysophanol

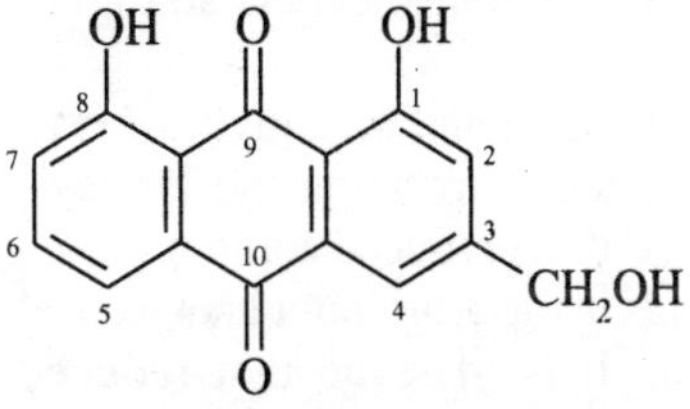

Aloe-emodin

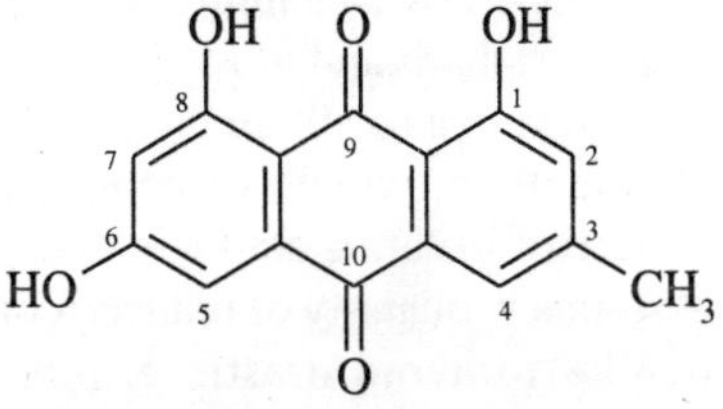

Emodin (Frangula emodin)

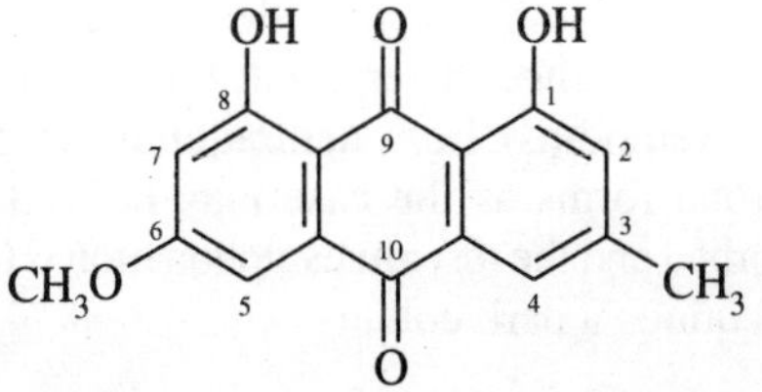

Physcion (Methoxy frangula emodin)

are O-glycosides and by their hydrolysis derivatives of 1 : 8 dihydroxy anthraquinone, anthranol, anthrone, or dianthrone are obtained. The common aglycones are aloe-emodin, emodin, rhein, chrysophanol and physcion, which may exist as anthraquinones, anthranols or anthrones. Dianthrones formed from two molecules of anthrones may be identical or different i.e. mixed or heterogenous. They as aglycones are of significant importance and are found in some species of *Cassia*, *Rheum* and *Rhamnus* (see individual drugs).

The sugars are usually arabinose, rhamnose and glucose. Further, aloin in aloe and cascarosides in cascara are C-glycosides. In the drug, originally glycosides are present as reduced derivatives or their dimers. During drying and storage by hydrolysis and oxidation free anthraquinones are produced.

Pharmacology

Anthracenosides are laxatives because of their irritating action on the large intestine. It is due to the stimulation of the muscular structure i.e. smooth muscles of the large intestine through which the peristaltic and large intestinal movements get accelerated. This results in the quick passage (evacuation) of intestinal contents. Since, simultaneously, the mucus secretion is stimulated and absorption of water is hindered, soft stools result. The action starts after 8–12 hours and the activity is possessed by the anthranols, anthrones and also dianthrones. Anthraquinones must first be reduced. Glycosides of reduced derivatives are much more active than oxidised aglycones (also called emodins). This is due to the fact that sugars take the glycosides to the site of action and thus they are more active. The important drugs containing these glycosides are senna leaflets and pods, cascara, rhubarb and aloe.

Most active of all are the sennosides, the rhein-anthrone glycosides as also the aloin, which, of course, could result in irritating the kidneys. Because of irritating action of anthrones and other reduced compounds on the stomach, quantity of reduced compounds in the drug should not exceed 30–40% to avoid drastic griping action. It is believed that reduced derivatives are irritating on skin and mucous membrane. *Chrysarobin* and *Cassia tora* seeds are used in ringworm and other skin diseases.

Biotransformation of anthrasennosides takes place through their hydrolysis under the influence of large intestinal bacteria (*E. coli*). The resultant aglycones (emodins) from anthraquinone type are reduced to anthranol or anthrone forms as the case may be. A smaller portion of aglycones is reabsorbed and the rest after sulphonation is eliminated through the urine, which acquires a dark colour.

Analysis of Anthracenosides

Chemical assay

In the chemical assay all anthracene compounds are oxidised to free anthra-quinones by ferric chloride and are by reaction with sodium hydroxide made into red alkali salts, which are estimated spectrophotometrically at max. 510–540 nm as the case may be using 1 : 8 dihydroxyanthraquinone as the standard.

First free anthraquinones are estimated by extraction with chloroform or ether, then O-glycosides are estimated usually by hydrolysis with a mixture of hydrochloric acid or periodate. After reaction with alkali in all the cases estimation in made as above.

After hydrolysis estimation may be carried out as magnesium chelate complex in 1 cm thick layer usually at max. 515 nm using methanol for comparison.

Bioassay

The chemical methods of estimation do not run parallel with biological activity and so bioassay is carried out on mice or rats by counting the number of wet faeces after administration of the drug according to the weight of animals for determining the activity.

CARDIOACTIVE GLYCOSIDES

A number of steroidal glycoside molecules are effective in the treatment of heart disease. These cardioactive glycosides occur in different plants, such as *Digitalis purpurea* Linn., *D. lanata* Ehrl., *D. ferruginea* Linn., *D. lutea* Linn., *D. thapsi* Linn., *Acokanthera friesiorum* Markgr., *Apocynum cannabinum* Linn., *Strophanthus gratus* Wall, et Hook., *S. kombe* Oliv., *Convallaria majalis* Linn., *Urginea burkei* Baker., *U. indica* Kuhth., *U. maritima* Baker., *Adonis murensis* Linn. and *A. verrialis* Linn.

The naturally occurring cardioactive steroids are classified into two groups: cardenolides and bufadienolides. The cardenolides are found in abundance in nature as C-23 steroids with a β-unsaturated γ-lactone ring while bufadienolides are C-24 steroids with an unsaturated 6-membered lactone ring.

Cardenolides   Bufadienolides

(R represents sugar moiety)

Different cardiotonic glycosides have the same sugar portion but different aglycones, whereas some glycosides have identical aglycones but different sugar moieties. The aglycones of these cardiotonic glycosides possess mostly the saturated tetracyclic carbon steroidal structures. In addition to this steroidal part there is an unsaturated lactone ring attached to C-17 in the steroidal aglycone, the fusion of the rings A and B is *cis* with the hydrogen at C-5, exhibiting a beta configuration. The ring C and D fusion is also *cis* and the hydrogen at C-8 is either beta or alpha in configuration. The methyl or ether group attached to C-10 and C-13 both show the beta configuration. These aglycones possess hydroxyl groups at C-3 and C-14, both in the beta configuration. In a number of these cardioactive glycosides, the aglycone may have additional hydroxyl groups at other positions. The C-1 sugar moiety is likely through the hydroxyl group at C-3 of the aglycones.

The different cardioactive glycosides may possess one or more mono-saccharide units in the sugar chain of the molecule. Beside glucose, the other sugars present are rhamnose, digitoxose, digitalose and cymarose.

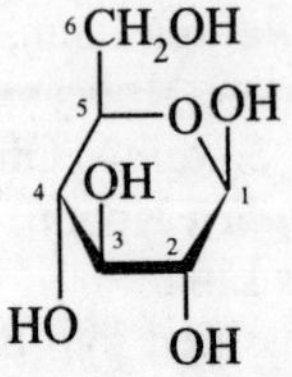

β-D-Glucose 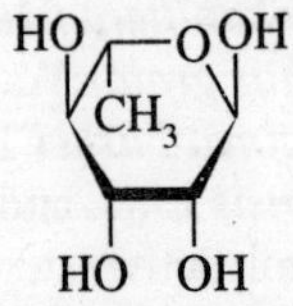   α-L-Rhamnose 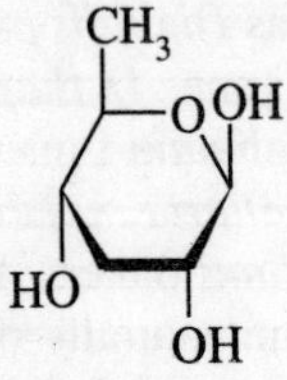   β-D-Digitoxose

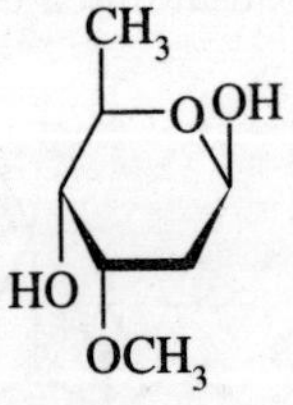

β-D-Cymarose 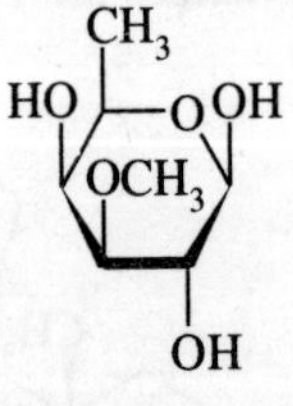   β-D-Digitalose

The last three are rarely occurring sugars. Out of these sugars only rhamnose is in the L-series whereas glucose, digitoxose and cymarose are in the D-series. The number and nature of the sugars in the glycoside determines its miscibility in water and other polar organic solvents. Individual glycosides with corresponding structures will be given under the drugs included in the syllabus.

SAPONIN GLYCOSIDES

Saponins, yet another class of plant glycosides, have long been in use throughout the world. This may have been due to their distinctive property to froth with detergent action. They are found widely distributed in higher plants.

The word **saponin** is derived from the Latin word *"sapo"* which means soap and hence plants containing saponins and saponins as such produce frothing in aqueous solution. Saponins have a bitter acrid taste and they and the drugs containing them are sternutatory and irritate the mucous membrane. Saponins also have haemolytic property i.e. they cause haemolysis of blood and prove highly toxic on being injected into the blood stream. However, when taken by mouth, saponins are quite harmless. **Saponins** have high molecular weight and their isolation in pure form may pose some difficulties.

Saponins give precipitate with alcoholic solutions of sterols and higher alcohols, emulsify oil and water and are toxic to lower organisms like earthworm and fish and kill them. Saponins are non-crystalline and dissolve in water with colloidal solutions. They are soluble in alcohol but insoluble in ether and light petroleum. Saponins are glycosides and give on hydrolysis aglycones, known as **sapogenins** and sugars. The **sapogenins** upon acetylization result in crystallizable compounds. This process can be successfully used to purify sapogenins.

On the basis of chemical structure of the aglycone or sapogenin the saponins are classified into two types viz. (1) **Steroidal saponins** (also commonly called tetracyclic triterpenoids), and (2) **Pentacyclic triterpenoid saponins** and their chemical structures are given below. In both of these types the glycosidal linkage is at position C-3 and it is known and well understood that both of these types have a common biogenetic pathway through mevalonic acid and isoprenoid units.

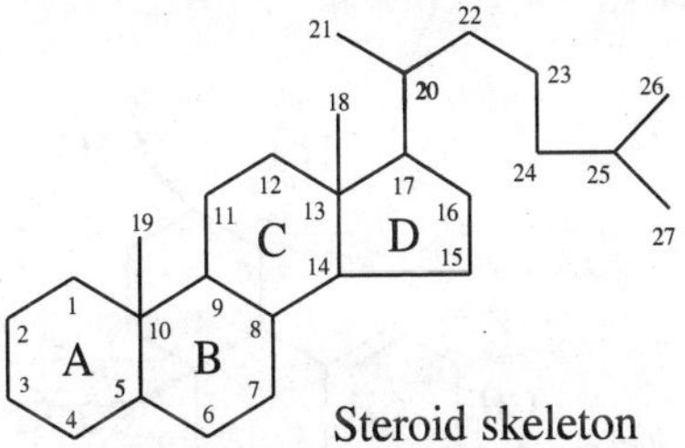

Steroid skeleton

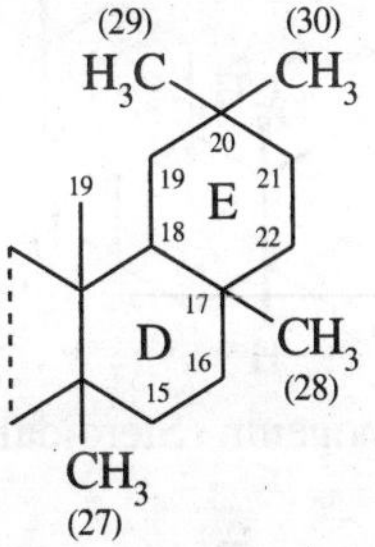

Pentacyclic triterpenoid skeleton

Steroid saponins are cyclopentanophenanthrene derivatives. Diosgenin is the important steroid sapogenin. Recently from these saponins steroid hormones like progesterone, cortisone, etc. are obtained by partial synthesis and thus their importance has increased considerably.

Triterpene saponins are usually β-amyrine derivatives and some are also α-amyrine and lupeol derivatives.

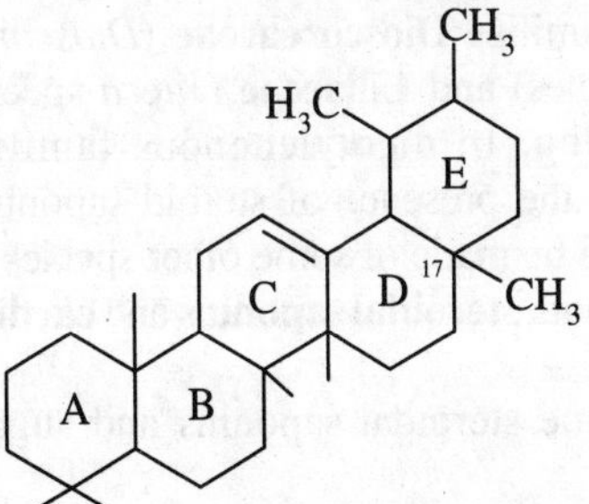

α-Amyrine type

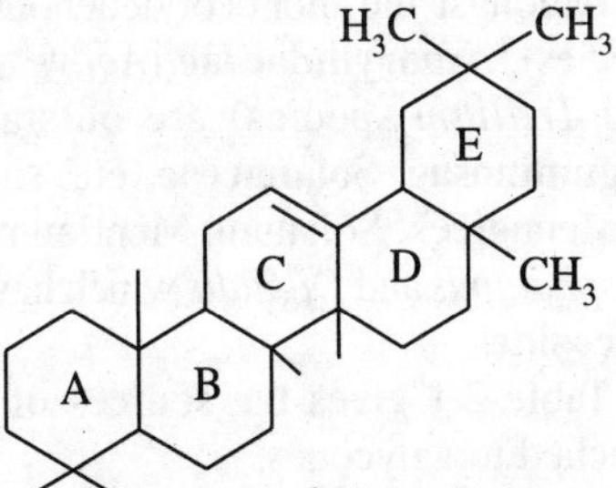

β-Amyrine type

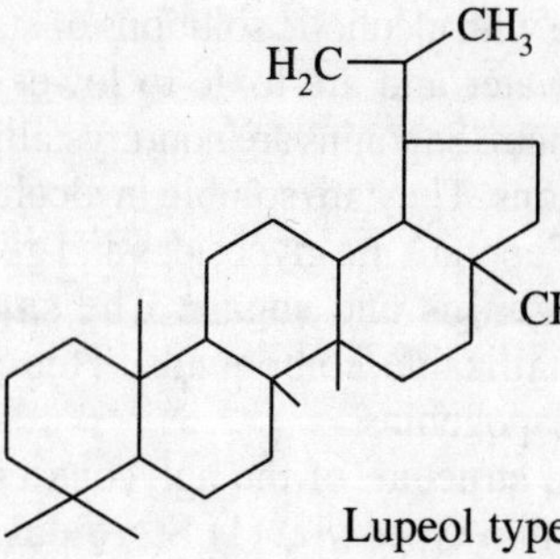

Lupeol type

An example of each of the above mentioned skeleton is shown below:

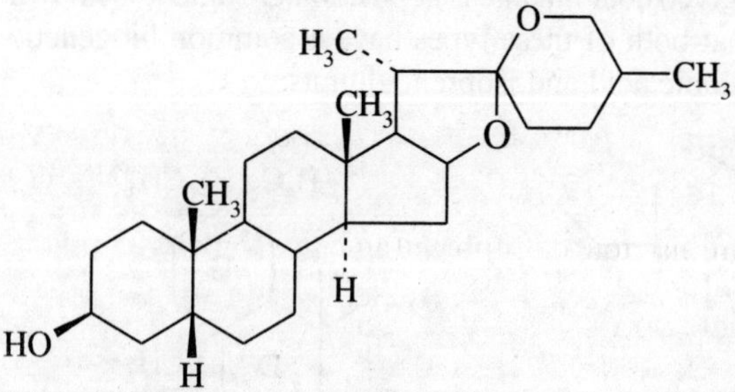

Sarsasapogenin (Steroidal sapogenin)

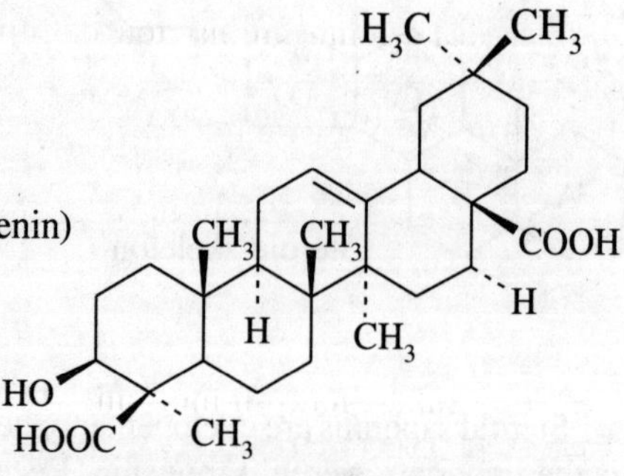

Gypsogenin (Triterpenoid sapogenin)

Steroid saponins

Steroidal saponins are known to occur in nature less commonly than as compared to the pentacyclic triterpenoids.

Amongst the monocotyledenous families **Dioscoreaceae** (*Dioscorea* species), **Amaryllidaceae** (*Agave* species) and **Liliaceae** (*Yucca* species and *Trillium* species) are outstanding. In dicotyledenous families **Leguminosae, Solanaceae**, etc. show the presence of steroid saponins, e.g. fenugreek, Solanum. Mention need be made of some other species of *Strophanthus* and *Digitalis* which have both **steroidal saponins** and **cardiac glycosides**.

Table 2.1 gives the sources of some steroidal saponins and sugars attached to aglycones.

Table 2.1. Sources of some steroidal saponins and sugars attached to aglycones

Botanical source	Steroidal saponin	Sapogenin (Aglycone)	Sugars attached (Glucones)
Smilax aristolochiaefolia	Sarsasaponin	Sarsasapogenin	2 glucose + 1 rhamnose
Digitalis purpurea Digitalis lanata	Digitonin	Digitogenin	2 glucose + 2 galactose + 1 xylose
Digitalis purpurea Digitalis lanata	Gitonin	Gitogenin	1 glucose + 2 galactose + 1 xylose
Dioscorea deltoidea	Dioscin	Diosgenin	1 glucose + 2 rhamnose
Jurubia species	Jurubin	Jurubidine	1 glucose
Digitalis purpurea	Gitonin	Gitogenin	1 glucose + 2 galactose + 1 xylose
Dioscorea species	Gracillin	Diosgenin	2 glucose + 1 rhamnose
Agave sisalana	Hecogin	Hecogenin	1 glucose + 1 rhamnose

Steroidal saponins are also found distributed amongst some other genera, such as *Nolina, Agapanthus, Chlorogalum* (Liliaceae), *Manfreda* (Amyryllidaceae), *Digitalis* (Scrophulariaceae), *Lycopersion* and *Centrum* (Solanaceae).

Steroidal saponins may have as such limited use, but they or their sapogenins having certain types of structure which are of great importance and medico-commercial interests, since they serve as starting materials for the synthesis and production of steroid hormones. These hormones are very important agents in medicine. This is because of the fact that they have close structure relationship with compounds like the sex hormones, cortisone, cardiac glycosides, diuretic steroids and vitamin D.

Triterpenoid saponins

Triterpene saponins are usually β-amyrine derivatives and some are also α-amyrine and lupeol derivatives.

Triterpenoid saponins have been isolated from different plant species and some of the examples are *Aesculus hippocastanum* Linn. (aescin), *Aralia japonica* Thunb. (aralin), *Cyclamen europaeum* Linn. (cyclamin), *Glycyrrhiza glabra* Linn. (glycyrrhizin), *Primula elatior* (L.) Hill, (primulasaponin), *Hedera helix* Linn. (hederacoside A), *Quillaia saponaria* Molina (quillaia saponin), *Bupleurum falcatum* Linn. (saikasaponin), *Platycodon grandiflorum* DC (platycodin D), Polygala tenuifolia Linn. (tenuifolin), *Akebia quinata* DC (akeboside), and *Zizyphus jujuba* Mill. (jujuboside A). A list of triterpenoid saponins, their sources, sapogenins and sugar moieties is given in Table 2.2.

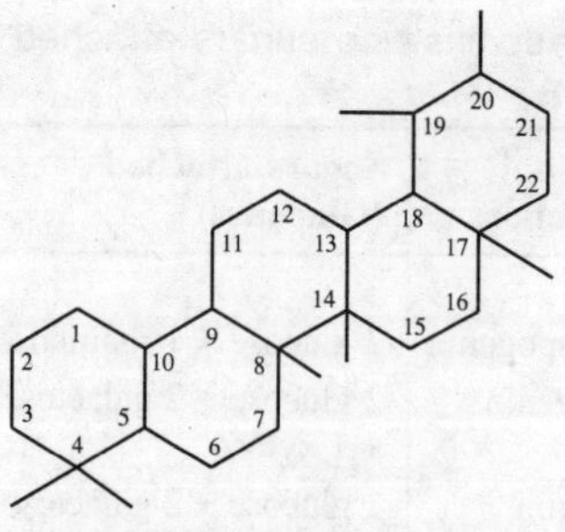

α-Amyrine type saponin

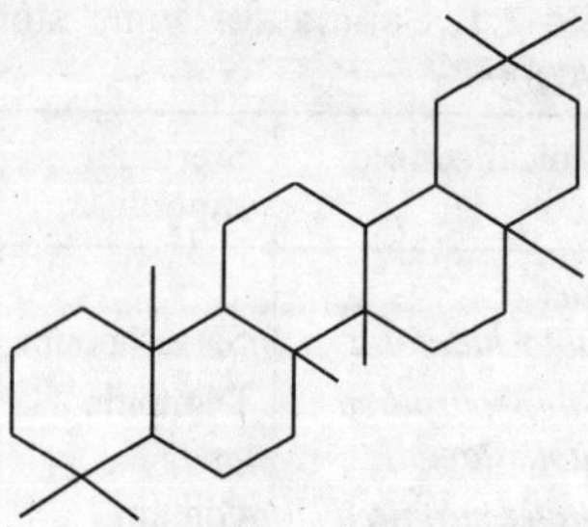

β-Amyrine type saponin

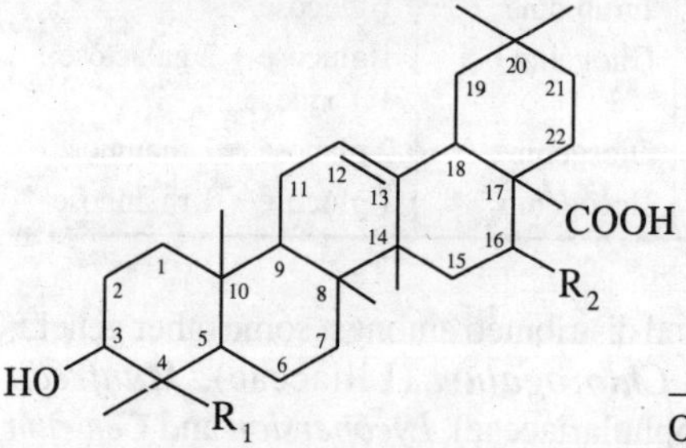

β-Amyrine sapogenins

	R_1	R_2
Oleanolic acid	CH_3	H
Hederagenin	CH_2OH	H
Gypsogenin	CHO	H
Quillaic acid	CHO	OH
Echinocystic acid	CH_3	OH

Some β-amyrine sapogenins are mentioned in Table 2.2. Glycyrrhetic acid from glycyrrhiza belongs also to this group. These saponins are used as expectorant. 18-β-glycyrrhetic acid has anti-inflammatory properties. Besides number of other actions like diuretic, anthelmintic, etc. are attributed to them. They are also used as foaming agents in the aerated waters and as fire extinguishers.

Some of the sugars associated with the above saponins are given below:

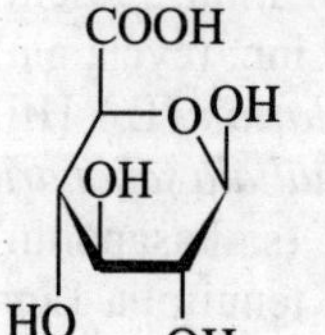

β-D-Glucuronic

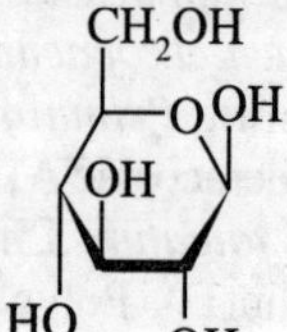

β-D-Glucose

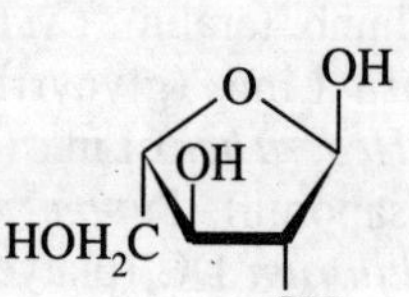

Arabinose
(furanose)

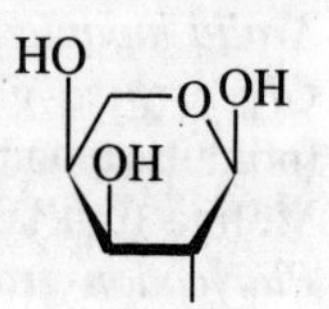

L-Arabinose
(pyranose)

Table 2.2. Some important triterpene saponins

Saponin	Source	Genin	Sugar portion
Aescin	*Aesculus hippocastanum*	Aescigenin	(Glucose)$_2$ + glucuronic acid + tiglic acid
Aralin	*Aralia japonica*	Aralidin	(Arabinose)$_2$ + glucuronic acid
Cyclamin	*Cyclamin europaeum*	Cyclamigenin	Xylose + (glucose)$_2$ + arabinose
Glycyrrhizin	*Glycyrrhiza officinalis*	Glycyrrhetinic acid	(Glucuronic acid)$_2$
Hederin	*Hedera helix*	Hederagenin	Glucose + arabinose
Primulasaponin	*Primula elatior*	Primulagenin	Rhamnose + glucose + galactose + glucuronic acid
Araloside A	*Aralia manschurica*	Oleanolic acid	Glucose + galacturonic acid + L-arabinose
Asiaticoside	*Centella asiatica*	Asiatic acid	(Glucose)$_2$ + rhamnose
Quinovin-glycoside A	*Cinchona calisaya*	Quinovic acid	6-Deoxyglucose (quinovose)
Quillaia-saponin	*Quillaia saponaria*	Hydroxy-gypsogenin	Glucuronic acid
Saikosaponin A	*Bupleurum falcatum*	Saikogenin-F	Fucose + glucuronic acid
Platycodin D	*Platycodon grandiflorum*	Platycodigenin*	Arabinose + rhamnose + xylose + apiose; glucuronic acid
Tenuifolin	*Polygala tenuifolia*	Presnegin*	Rhamnose + xylose + galactose + fructose; glucose
Akeboside	*Akebia quinata*	Oleanolic acid	Rhamnose + glucose + arabinose
Ginsenoside	*Panax ginseng*	Oleanolic acid	(Glucuronic acid)$_2$

* Sugars attached at two different places on the aglycone.

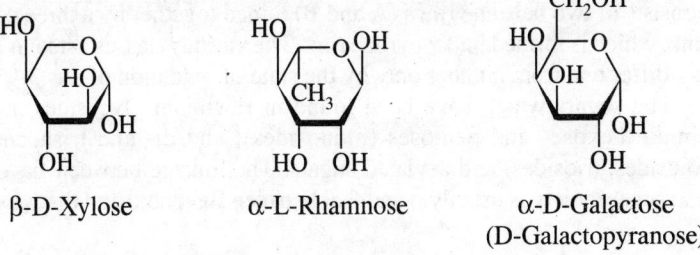

β-D-Xylose   α-L-Rhamnose   α-D-Galactose (D-Galactopyranose)

FLAVONE GLYCOSIDES

Flavones are phenyl benzo-γ-pyrone derivatives and occur as flavone, flavonol, flavanone, isoflavone and chalcone. Flavones occur free or as O-glycosides and C-glycosides.

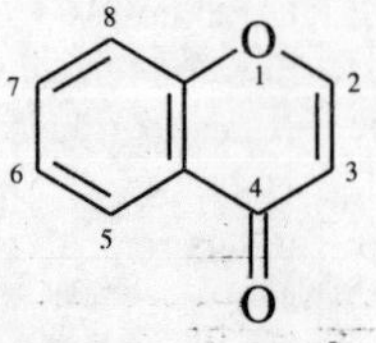

Benzo-γ-pyrone
(Chromone)

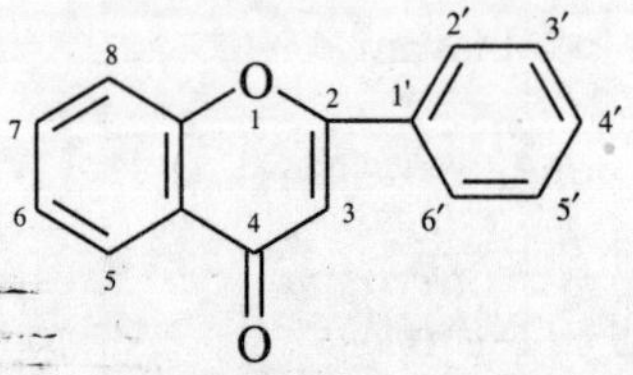

Flavone
(2-Phenyl benzo-γ-pyrone)

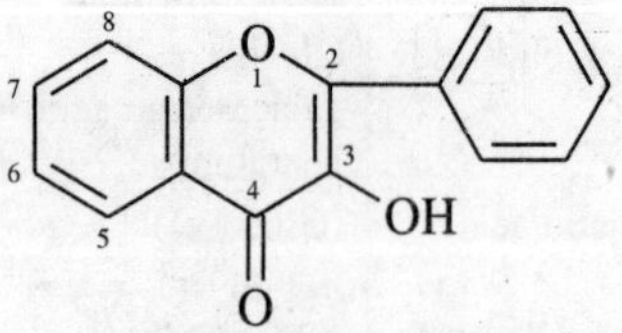

Flavonol

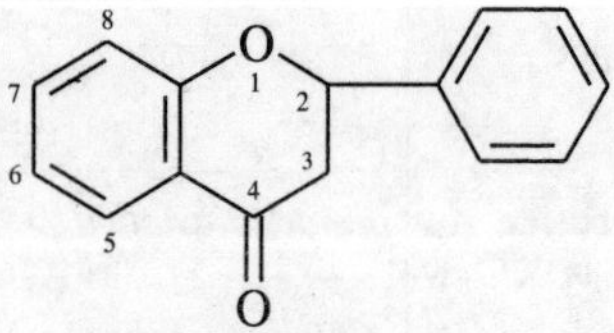

Flavanone

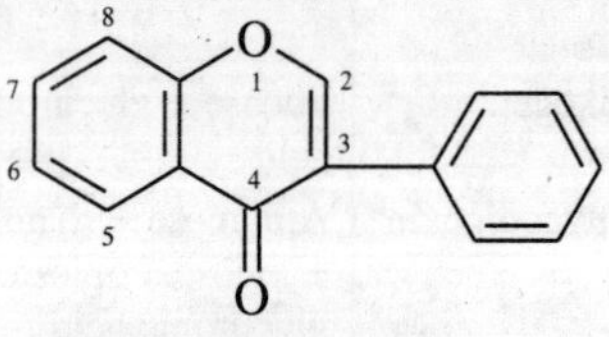

3-Phenylbenzopyrone
Isoflavone

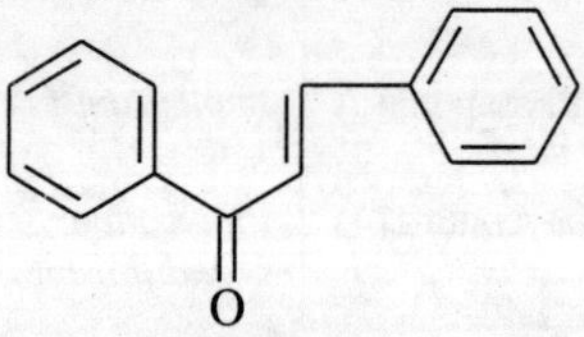

Chalcone

The flavonoids are a group of compounds comprising the derivatives of flavone and flavanones, isoflavonones, flavanols and isoflavones The chemical structure of these compounds is derived from the aromatic nucleus of flavan or 2-phenyl benzopyran. The flavonoids are found either in the free state or as glycosides in a variety of plants. It can be seen that flavone consists of two benzene rings (A and B) joined together by a three carbon link, which is formed into γ-pyrone ring. The various classes listed in Table 2.1 differ one from another only by the state of oxidation of this 3-C link.

The sugars which have been found in flavonoid glycosides include simple hexoses and pentoses (monosides); and di- and trisaccharide (biosides, triosides) and acylated sugars. The linkage between flavonoid and sugar moiety is usually β and that between flavonoid and rhamnosides

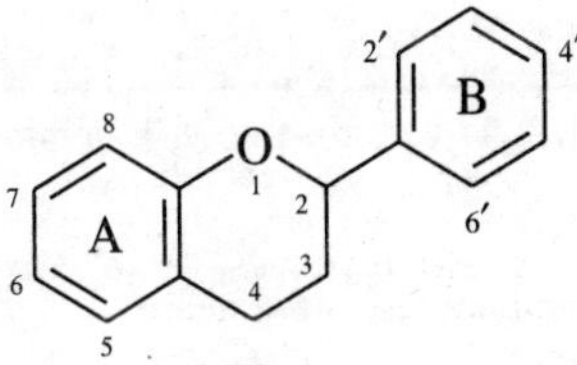

Flavan

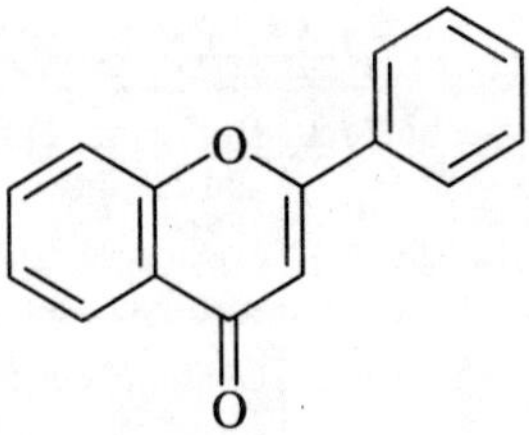

Flavone

and between flavonoid and arabinosides is α. Some of the sugars linked to flavonoids are given in Table 2.2. A list of a number of flavonoid glycosides is given in Table 2.3.

Table 2.3. Classes of commonly occurring flavonoid compounds

Name	Structure of 3-C compound	OH
Flavone	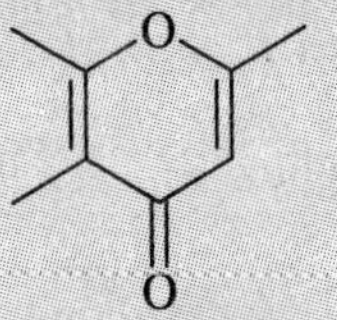	Apigenin: 5, 7, 4' Luteolin: 5, 7, 3', 4'
Flavanone	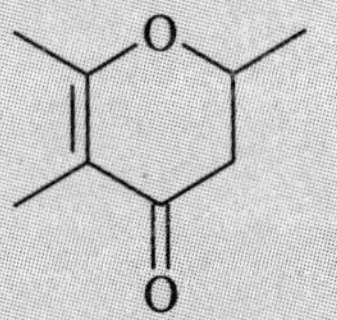	Naringin: 5, 7, 4' Butin: 7, 3, 4' Eriodictyol: 5, 7, 3', 4'
Isoflavanone	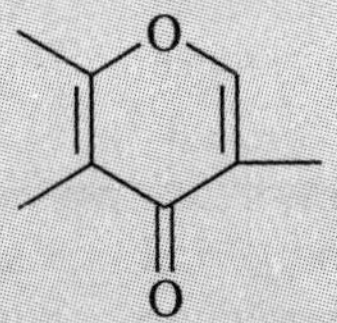	Padmakastein: 5, 4' Dihydroxy, 7-methoxy
Flavonol	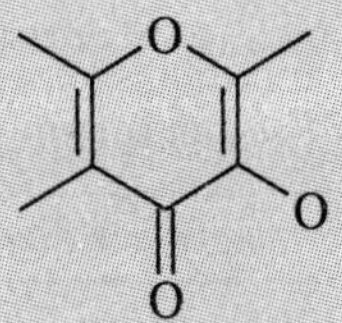	Kaempferol: 5, 7', 3 Quercetin: 5, 7, 3', 4'
Isoflavone	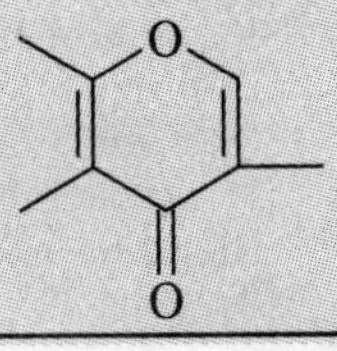	Genistein: 5, 7, 4' Orobol: 5, 7, 3', 4'

Table 2.4. Sugar linked to flavonoid compounds

Monosaccharides	D-glucose, D-galactose, D-xylose, L-rhamnose, L-arabinose and D-glucuronic acid
Disaccharides	Sophorose (glucose-1 → 2-glucose), gentiobiose (glucose-1 → 6-glucose), rutinose (rhamnose-1 → 6-glucose)
Trisaccharides	Gentiotriose (glucose-1 → 6-glucose-1 → 6-glucose), sorborose (glucose-1 → 6-glucose-1 → 4-glucose)
Acylated sugars	2-acetylglucose, 6-p-coumaroylglucose, 4-p-coumaroyl-rutinose, p-coumaroylsophorose, 2-feruloylsophorose

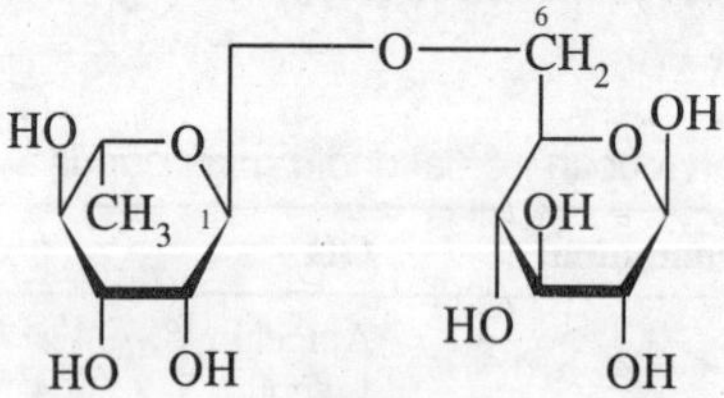

Rutinose
(α-L-Rhamnosyl-6-(6-1)-β-D-glucose)

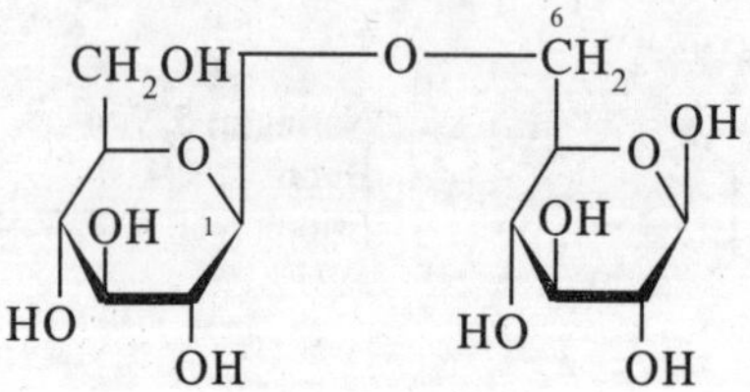

Gentiobiose
(β-D-Glucopyranosyl-(6-1)-β-D-glucose)

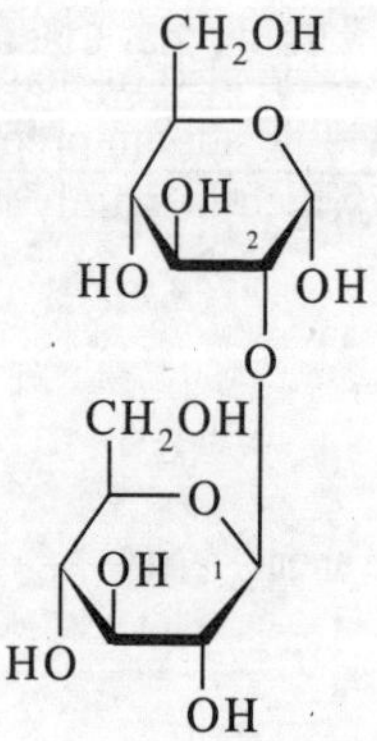

Sophorose
(β-D-Glucopyranosyl-(2-1)-β-D-glucose)

Among the flavonoid glycosides, which possess some biological and pharmacological activity, rutin and hesperidin, and some of their derivatives are used as a medicinal agents. However, mention is being made hereunder about some other flavonoids contained in other drugs (see Table 2.5).

Table 2.5. List of some flavonoid glycosides

Glycoside	Source	Aglycone and sugar moiety
Astragalin	*Astragalus sinicus*	Kaempferol-3-glucoside
Kaempfertin	*Indigofera erecta*	Kaempferol-3,7-dirhamnoside
Quercetrin	*Quercus infectoria*	Quercetin-3-rhamnoside
Rutin	*Ruta graveolens*	Quercetin-3-rutinoside
Myricitrin	*Myrica rubra*	Myricetin-3-rhamnoside
Hesperidin	*Fagopyrum esculentum*	Hesperitin-7-β-rutinoside
Vitexin	*Vitex* species	Apigenin-7-O-β-D-glucopyranoside

COUMARIN GLYCOSIDES

They are benzo-α-pyrone derivatives having aromatic smell and their alcoholic solutions, when made alkaline, show blue or green fluorescence. Umbelliferon is 7-OH coumarin and is present in free state in galbanum and in combined state in asafoetida. Aesculetin is 6 : 7 dihydroxy coumarin. Aesculetin and its glycoside aesculin are present in species of Rosaceae including *Crataegus oxyacantha*. Aesculin, similar to rutin, has Vit. P like activity and is official in French Pharmacopoeia. Scopoletin is 6-methoxy, 7-hydroxy coumarin and its glycoside scopolin or methyl aesculin is present in belladonna, datura, wild cherry bark and jalap. Coumarins have flavouring property but they cause damage to liver. Coumarin drugs also cause drug interactions with many other drugs and possess carcinogenic properties. As a result their use in U.S.A. as flavouring agents is banned. They are also of diagnostic importance. Umbelliferon and aesculetin are added in sun tan preparations as they absorb rays of wavelength 280–315 nm which is mainly responsible for erythema formation.

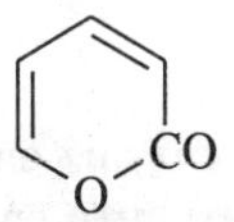

α-Pyrone 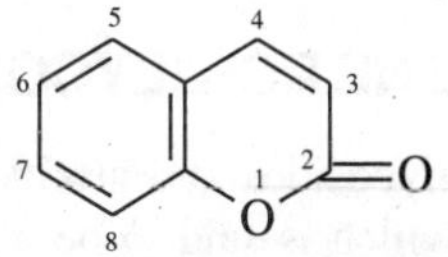   Benzo-α-pyrone (Coumarin)

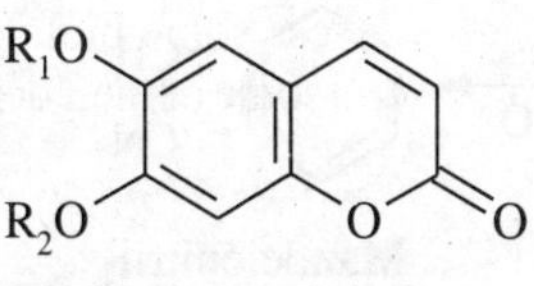

	R
Umbelliferon	H
Herniarin	CH_3

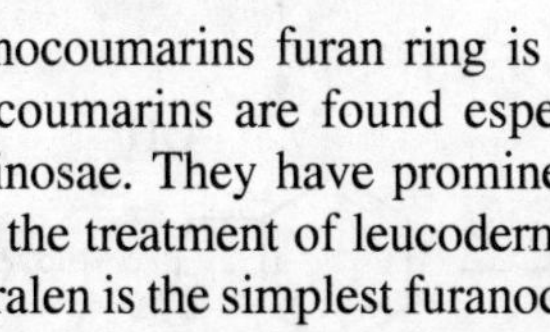

	R_1	R_2
Aesculetin	H	H
Aesculin	Glucose	H
Scopoletin	CH_3	H
Scopolin	CH_3	Glucose

FURANOCOUMARINS

In furanocoumarins furan ring is joined at 6 : 7 or 7 : 8 to coumarins. Furanocoumarins are found especially in Rutaceae, Umbelliferae and Leguminosae. They have prominent photosensibilising property and are used in the treatment of leucoderma.

Psoralen is the simplest furanocoumarin and is present in Bavchi fruits. Xanthotoxin is 8-methoxy psoralen and is present in *Ammi majus* fruits. Bergapten is 5-methoxy psoralen and is present in bergamot, *Citrus*

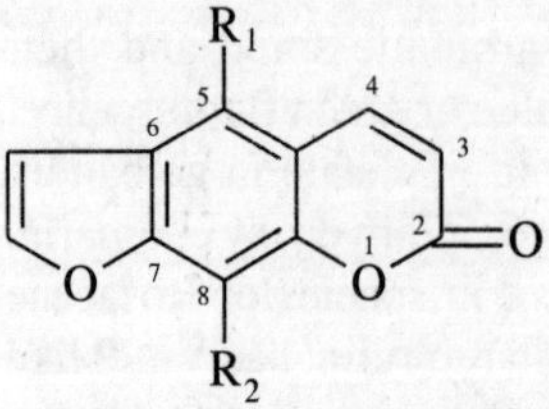

	R_1	R_2
Psoralen	H	H
Xanthotoxin	H	OCH_3
Bergapten	OCH_3	H
Imperatorin	H	$OCH_2CH=C\begin{smallmatrix}CH_3\\CH_3\end{smallmatrix}$

bergamia (Rutaceae). If Eau de Cologne containing bergamot oil is applied to the skin and exposed to sun light, pigmentation occurs. Imperatorin is 8-dimethyl allyloxy psoralen. Marmelosin found in *Aegle marmelos* fruits is the same substance as imperatorin. Furanocoumarins absorb rays of 315–400 nm wavelength at which pigmentation occurs. Recently xanthotoxin is used in psoriasis. After application, irradiation with long UV rays max 360 nm should be carried out. According to recent findings xanthotoxin has carcinogenic properties.

CYANOGENETIC GLYCOSIDES

They are β-glycosides and are hydrolyzed by an enzyme emulsin, a β-glycosidase which is said to be a mixture of two or three enzymes. The hydrolysis of cyanogenetic glycosides takes place in two or three stages and ultimate products of hydrolysis are benzaldehyde, sugars and hydrocyanic acid. The medicinal action of cyanogenetic glycosides is due to hydrocyanic acid and so action of enzyme is desirable. Amygdalin is well-known and widely distributed cyanogenetic glycoside. It is present in bitter almond and its hydrolysis takes place as follows:

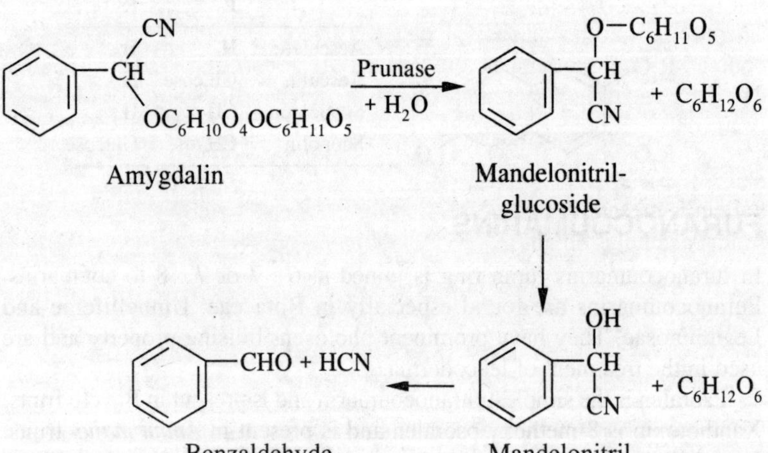

Amygdalin $\xrightarrow[+ H_2O]{\text{Prunase}}$ Mandelonitril-glucoside $+ C_6H_{12}O_6$

Mandelonitril-glucoside $\longrightarrow$ Mandelonitril $+ C_6H_{12}O_6$

Mandelonitril $\longrightarrow$ Benzaldehyde (CHO) + HCN

The cyanogenetic glycosides may be identified by the following tests which depend on the liberation of volatile hydrocyanic acid.

1. Grignard reaction or sodium picrate test: Dip a strip of white filter paper in 10% aqueous solution of picric acid, drain it and dip in a 10% sodium carbonate solution and drain again. Bruise or powder the drug, moisten it with water and put into a conical flask. Trap the sodium picrate paper on the neck of flask with cork. Because of volatile hydrocyanic acid, the paper will become brick red or maroon-coloured.
2. With 3% aqueous solution of mercurous nitrate reduction to metallic mercury takes place. This test can be used as localization test.

BITTER GLYCOSIDES

Bitter glycosides are characteristic of species of Gentianaceae. According to Korte gentiopicrin is characteristic glycoside of Gentianaceae. Bitter drugs and bitter constituents are used since a very early period as stomachics, febrifuges, bitter tonics and in digestive disturbances. In different countries different species of Gentianaceae are used. Bitter substances usually containing lactone group are soluble in water and their evaluation is carried out by bitter limit which is the maximum dilution in which they still taste bitter.

Bitter substances increase the digestive secretion by reflex action and are used as stomachics and digestives. Because of bitter taste they are used as bitter tonics and antipyretic. Bitter drugs or their preparations should be taken before or during meals, otherwise they cause digestive disturbances like diarrhoea, vomiting and pain in the stomach.

ALCOHOL AND OTHER GLYCOSIDES

There are some other alcoholic (phenolic) glycosides, other than the tannins, coumarins, anthraquinones, etc., which are found distributed in nature. They are mentioned hereunder with sufficient information about their occurrence, nature, uses, etc.

Salicin

Salicin is present in barks of *Salix* species. By its hydrolysis saligenin or salicyl alcohol is obtained, which contains alcohol as well as phenol group

Salicin   Saligenin

and it can be considered also phenol glycoside. Salicin is bitter tonic, febrifuge, analgesic and antirheumatic. Its action is attributed to salicylic acid produced by oxidation. Coniferin is also alcohol glycoside and on oxidation yields vanillin. Further, phenol glycoside arbutin, aldehyde glycoside vanilloside and ester glycoside monotropitoside also occur.

Arbutin

Arbutin is the phenol glycoside present in leaves of Uva ursi (*Arctostaphylus uva ursi*) and in other species of Ericaceae and in species of Rosaceae. Arbutin on hydrolysis yields glucose and hydroquinone.

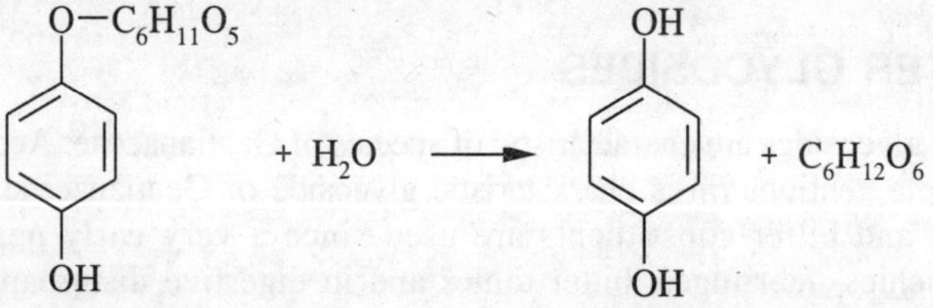

Arbutin + H_2O ⟶ Hydroquinone + $C_6H_{12}O_6$

$O-C_6H_{11}O_5$

Arbutin is used as a diuretic and urinary antiseptic for which hydroquinone is considered responsible for the activity. Even though the drug has great reputation and is used since a very early period, it has been shown that for activity of arbutin or arbutin-containing drugs, alkaline reaction of urine and a high dose of drug are necessary which is rarely the case. The drug contains hyperoside (quercetin-3-galactoside) and myricetin (5,7,3',4',5'-pentahydroxyflavonol) which may be responsible for the above activity.

Vanilloside is the aldehyde glycoside and occurs as glucovanillin and is present in vanilla pods. On its hydrolysis vanillin and glucose are obtained.

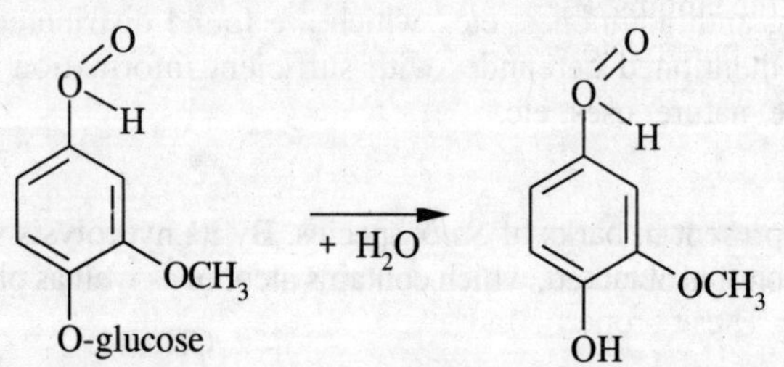

Vanilloside + H_2O ⟶ Vanillin

Monotropitoside

Monotropitoside is present in the leaves of *Gaultheria procumbens* (Ericaeae) and bark of *Betula lenta* (Betulaceae). It is an ester glycoside of methyl salicylate and sugar primeverose consisting of two sugars, xylose and glucose. By partial hydrolysis an intermediary glycoside gaultherin and xylose are obtained. Gaultherin is present also as an independent glycoside. Gaultherin on hydrolysis yields methyl salicylate and glucose. By steam distillation of the above drugs oil, called wintergreen oil, is obtained. Wintergreen oil contains 99% methyl salicylate. Methyl salicylate is also obtained synthetically. Methyl salicylate is used as a flavouring agent, as internal antiseptic and as an aromatic in Cascara preparations. It has irritant property and is used externally in rheumatism. Methyl salicylate is popularly used in dental preparations.

COOCH₃
O-Primeveyose
glucose + xylose
Monotropitoside

COOCH₃
O-glucose
Gaultherin

COOCH₃
OH
Methyl salicylate

TANNINS

Tannins constitute a large group of complex organic, non-nitrogenous, phenolic compounds of high molecular weight and are widely distributed in plant kingdom. They possess the property to 'tan', i.e. to convert hide and skin into leather. This property of these chemical substances of vegetable origin was first described by Sequin in 1976. Tannins are soluble in water and alcohol, have astringent taste, precipitate proteins, and produce acidic reaction. The acidic reaction is attributed to polyphenols or carboxyl group. Tannins with ferric salts give deep blue, green, black or violet colour or precipitate. Tannins give precipitate with antipyrine or gelatin. This is the test of true tannins. Pseudotannins like catechins do not show this test. Tannins give precipitate with heavy metallic salts, alkaloids and proteins and are used as antidotes in alkaloid and heavy metal poisonings. They are used as reagents for identifying gelatin, alkaloids and proteins. The reaction with potassium dichromate or 1% chromic acid is used in the manufacture of 'Chrome leather'. Tannins give precipitate with alkaloids and produce tannates, many of which are insoluble in water and are used in alkaloidal poisonings. These properties are enumerated below:

1. They have sharp puckering taste (astringent taste).
2. Both kinds of tannins are non-crystallizable compounds.
3. With water they form colloidal solutions possessing an acid reaction (test for acidity of the solution).
4. Precipitation of solution of gelatin takes place.

5. Precipitation of solution of alkaloid takes place.
6. With $FeCl_3$ they form dark blue or greenish black soluble compounds.
7. They produce deep red colour with potassium ferricyanide and ammonia.
8. They are precipitated by salts of copper, lead and tin.
9. They are precipitated by a strong aqueous potassium dichromate or 1% chromic acid solution.
10. In alkaline solution, many of their derivatives readily absorb oxygen.
11. They have ability to combine with the protein rendering them resistant to proteolytic enzymes.

Note: The above physical and chemical properties are common in this group of complex chemical substances i.e. tannins, but they are not structurally alike.

Classification of tannins

Tannins are classified as follows:

1. Hydrolysable tannins
2. Condensed tannins
3. Pseudotannins.

Hydrolysable tannins

These tannins undergo hydrolysis by acids or enzymes and produce gallic acid or ellagic acid and according to the acid produced they are known as gallitannins or ellagitannins. Gallic acid and ellagic acid are found united by ester linkages to a central glucose residue. These tannins were formerly known as pyrogallol tannins as on dry distillation gallic acid and other similar components yield pyrogallol. Ellegic acid mostly occurs as a diester of its open-ringed form, hexahydroxydiphenic acid. These tannins show the following tests:

1. With ferric chloride blue or black colour or precipitate is produced and thus they are used in the manufacture of inks.
2. When these tannins are heated pyrogallol is produced.
3. When heated with hydrochloric acid the corresponding acid like gallic acid is produced.

Galls and tannic acid are hydrolysable tannins.

Condensed tannins

Condensed tannins are formed by condensation of many catechin units. These tannins are also known as catechol tannins or phlobatannins. These tannins show the following reactions:

1. When these tannins are heated catechol is produced.

2. With ferric chloride they show green colour.
3. These tannins produce phloroglucinol by reaction with dilute hydrochloric acid. Because of this reaction these tannins show match-stick test where the lignin of the match-stick shows red colour.
4. With vanillin–alcohol–dilute hydrochloric acid (1 : 10 : 10) they show red colour.
5. When heated with hydrochloric acid or on oxidation the soluble light-coloured phlobatannins are converted into insoluble, dark-coloured decomposition products phlobaphenes. Thus, cinchotannic acid in cinchona bark is converted into phlobaphene cinchona red.
6. With bromine water these tannins give precipitate.

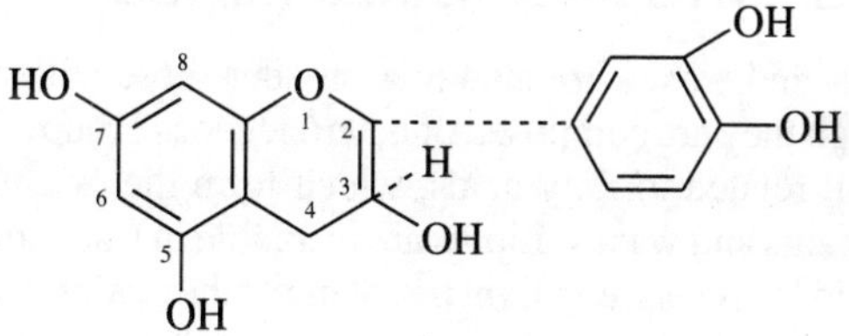

(+) – Catechin

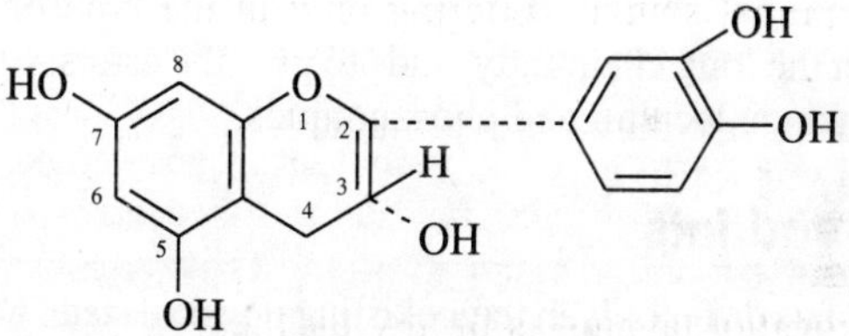

(+) – Epicatechin

Pale and black catechu, cinchona, cinnamon and wild cherry bark contain condensed tannins.

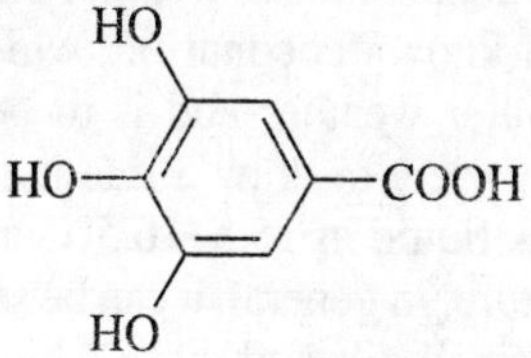

Gallic acid

Tannins are used as antiseptic on skin and mucous membrane because proteins are precipitated and microorganisms starve as protein is not available as food and they are used as healing agents in inflammation, leucorrhoea, gonorrhoea, piles, burns, etc. Phenol groups are also responsible for the antiseptic activity. Tannins are also used in gastro-intestinal diseases like diarrhoea.

Recent studies have shown that certain tannin-rich plant materials on prolonged use may act as potential carcinogenic agents. Thus, habitual chewing of betel nut (*Areca catechu*) containing besides alkaloids, condensed tannins, has been linked with high incidence of oral and esophageal cancer in South Africa and India. Even tea taken without milk may cause cancer. Milk precipitates tannins and incidence of cancer may not take place. Extracts of *Areca catechu* when injected subcutaneously in mice caused malignant tumours.

FIXED OILS, FATS AND WAXES (LIPIDS)

Fixed oils, fats and waxes are also in a broader sense collectively called **lipids**. Although they are composed of heterogeneous group of compounds, yet they are all related to fatty acids, which form the essential structural entities of oils, fats and waxes. Lipids are insoluble in water and are soluble in organic "lipid" solvents, e.g. light petroleum, ether, chloroform, benzene, etc. For the sake of convenience, the oils and fats and waxes can be considered here separately, even though they are substances of either vegetable or animal source, differing only in the type of alcohol that combines with the long chain fatty acids to give the esters. Lipids, besides waxes, also include lecithin and phospholipids.

Fixed oils and fats

Fixed oils and fats differ only in their existing physical state, which depends upon the temperature. The fluids are known as oils, while the solids or semisolids are known as fats. Further, an oil at a lower temperature may attain the state and status of fats, while reverse is possible for a fat taking shape or state of an oil at higher temperature. Thus, a lipid which is an oil, e.g. chaulmoogra oil in Dubai in the hot weather of May is a fat in Kashmir, in cold season. The well-known coconut oil, which is normally a liquid, solidifies in the cold winter weather and is to be warmed before being used as a hair oil. With a view to draw a line it can be safely said that a lipid is a fixed oil, if it is liquid at 15.5–16.5°C and a fat, if it is solid or semisolid at this temperature. In general, it can be said that liquids at normal temperature are fatty or fixed oils and those which are solid or semisolid are fats. Another generalised view is that the vegetable lipids are liquids at ordinary temperature, while the lipids obtained from animals are fats. Exceptions do exist. Cocoa butter, a vegetable lipid, is a solid oil and cod liver and shark liver oils, the animal lipids, are liquid fats.

Fixed oils and fats belong to a larger group of natural organic polar compounds, which are of common occurrence in food materials. Hence, they, along with carbohydrates and proteins, are of great nutritional value. Besides, they are important materials in pharmaceutical and other industries and as such they are very much utilised.

Most of the fixed oils are obtained by direct expression of the material. In other cases the material is grounded and then subjected to hydraulic pressure. Another method is to extract the fixed oil with organic solvents. These methods are given under each oil.

Fixed oils can also be grouped into three categories according to their behaviour on exposition to air, such as drying oils, semi-drying oils and non-drying oils. This grouping is based upon their ability to absorb oxygen from the air, and as such oxygen saturates the double bonds to form oxides which may be polymerized to form hard and/or elastic films on surfaces, especially woody, on which they are applied.

Fixed oils may be hydrogenated by passing hydrogen gas in the presence of finely divided nickel through the oil heated to 160–200°C. In this process the unsaturated fatty acids are more or less completely converted into saturated acids, which are usually solid at room temperature and very stable. Sulphonated oils are produced by reacting fatty acids and sulphuric acid under low temperature, resulting in the sulphates of fats. Sulphonated oils find their wide use in textile, leather and metal industries.

Chemically fixed oils and fats are the glycerides (or Glyceryl 1 esters) of fatty acids having the following general formula:

$$
\begin{array}{l}
CH_2-O-CO-R \\
\;\;| \\
CH-O-CO-R \\
\;\;| \\
CH_2-O-CO-R
\end{array}
$$

Glycerine has three alcoholic hydroxy (OH) groups. If the same fatty acid is combined with all the three OH groups the fat is a simple glyceride, but if three different fatty acids are combined it is called a mixed glyceride. Fats usually contain mixed glycerides.

CH_2OH	CH_2OCOR	CH_2OCOR_1
$CHOH$	$CHOCOR$	$CHOCOR_2$
CH_2OH	CH_2OCOR	CH_2OCOR_3
Glycerine	Simple glycerides	Mixed glycerides

Thus if R_1, R_2 and R_3 are having the same fatty acid radical, e.g. $C_{15}H_{31}$ tripalmitin will result; if the radicals are $C_{17}H_{35}$ and $C_{17}H_{33}$ the resultant glycerides are called tristearin and triolein, respectively. Examples of two simple triglycerides (now preferably called triacylglycerols) are given below.

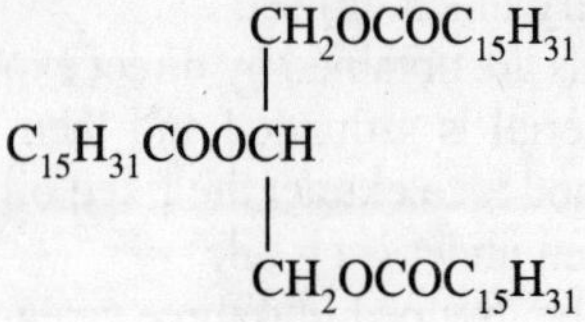

$$CH_2OCOC_{15}H_{31}$$
$$C_{15}H_{31}COOCH$$
$$CH_2OCOC_{15}H_{31}$$

Tripalmitin
Simple triglycerol or lipid with saturated fatty acid*
$$CH_3 . (CH_2)_{14} . COOH]$$

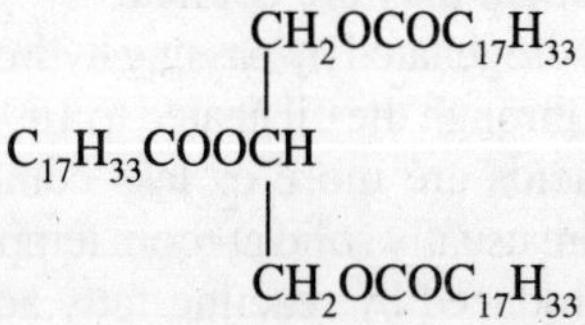

$$CH_2OCOC_{17}H_{33}$$
$$C_{17}H_{33}COOCH$$
$$CH_2OCOC_{17}H_{33}$$

Triolein
Simple triglycerol or lipid with unsaturated fatty acid*
$$[CH_3 . (CH_2)_7 . CH=CH-(CH_2)_7 . COOH$$

* Fatty acids are called fatty acids as they were discovered as a result of hydrolysis of glyceryl esters in fats.

Besides, glycerol can also react partially and yield monoglycerides, diglycerides or triglycerides depending upon whether its one, two or all the three alcoholic hydroxy groups react with one, two or all the three molecules of monobasic fatty acids. In the above two examples triglycerides are shown. Examples of mono- and diglycerides are:

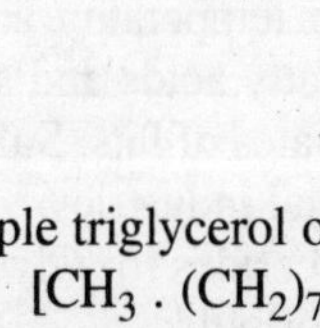

$$CH_2OCOR$$
$$HOCH$$
$$CH_2OH$$

$$CH_2OCOR$$
$$R'COOCH$$
$$CH_2OH$$

D-α-monoglyceride 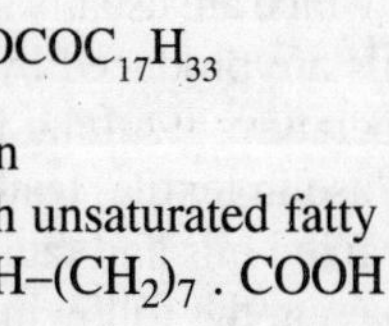   D-α-β-diglyceride

Normally the plant lipids have saturated straight chain of even number of carbons. These acids, therefore, represent homologous series viz. $CH . (CH)_n . COOH$ wherein n is even number. But recent gas liquid chromatographic (GLC) analysis has shown the occurrence of odd number of fatty acids. An example of such acid is "isovaleric acid" with five carbons (C) which is found in the hydrolysate of dolphin oil and shows the following branched chain formula:

$$
\begin{array}{l} H_3C \\ \diagdown \\ CHCH_2COOH \\ \diagup \\ H_3C \end{array}
\qquad
\begin{array}{l} CH=CH \\ | \diagdown \\ CH[CH_2]_{12}COOH \\ | \diagup \\ CH_2-CH_2 \end{array}
$$

    Isovaleric acid   Chaulmoogric acid

Some other fatty acids of plant origin (like gorlic, hydnocarpic and chaulmoogric acids) have a hydrocarbon chain which terminates in a cyclopentene ring.

In the mixed glycerides usually saturated acids like stearic acid and palmitic acid or unsaturated acids like oleic acid or linoleic acid are found. If the unsaturated acids are more, usually it is an oil and if saturated acids are more than it is a fat. In the fixed oils and fats, besides glycerine and fatty acids 2–5% other substances like phosphatides and in unsaponifiable part phytosterols (β-sitosterol, stigmasterol), hydrocarbons, fat-soluble vitamins as A, D and E and other substances possessing smell are present. Fixed oils and fats cannot be distilled without their decomposition. On distillation of oils or fats acrolein, an aldehyde, possessing a smell of scorched fat, so often found in scorched milk, is produced. Acrolein is produced by loss of water from glycerine.

$$
\begin{array}{l} CH_2OH \\ | \\ CHOH \\ | \\ CH_2OH \end{array}
\quad \xrightarrow{-H_2O} \quad
\begin{array}{l} CH_2 \\ || \\ CH \\ | \\ CHO \end{array}
$$

    Glycerine   Acrolein

If fats are hydrolyzed with alkali, salts of fatty acids, which are nothing but soaps and glycerine are produced. As soap is formed in this hydrolysis, this process is called saponification. If saponification is carried out with sodium hydroxide hard sodium soaps, used for washing clothes, are produced. With potassium hydroxide soft soaps are produced. Lead soaps formed with lead monoxide are used as plasters.

Rancidity

Many fixed oils and fats become rancid because of the effect of moisture, air, light and microorganisms and are characterized by unpleasant smell and bad taste. These rancid oils are unsuitable as food or as vehicle in pharmaceuticals. In contact with moisture hydrolysis of fats by lipase takes place and free fatty acids are produced. Microorganisms in the presence of oxygen produce ketone and ketone acids and oxygen of the air in the presence of light produces oxides and peroxides and all these substances produce rancidity. Hence fats should be stored in air-tight containers protected from moisture, light and air to prevent rancidity.

Hydrogenated fats

Fixed oils contain unsaturated fatty acids and hydrogenation of unsaturated acids is carried out with nickel as a catalyst and hydrogen is added to the double bonds of fatty acids and fixed oils become solid. In India mainly groundnut oil is used for hydrogenation. Margarine used in Europe is also a hydrogenated fat. Though hydrogenated fat is less digestible than natural fats and its absorption is less, yet it is more convenient to use and has a better taste. According to one belief the cholesterol in the blood in solid hydrogenated fat is not transported easily, it accumulates in the blood and its increase in blood is one of the causes of heart diseases.

Polymerisation

As stated above fixed oils are also classified as drying oils, semi-drying oils and non-drying oils. If a thin layer of drying oil is applied and exposed to air, it resinifies, dries and forms a hard transparent film. Linseed oil is an example of drying oil and because of this property it is used in the manufacture of paints and varnishes. Drying oils contain unsaturated acids with two or more double bonds and add oxygen at the double bonds and this additive compound polymerizes and resinifies. Semi-drying oils like cottonseed oil resinify and dry out but do not form the film. Non-drying oils neither dry nor form a film. Olive oil is an example of non-drying oil.

In the following pages are given some tables listing the fatty acids, both saturated and unsaturated, as also those which have cyclic structures, along with certain specifications some of which are also included in pharmacopoeias, like iodine values, saponification value, etc. which are used for the analysis affixed oils. These specifications are also briefly mentioned below and for details pharmacopoeias and other reference books may be consulted by the readers.

Fixed oils can often be identified by their physical properties such as melting point, refractive index, specific gravity, etc. Apart from determining the physical constants, a number of chemical tests are carried out on fixed oils to determine their identity, quality and purity.

Saponification value or number is the number of milligrams of potassium hydroxide required to saponify one gm of oil or fat.

Iodine value or number is a measure of the degree of unsaturation of fat or oil and is defined as the number of grams of iodine absorbed by 100 gm of fat or oil.

Acid value or Acid number indicates the amount of free fatty acids present in the oil i.e. number of milligrams of potassium hydroxide required to neutralize free fatty acids in 1 gm of the substance.

Riechert-Meissl number is defined as the number of millilitres of 0.1 N potassium hydroxide solution required to neutralize the volatile water-soluble acids obtained by the hydrolysis of 5 gm of fat or fixed oil.

Uses

Unsaturated fatty acid, linoleic acid, containing two double bonds is not synthesised in the organism and its absence in the food causes certain deficiency symptoms like skin lesions. Linolenic acid containing three double bonds however can be synthesised from linoleic acid and has the same action as linoleic acid. These symptoms disappear when the above two acids are administered and so are called essential acids. These acids lower the cholesterol level in the blood and are used as cholesterol suppressants. These essential acids are precursors of physiologically very active substances, prostaglandins. These acids are also used as antifungal agents.

The fats and oils are emollients when used externally and have protective action on skin and mucous membrane and are used in the treatment of wounds, burns, sunburns, eczema and dandruff of hairs. Internally oils are indifferent substances and so olive oil is used as a mild laxative and has also cholagogue action.

Certain oils and fats have their own therapeutic action. Castor oil is used as laxative and chaulmoogra oil is used in leprosy. Fats along with carbohydrates and proteins are important articles of food rich in calories and are used as dietary supplement. Fats and oils are used as vehicles for other medicaments and are used in the preparations of ointments, liniments and suppositories. Certain oils and fats contain fat-soluble vitamins A, D and E and are used in avitaminoses of these vitamins.

Further fats and oils are used in the manufacture of soaps, glycerine, paints and varnishes and as lubricants.

Waxes

Waxes have physical properties similar to fats and are solid, semi-solid or occasionally liquid. Chemically waxes are esters or mixtures of esters of higher fatty acids and higher alcohols. The fatty acids in wax are the same as the fatty acids in fats. Alcohols are monohydroxy alcohols of high molecular weight especially ceryl alcohol and myricyl alcohol. Sometimes cholesterol or phytosterols are also combined.

Fats can he hydrolyzed by aqueous alkali while waxes are not hydro-lyzed by aqueous alkali but by alcoholic alkali solutions.

Hydrolyzing enzymes of wax are not present in our alimentary system and as such they are not suitable as food similar to fats.

Table 2.6. Some common fatty acids of plants

Saturated acids

Caproic	$C_5H_{11}COOH$	$CH_3(CH_2)_4COOH$	n-Hexanoic
Caprylic	$C_7H_{15}COOH$	$CH_3(CH_2)_6COOH$	n-Octanoic
Capric	$C_9H_{19}COOH$	$CH_3(CH_2)_8COOH$	n-Decanoic
Lauric	$C_{11}H_{23}COOH$	$CH_3(CH_2)_{10}COOH$	n-Dodecanoic
Myristic	$C_{13}H_{27}COOH$	$CH_3(CH_2)_{12}COOH$	n-Tetradecanoic
Palmitic	$C_{15}H_{31}COOH$	$CH_3(CH_2)_{14}COOH$	n-Hexadecanoic
Stearic	$C_{17}H_{35}COOH$	$CH_3(CH_2)_{16}COOH$	n-Octadecanoic
Arachidic	$C_{19}H_{39}COOH$	$CH_3(CH_2)_{18}COOH$	n-Eicosanoic

Unsaturated acids

Oleic	$C_{17}H_{33}COOH$	$CH_3(CH_2)_7CH = CH(CH_2)_7COOH$
Linoleic	$C_{17}H_{31}COOH$	$CH_3(CH_2)_4CH = CHCH_2CH = CH(CH_2)_7COOH$
Linolenic	$C_{17}H_{29}COOH$	$CH_3(CH_2)CH = CHCH_2CH = CH(CH_2)_7COOH$
Arachidonic	$C_{19}H_{31}COOH$	$CH_3(CH_2)_4(CH = CHCH_2)(CH_2)_2COOH$

Acetylenic acids

Tariric	$C_{17}H_{31}COOH$	$CH_3(CH_2)_{10}C = C(CH_2)_4COOH$
Stearolic	$C_{17}H_{31}COOH$	$CH_3(CH_2)_7C = C(CH_2)_7COOH$

Hydroxy acids

Ricinoleic	$C_{17}H_{32}(OH)COOH$	$CH_3(CH_2)_5CHOH . CH_2CH = CH(CH_2)_7COOH$

Cyclic acids

Sterulic	$C_{19}H_{31}COOH$	CH_2 over $CH_3(CH_2)_7C = C(CH_2)_7COOH$
Hydnocarpic	$C_{15}H_{27}COOH$	$CH=CH$ / CH_2-CH_2 ring $CH[CH_2]_{10}COOH$
Chaulmoogric	$C_{17}H_{31}COOH$	$CH=CH$ / CH_2-CH_2 ring $CH[CH_2]_{12}COOH$
Gorlic	$C_{17}H_{29}COOH$	$CH=CH$ / CH_2-CH_2 ring $CH[C_{12}H_{22}]COOH$

PROTEINS

Proteins, carbohydrates and fats are essential groups of compounds which occur in plants and animals. Hence they are of immense biochemical importance. Of these groups, proteins, which are always present in all living matter, can be easily singled out as substances of great significance in biochemistry. Important sources of animal proteins are flesh and meat of all kinds and eggs, while the plant sources rich in proteins are organic nitrogenous substances (compare with alkaloids, another group referred to as organic nitrogenous substances) made up of amino acids or in other words amino acids are the structural units of proteins. As many as twenty amino acids of L-configuration are known to build up a molecule of proteins or peptides. Amino acids combine by a peptide linkage, CONH, which results through the combination of carboxylic (COOH) group of one amino acid with the amino (NH_2) group of another amino acid with elimination of water (HOH), as exemplified below.

$$R-CH(NH_2)CHOOH \quad + \quad R-CH(CH_2).COOH$$

Amino acid $\qquad \downarrow \qquad$ Amino acid

$$R-CH(CH_2)-CO-NH-CH-R+H_2O$$

$$COOH$$

Dipeptide

By successive combination of amino acids, tri-, terra-, penta- and polypeptides are formed, leading to the formation of proteins. The peptides and proteins represent a wide variety of compounds having low to very high molecular weight and exhibiting different physical, chemical and therapeutic properties. Proteins are usually classified into three main groups: (1) simple proteins, (2) conjugated proteins, and (3) derived proteins. Simple proteins on being hydrolysed give rise to amino acids and are exemplified by albumins, globulins, glutalins and protamines. Conjugated proteins are rather more complex proteins and are composed of a protein and a non-protein group (called prosthetic group) and are exemplified by mucoproteins (in combination with carbohydrate); casein (phosphorous-containing protein); nucleoproteins (protein in combination with lipids). Besides, there are some cyclic polypeptide structures with lower molecular weight, such as antibiotics (bacitracin, gramicidin, polymisin); peptide hormones (oxytocin, vasopressin); and glutathione (found in almost all living cells) which belong to the conjugated proteins group. The derived proteins are the degradation products of the proteins.

Proteins have multiple functions to perform. Both plant and animal proteins are essential foodstuffs and supply essential amino acids. The enzymes are proteins and they act as catalysts in most biochemical reactions. Peptide hormones e.g. insulin carry out the regulatory functions in the organism. As antibodies they are a part of immune system of the animals.

Serum albumin acts as a buffer in blood, and the iron-containing hemoglobin transports oxygen in organism. Scleroproteins are constituents which support skeletal substances of the body. The contraction of the muscle is due to two proteins known as myosin and actin. Biologically, as stated above, the most important proteins are nucleoproteins in which proteins are combined with nucleic acid present in the living cell in nucleus and cytoplasm. They play important role in genetics. Nucleoproteins are also present in viruses.

There are also some proteins which are very poisonous. Ricin in castor oil, robin from locust bark and abrin in jequirity seeds are poisonous plant proteins. Likewise, poisonous animal proteins are hemolysins from salamanders (*Triturus* species) and neurotoxins from snake venoms. The venom is a complex mixture of protein comprising of two fractions, one with enzymatic activity and another with nonenzymatic activity, the latter having the neurotoxins.

Amino acids

It is relevant to state here about amino acids, as they have been repeatedly referred to above as not only the basic units of proteins, but otherwise also as essential substances of metabolic and biochemic importance. Amino acids, besides being the basic units, are also found in free state. They have four regular elements – carbon, hydrogen, oxygen and nitrogen – which build their structure. However, some amino acids may contain atoms like sulphur, iodine and phosphorus. An amino acid may contain more than one amino group (NH_2) as also more than one carboxylic group (COOH). Although most of the amino acid are straight-chained aliphatic compounds, yet some have aromatic as well as heterocyclic structures (see structures below).

Amino acids are usually freely soluble in water and only slightly soluble in alcohol. They give pink, violet or blue colour on being warmed with ninhydrin, a test which is also utilised in paper and thin layer chromatographic visualization and identification of amino acids. As an exception the amino acid proline gives only a yellow colour with ninhydrin. The famous biuret test given by peptides and proteins is not given by amino acids. Besides, some amino acids give a few other special tests which help in detecting and distinguishing these amino acids e.g. histidine colour reaction with diazonium salts. Given below are some structures of amino acids which will show certain variations mentioned above. Also these amino acids are the ones which are commonly met within protein molecules.

$$H_3C-CH(NH_2)-COOH$$
Asparagine

$$H_2N-OC-CH_2(NH_2)-COOH$$
Alanine

$$H_2N-\overset{\overset{NH}{\|}}{C}-NH-(CH_2)_3-CH(NH_2)-COOH$$
Arginine

$$HOOC-CH(NH_2)-CHOH$$
Aspartic acid

$$HOOC-CH(NH_2)-CH_2-SH$$
Cysteine (has sulphur)

$$HOOC-CH(NH)-CHOH$$
Serine

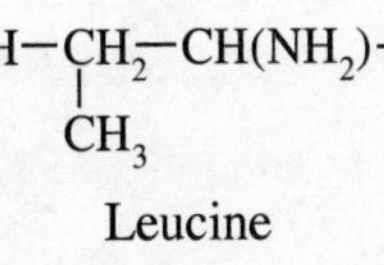

Proline

$$H_3C-CH-\underset{\underset{CH_3}{|}}{CH_2}-CH(NH_2)-COOH$$
Leucine

There are several hundred amino acids which are known to occur in nature. They have been characterized as free amino acids as they are not found in proteins. However, only some of them are met with commonly and the larger number of them, found in plant organs, act only as nitrogen reserve.

Amino acids are very essential for the biosynthesis of enzymes, storage proteins, hemoglobin, actin, myosin, antibodies, clotting factors and hormones. Protein deficiency leads to malnutrition and affects the growth and development of the body.

Qualitative test for protein

Biuret test

To 2–3 ml of protein solution in a test tube is added an equal volume of 10% sodium hydroxide solution. The solution is mixed thoroughly followed by the addition of a 0.5% copper sulphate solution drop by drop until a purplish violet colour is produced. Biuret test is positive for those molecules which contain two carbamyl groups (–CONH) joined either directly together or through a single atom of nitrogen or carbon.

Ninhydrin reaction

To 5 ml of a dilute protein solution (pH between 5 and 7) is added 0.5 ml of a 0.1 % solution of ninhydrin. The solution is heated to boiling for two minutes and allowed to cool. Blue colour indicates the presence of protein.

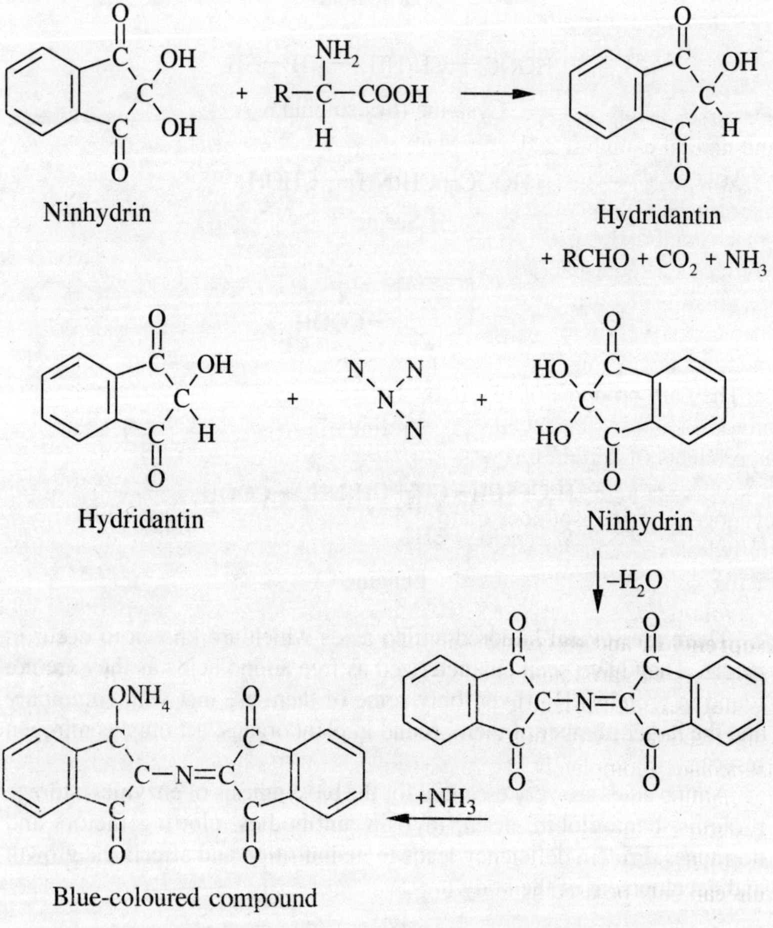

Ninhydrin

Hydridantin

+ RCHO + CO$_2$ + NH$_3$

Hydridantin

Ninhydrin

$-H_2O$

$+NH_3$

Blue-coloured compound

VOLATILE OILS

ESSENTIAL OILS, ETHEREAL OILS

Volatile oils are odorous constituents of plants. They are liquid, lipophile and volatile with a characteristic smell. Volatile oils volatize or evaporate on being exposed to atmosphere at an ordinary temperature and so they are called ethereal oils. They are also called essential oils as they are essences or concentrated constituents of the plants. Volatile oils are nearly insoluble in water. However, they dissolve in 1 : 200 parts of water, which concentration is sufficient to impart the characteristic taste and smell to the water. This property is utilised in the preparation of aromatic waters in pharmacy, e.g. rose water. Volatile oils are soluble in alcohol, ether and other lipide solvents. Volatile oils are usually lighter than water and their specific gravity is less than one. However, some volatile oils, like clove oil, have specific gravity more than one.

Volatile oils have high refractive index and show optical rotation. Optical rotation often gives useful information. Synthetic menthol and camphor are optically inactive or racemic, while natural menthol is levorotatory and natural camphor is dextrorotatory.

Volatile oils are present in the entire plant or almost in any part of the plant, as leaf, flower, bark, seed, fruit, wood and subterranean parts. They are characteristic of certain natural orders, such as Labiatae, Rutaceae, Myrtaceae, Lauraceae, Piperaceaei, Zingiberaceae and Umbelliferae.

Volatile oils are present in large modified parenchyma cells and in specialized well-defined secretory structures, such as glandular trichornes, endogenous oil containers and shizolysigenous oil ducts and oil canals.

They are products of plant metabolism, being formed directly by the protoplasm or by the decomposition of resinogenous layer of cell walls or as products of certain types of glycosides. Thus most volatile oils occur free or as such, but some are in glycosidal combination, as volatile oils in cyanogenetic and isothiocyanate glycosides, and are liberated subesquent to hydrolysis. Volatile oils are also present in oelo-resins and oelo-gum-resins, combined with resins and gums respectively.

Volatile oils belong to a chemical group known as **Terpenoids** or **Isoprenoids**, and as constituents of essential oil, the monoterpenes and sesquiterpenes are found in extremely high frequency. Monoterpenes may be defined as molecules containing ten carbon atoms derived by dimerization of two molecules of isoprene (2-methylbuta-1,3-diene) or isopentane (completely saturated form of five carbon units of isoprene) residue usually joined in a head to tail fashion, sometimes followed by oxidation-reduction rearrangement or other chemical reaction. Whereas sesquiterpenes form the higher boiling fraction of volatile oil, the isoprene rule can only be used as a guiding principle rather than a fixed rule. The isoprene rule together with modern carbonium ion chemistry can explain a large variety of monoterpene and sesquiterpene structures.

Chemically a volatile oil, as stated above, is a mixture of several constituents in which certain types of constituents are more predominating than the others, as hydrocarbons, alcohols, acids, ethers, esters, aldehydes, ketones or oxides. The chemical constituents present are complex and are mixtures of terpenes, as monoterpenes, sesquiterpenes or diterpenes and their derivatives and phenyl propane derivatives. Some volatile oils show one or two components in higher percentages, e.g. linalool in coriander, eugenol in clove and carvone in caraway. This predominance of one or two components determines the odour and use of a particular drug or its oil. In general otherwise a volatile oil has some 50 to 150 components of terpene derivatives and these all together are responsible for the odour of a particular oil. Some volatile oils containing plants are known to show qualitative and quantitative variations when they grow at different places and this phenomenon has been well documented by Stall and co-workers, who referred to this as chemical races.

Chemical constituents of volatile oils may also be divided into two broad classes on the basis of their biosynthetic origin:

1. Terpene derivatives formed via the acetate-mevalonic acid pathway.
2. Aromatic compounds formed via the shikimic acid-phenyl propanoid route.

As stated above, many volatile oils consist largely of terpenes, which are defined as natural products whose structures may be divided into (as they are built up of) isoprene (C_5H_8) units. These units arise from acetate via mevalonic acid and are branched-chain five carbon units containing two unsaturated bonds.

$$\underset{\text{Isoprene}}{CH_2-\overset{\overset{\displaystyle CH_3}{|}}{C}-CH=CH_2}$$

In terpenes formation the isoprene units are linked in a head to tail fashion and the number of units incorporated into a particular terpene serves as a basis for the classification of these compounds. Monoterpenes are composed of two isoprene units and have molecular formula, $C_{10}H_{16}$. Sesguiterpenes, $C_{15}H_{24}$, contain three isoprene units, diterpenes, $C_{20}H_{32}$, have four isoprene units and triterpenes, $C_{30}H_{48}$, are composed of six isoprene units.

Most of the terpenes found in volatile oils are monoterpenes. A few examples showing the number of isoprene units involved are given below (with zig-zag lines).

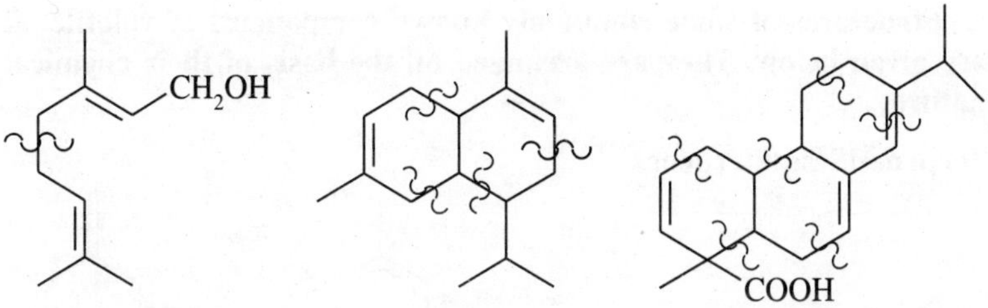

Geraniol
(monoterpene)

Cadinene
(sesquiterpene)

Abietic acid
(diterpene)

A second larger group of volatile oil constituents consists of phenyl propanoids, which contain the C_6 phenyl ring with an attached C_3 propane side chain, as shown below:

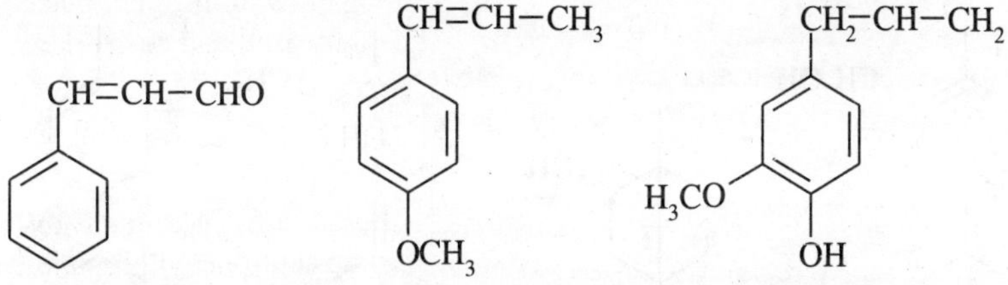

Cinnamaldehyde

Anethole

Eugenol

Preparation of volatile oils

Volatile oils may be prepared by steam distillation, by mechanical methods as sponge or Écuelle à piquer process, by extraction with non-volatile solvents or by extraction with volatile solvents. Details of these methods are considered outside the scope of this book.

Medicinal and commercial uses

Many crude drugs are used medicinally because of their volatile oil content. However, in numerous cases, volatile oils separated from drugs are used as drugs themselves. Similarly, various crude drugs are powdered and are employed as spices and condiments (anise, clove, etc.). The most common use of volatile oil is flavouring agents.

They are used externally as counter-irritants in inflammation, swelling and rheumatism as turpentine oil. They are used as carminative, digestive, spasmolytic, stimulant, bactericidal, antiseptic, disinfectant, diuretic, expectorant and as anthelminitic according to the active constituents present in them.

They are also used in perfumery, manufacture of soaps, toiletries, deodorizers and for masking or providing odour to household cleaners, polishes and insecticides.

Structures of some commonly known components of volatile oil are given below. They are arranged on the basis of their chemical nature.

Terpenes/Sesquiterpenes

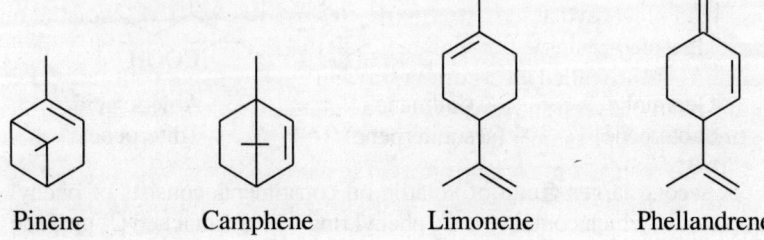

Pinene   Camphene   Limonene   Phellandrene

Alcohols

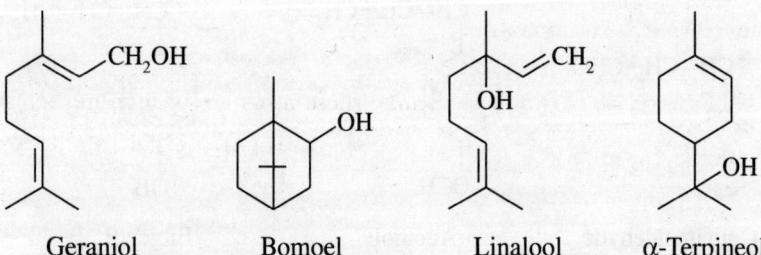

Geraniol   Bomoel   Linalool   α-Terpineol

Aldehydes and Ketones

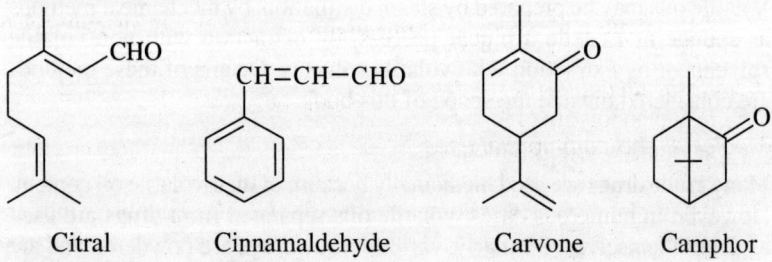

Citral   Cinnamaldehyde   Carvone   Camphor

Esters

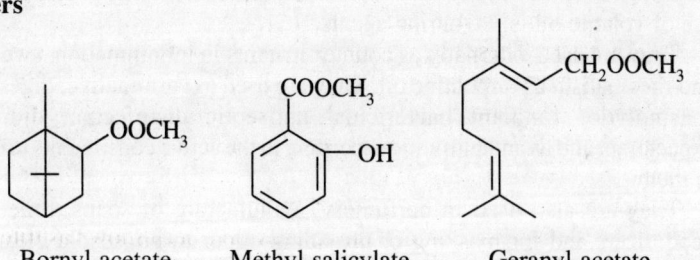

Bornyl acetate   Methyl salicylate   Geranyl acetate

RESINS

These are formed in schizogenous, lysigenous or schizlysigenous ducts or cavities. Resin is also found present differently, as in cells, ducts, cavities or glands. In **guaicum wood** all cells and tissues of heartwood are full of resins. Some resins, like **benzoin**, occur alone, while others are found in association with volatile oils or gums. Resins associated with volatile oil are called **oleo-resins**, e.g. **copaiba**. Resins in association with both volatile oil and gum are called **oleo-gum-resins** and those with gum only are called **gum-resins**. **Myrrh** and **asafoetida** are examples of oleo-gum resins, while **gamboge** is an example of gum-resins.

If the resins contain benzoic acid and/or cinnamic acid and/or their esters, they are called **balsams**. **Benzoin, storax, balsams of Tolu and Peru** are examples of balsams. Resins are considered as the end products of destructive metabolism or oxidation products of terpenes.

Resins are chemically not pure substances but are complex mixtures of several resinous substances. The resinous substances present in the resins are as follows:

1. *Resin acids or Resinolic acids:* These acids are of high molecular weight. They combine with alkali and their metallic salts and are called resinates. With aqueous solutions of alkali they form soap-like solutions or colloidal suspensions and are used in the preparation of varnishes and cheap phenyles. Resin acids contain a large proportion of diterpenoid oxyacids and show the properties of both carboxylic acids and phenols. Abietic acids in colophony and copaivic acids in capaiba are diterpenoid acids. Further, triterpene acids like boswelic acid, siaresinolic acid and elemic acid are met with. Resin acids may occur free or combined as esters.

2. *Resin alcohols (Resinols) and resinotannols:* Resin alcohols and resinotannols are of high molecular weight and occur free or combined as esters with balsamic acids or resin acids. Resin alcohols are tetracycline alcohols or pentacylic alcohols and are usually α-amyrine and β-amyrine derivatives. Sometimes tannins having phenolic groups are combined with iron salts. Storesinol in storax is resin alcohol and peruresinotannol in Peru balsam and toluresinotannol in tolu balsam are resinotannols.

3. *Resin esters:* These esters are of resin alcohol or resinotannol combined with resin acids or balsamic acids.

4. *Resenes:* They are complex neutral inert substances and do not show any characteristic chemical properties. These substances are insoluble and do not form salts or esters and are not hydrolyzed by alkalies. These substances are not affected by moisture, light and many other chemical reagents. Some of the resenes have been shown as triterpene alcohols. Usually they are of high molecular weight. Colophony and asafoetida contain resenes.

5. *Glycoresins:* This group consists of glycosidal resins. Glycoresins on hydrolysis yield sugars and complex acids. Resins of Convolvulaceae, like jalap resin and ipomoea resin are glycoresins.

If the above resins contain greater proportion of acid, ester or resenes, they are called acid resin, ester resin or neutral resin, respectively. Some resins, in addition to ferulic acid, cinnamic acid and coniferyl alcohol, also contain lignans, xanthones and higher condensed coumarins. Pharmaceutical resins are obtained by (1) extracting the drug with alcohol and precipitating the resin in water, e.g. podophyllum resin; (2) separating the oil from oleoresin by distillation, e.g. colophony from turpentine oil; or (3) collecting the product, which exudes or allowed to exude as oleoresin from the plant by natural or artificial punctures. In such cases the oil partially gets evaporated into the atmosphere, as in mastic. Mostly resins are considered plant exudates, except shellac or lac, which the lac insect prepares from plant juices.

A classification of resins, with examples, based on above consideration is as follows:

1. Acid resin   Colophony
2. Balsams   Tolu balsam, storax, benzoin
3. Oleo-resin   Copaiba
4. Oleo-gum-resins   Myrrh, asafoetida
5. Gum resin   Gamboge

ALKALOIDS

The alkaloids represent a group of natural products that has had a major impact throughout history on the economic, medical, political and social affairs of humans. Many of these agents have potent physiological effects on mammalian systems as well as other organisms and, as a consequence, some constitute important therapeutic agents.

Definition

Alkaloids are difficult to define because they do not represent a homogenous group of compounds from the chemical, biochemical or physiological viewpoint. However, alkaloids can be considered as organic nitrogenous substances, usually found in plants and are more or less alkaline in reaction. Many alkaloids show prominent pharmacological action in small doses, some are obtained from animal kingdom, practically all are synthesisable and a few are not basic as colchicine. A larger number of drugs, that too more important ones, are obtained from alkaloids-containing plants.

The word alkaloid or *"alkali-like"*, which refers to the basic nature of these compounds, was coined by the pharmacist W. Meissner in 1818. With the accumulation of chemical and biological data, more physicochemical features have been added to define alkaloids. Although there is no completely satisfactory definition of alkaloids, several common features can be attributed to them. Among the known alkaloids, a number of cases can be cited which are exceptions to one or more of these features. Generally speaking, alkaloids have following features:

1. They possess a complex molecular structure and contain nitrogen in the molecule.
2. They are usually basic (alkaline) in nature.
3. They are biosynthetically derived, at least in part, from various amino acids.
4. They manifest significant pharmacological activity.

In addition to these salient features, some more qualifications that are usually added to describe alkaloids are:

1. Alkaloid bases are soluble in a number of organic solvents, but they are rather insoluble in water.
2. A number of them give characteristic colour reaction with certain reagents.
3. Many of them are precipitated by certain reagents.
4. A number of them are either decomposed or degraded by exposure to air and/or light and heat.
5. Most of them are well-defined crystalline compounds and, with few exceptions, are colourless substances.

Nitrogen in the molecule of alkaloids

Alkaloids possess one or more nitrogen atoms in the molecule. A large number of alkaloids contain at least one nitrogen atom in a heterocyclic ring e.g. nicotine, atropine, morphine, tubocurarine and strychnine. However, in a numberof alkaloidal amines e.g. ephedrine, mescaline and colchicine, the nitrogen in the molecule is not in the ring. Alkaloids possess nitrogen atoms which are primary (RNH_2) e.g. mescaline, secondary (R_2NH) e.g. ephedrine, tertiary (R_3N) e.g. atropine, or quaternary e.g. tubocurarine.

Nitrogen in mescaline is as primary amine (RNH_2) and is in side chain. Such alkaloids are not true alkaloids and are called pseudoalkaloids.

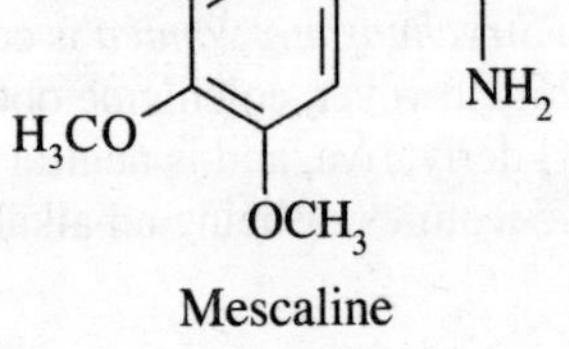

Mescaline

In ephedrine, nitrogen is in the form of secondary amine (R_2NH) and is also in the side chain and not in the ring. Hence ephedrine is also a pseudoephedrine alkaloid.

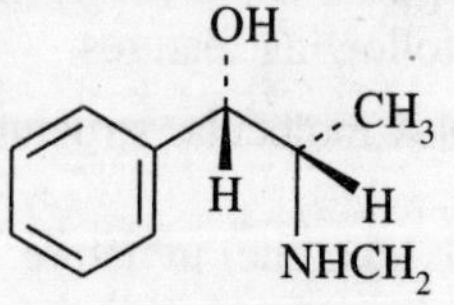

Ephedrine

In atropine, nitrogen is as tertiary amine (R_3N). It is also in the ring and hence a true alkaloid.

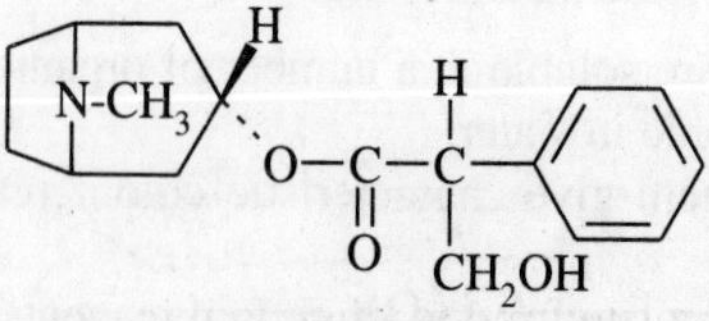

Atropine

In D-tubocuraine nitrogen is present as quarternary ammonium compounds, which are not alkaloids in the true sense of the term.

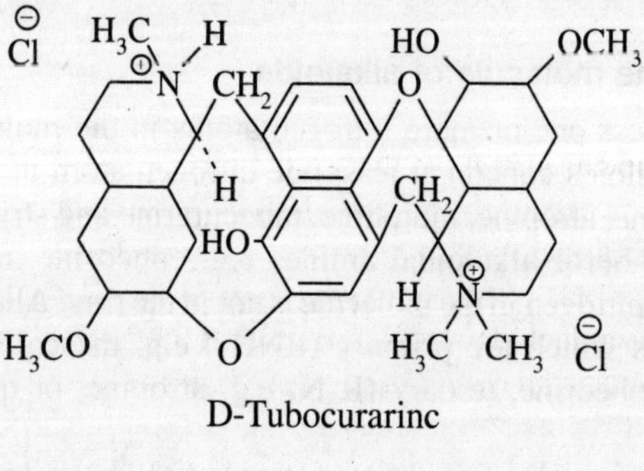

D-Tubocurarinc

Alkalinity

The alkaloids are basic (alkaline) in reaction, which is due to the presence of a lone pair of electrons on the nitrogen present in the molecule. The strychnine isolated from *Strychnos nux vomica* is considered a strong base having pKa value of 8.26. However, colchicine obtained from *Colchicum autumnale* is an N-acetyl derivarive, and is neutral in reaction; but it does show other characteristic features of being an alkaloid.

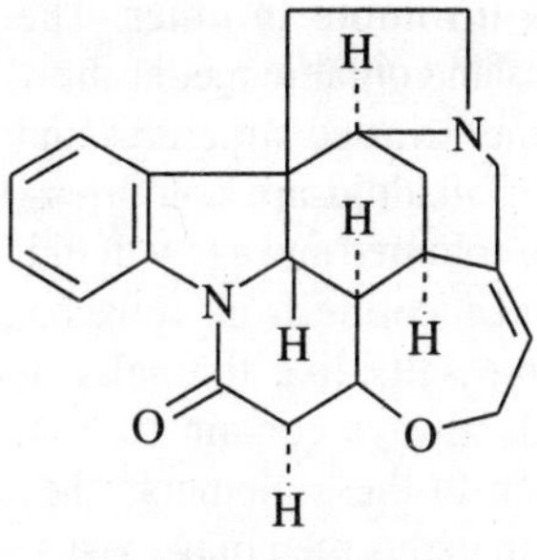

Strychnine 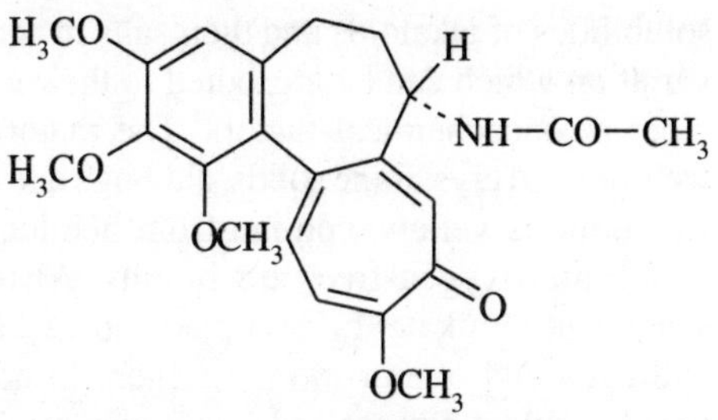   Colchicine

Amino acids as biosynthetic precursors of alkaloids

Alkaloids are derived from relatively simple precursors, such as phenyl-alanine, methionine, tyrosine, lysine, ornithine, histidine, tryptophan and anthranilic acid, besides "acetate units" and "terpene units". Biosynthetic studies are carried out by administering a suitably labelled precursor to a plant or microorganism. After a suitable period of growth, the intermediate and end products are isolated and studied. In this way, it was possible to show that alkaloids such as morphine, nicotine, hyoscyamine, papaverine, colchicine, and some others are derived from amino acids. On the other hand, the steroidal alkaloids are derived from terpenoid or other precursors of carbohydrate metabolism.

Pharmacological activity of alkaloids

The exploration of natural products, both plants and animals, for alkaloids of medicinal value has surpassed that of the other categories of chemical compounds. This is because the alkaloids have pronounced physiological and pharmacological activity and many of these are the sources of very useful drugs. Examples of alkaloids and their principal pharmacological and therapeutic uses include atropine (mydriatic), quinine (antimalarial), ephedrine (expectorant), morphine (strong analgesic), reserpine, (hypotensive), vinblastine, vincristine (antimitotic), ergometrine (oxytocic), tubocurarine (muscle relaxant), etc.

General consideration

1. Solubility

Most alkaloids (free bases) are insoluble (some sparingly soluble) in water, but are miscible with organic solvents such a chloroform, ether, benzene, etc. Alkaloids are alkaline in nature; therefore they form salts with acids. These alkaloidal salts are soluble in water and alcohol, but for the most part insoluble in water immiscible organic solvents. However, there are exceptions, such as ephedrine, colchicine and ergonovine which are water soluble, whilst morphine and colchicine are insoluble in ether. The solubilities of alkaloids and their salts in aqueous and organic media show variation which can be attributed to their extremely varied structures and other physicochemical factors. The majority of alkaloid are colourless, well-defined crystalline solids, although a few are coloured and a few liquid. Berberine is yellow, coniine from hemlock and nicotine from tobacco, which are oxygen-free, are liquids. Also some salts like the salts of sanguinarine alkaloid are copper red. Alkaloids always contain carbon, hydrogen and one or more nitrogen. In addition to these elements they mostly contain oxygen and sometimes sulphur. In plants they may exist as bases in free state (less frequent as compared to salt forms), as salts or as N-oxides, called alkaloid N-oxides. Alkaloid N-oxides are the N-oxidation products of alkaloids. N-oxides of tertiary alkaloids can be easily prepared in the laboratory from the original alkaloidal base. N-oxides have evinced interest as they are said to show delayed-release properties, low toxicities and low additive properties when compared with their corresponding tertiary alkaloids.

2. Detection and characterization

The alkaloid reagents used for detection and characterization are roughly divided into precipitants and colour reagents. Most alkaloids are precipitated from a neutral or acidic solution with different reagents, such as a potassium mercuric iodide solution (*Mayer's reagent*), a solution of iodine in potassium (*Dragendorff's reagent*) and a potassium bismuth iodine (*Wagner's reagent*) as well as from a solution of tannic acid, and a saturated solution of picric acid (*Hager's reagent*).

Certain groups of alkaloids give characteristic colour with certain reagents and this property may be utilized to quantify such alkaloids. The blue colour given by ergot alkaloids with *p*-dimethyl-amino benzaldehyde in hydrochloric acid (*Van Urk reagent*), the bright purple colour produced by some solanaceous alkaloids with fuming nitric acid and alcoholic potassium hydroxide (*Vitali-Morin reagent*) are examples of special colour reactions of individual alkaloids.

3. Extraction and separation

Alkaloid extraction techniques vary with the type of alkaloid group and the nature of the material. However, there are usually two general methods which are adopted with some modification for the extraction of alkaloids.

Procedure A: The powdered drug material is moistened with an aqueous solution of ammonia or sodium carbonate, which combines with the acids and phenolic substances and release the free alkaloidal bases which can be then extracted by a suitable solvent such as benzene, chloroform, etc.

Procedure B: The plant material is first defatted with hexane, diethyl ether or ethyl acetate; and thereafter it is extracted with ethyl alcohol containing dilute acid. Pigments, and other neutral substances are removed by shaking with cholorform or a suitable organic solvent. The free alkaloids are then precipitated by excess of sodium bicarbonate or ammonia. The alkaloids are then extracted with a suitable organic solvent.

Further purification of the alkaloids can be effected by using a variety of chromatographic techniques which are fast and reliable. Some of the chromatographic techniques are:

1. Paper chromatography
2. Column chromatography
3. Thin layer chromatography (analytical and preparative)
4. Counter-current distribution
5. Gas liquid chromatography
6. High pressure liquid chromatography (analytical and preparative).

Either alone, or in combination, paper chromatography, thin layer chromatography, gas liquid chromatography, and high pressure liquid chromatography will indicate the number and relative proportions of the constituents in the crude mixture. Quantitative separation of alkaloids is most frequently achieved by column chromatography and high pressure liquid chromatography, radial centrifugal chromatography (chromatotron), and less often by preparative thin layer chromatography. Paper chromatography and gas liquid chromatography are no longer used for the routine isolation of alkaloids. Counter-chromatography has recently been used to separate certain types of alkaloids.

Structure elucidation of alkaloids

The structure elucidation of an alkaloid is one of the most fascinating and interesting aspects of phytochemical investigation and chemical learning. Until 1950, the structure characterization of an alkaloid depended on chemical degradation, but with the increasing application of instrumental techniques such as ultraviolet (UV), infrared (IR), nuclear magnetic resonance (NMR), mass spectroscopy (MS), and x-ray crystallography, there has been a decline in the pure chemical approach. Now-a-days, a combination of classical (e.g. chemical degradation) and modern (e.g. spectroscopy) is widely adopted for structural determination work.

The first step in the structural determination of an alkaloid is the determination of its molecular formula. This can be carried out by a combustion analysis of elements such as carbon, hydrogen, nitrogen and often oxygen, together with molecular weight determination. Alternatively, the molecular formula can be conveniently determined by the high resolution mass spectroscopy. This method has to be made use of when only a small amount of the compound is available. This is followed by the determination of the functionality of oxygen and nitrogen. Oxygen may be present in one or more of the following groups:

Hydroxyl or phenol (–OH), methoxyl (–OCH₃), acetyl (–OCOCH₃), benzoxyl (–OCOC₆H₅); carboxyl (–COOH), aldehyde (CHO), ketone (C=O), etc.

Classification of alkaloids

There are a couple of ways of classifying the alkaloids. These are loudly three:

1. Proto alkaloids: These include tyramine, histamine, ephedrine, mescaline and choline.
2. Pseudo alkaloids: This class includes steroidal alkaloids and diterpene alkaloids.
3. True alkaloids: They are those alkaloids which are derived bio-synthetically from amino acids.

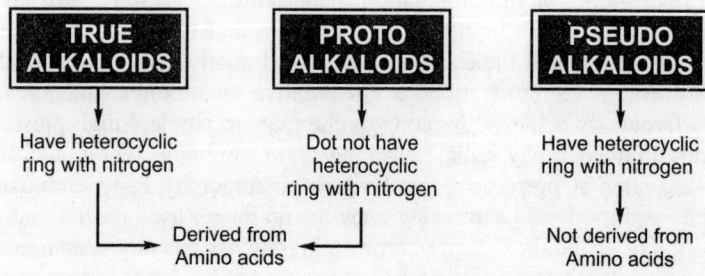

In general alkaloids are classified on the basis of their ring structure; more so they are grouped as non-heterocyclic and heterocyclic alkaloids, on the basis of the fact whether the nitrogen atom is present in the exocylic or cyclic structure, respectively. Also now-a-days one calls the heterocyclic alkaloids (with –N in the ring) as the true alkaloids, while the non-heterocyclic alkaloids (with –N in the side chain) are called pseudo-alkoloids.

Ring structures met with the alkaloids are pyridine, piperidine, indole, tropane, imidazole, pyrrolidine, isoquinoline, quinoline, quinazoline, purine, steroidal, phenylethyl amine (Ephedra alkaloids), colchicine alkaloids, and diterpene alkaloids. On the basis of the above two classes of alkaloids, therefore, ephedrine, mescaline, hordenine and colchicine are placed under non-heterocyclic (pseudo) alkaloids, while nicotine, ajmaline, vinblastine, ergometrine, hyoscyamine, atropine, pilocarpine, morphine, codeine, emetine, tubocurarine, quinine, protoveratrine and aconitine fall under heterocyclic (true) alkaloids.

The common ring structures that we come across amongst the alkaloids are given below, while the structures of some of the alkaloids will be given at appropriate places in the pages that follow.

From the foregoing pages it must have been noted that full advantage is taken from the solubility of alkaloids and their salts for the purpose of their extraction, isolation, characterisation, purification, etc. The alkaloids (as bases) are insoluble in water but their salts are usually freely soluble in water. The free alkaloids (alkaloidal bases) are on the other hand soluble in ether, chloroform and other relatively non-polar solvents in which solvents the alkaloidal salts are insoluble. This difference affords us a good means for the isolation of alkaloids as well as for their quantitative estimation.

Summarised method of extraction of alkaloids

The crude drug is powdered and then moistened with an aqueous alkali such as Na_2CO_3, $NaHCO_3$ or lime. This results in the liberation of alkaloidal bases in the free form (as they are mostly present in the form of salts). The free bases are then extracted exhaustively with chloroform or some other

Simplified flow diagram of extraction of alkaloids

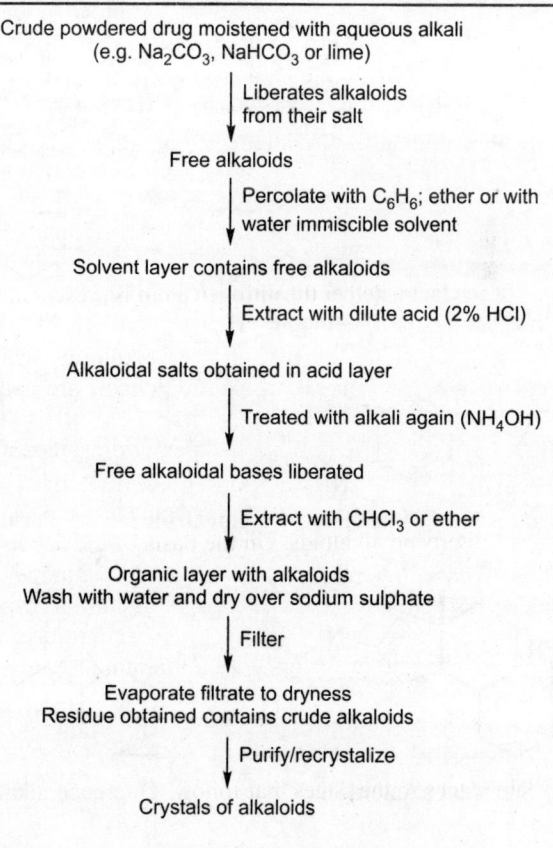

Crude powdered drug moistened with aqueous alkali
(e.g. Na_2CO_3, $NaHCO_3$ or lime)

↓ Liberates alkaloids from their salt

Free alkaloids

↓ Percolate with C_6H_6; ether or with water immiscible solvent

Solvent layer contains free alkaloids

↓ Extract with dilute acid (2% HCl)

Alkaloidal salts obtained in acid layer

↓ Treated with alkali again (NH_4OH)

Free alkaloidal bases liberated

↓ Extract with $CHCl_3$ or ether

Organic layer with alkaloids
Wash with water and dry over sodium sulphate

↓ Filter

Evaporate filtrate to dryness
Residue obtained contains crude alkaloids

↓ Purify/recrystalize

Crystals of alkaloids

organic solvent immiscible with water, till the last extract does not give any reaction or test for the presence of alkaloids. The solvent is recovered under reflux and the concentrate is treated with 2% aqueous hydrochloric acid. This results in the formation of alkaloidal salts in the aqueous layer, while the organic layer contains the non-alkaloidal components which may be rejected if so desired. The aqueous acidic layer is then made alkaline (basified) with NH_4OH in order to liberate the free alkaloidal bases which are then extracted with chloroform or ether. The organic layer is then separated, washed with water, dried over sodium sulphate, filtered and evaporated to dryness. The residue consists of the alkaloids in the crude form which may be separated either by fractional crystallisation or by column chromatography, etc.

Alkaloids are usually classified according to the nature of the basic chemical structures from which they are derived. A number of these structures are shown hereunder.

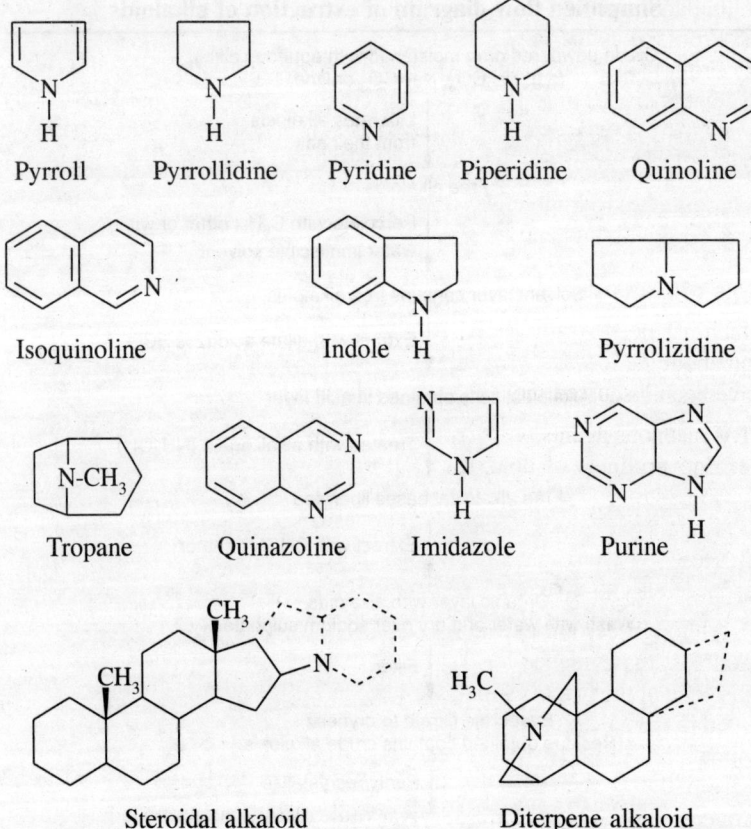

| Pyrroll | Pyrrollidine | Pyridine | Piperidine | Quinoline |

Isoquinoline   Indole   H   Pyrrolizidine

Tropane   Quinazoline   Imidazole   Purine

Steroidal alkaloid   Diterpene alkaloid

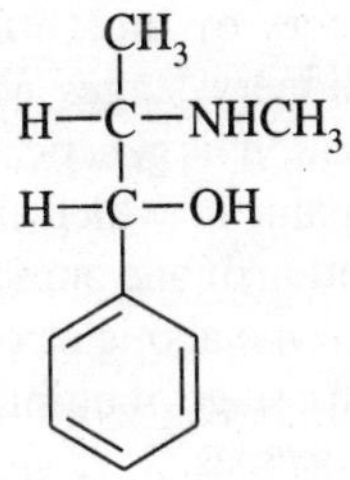

CH₃
H—C—NHCH₃
H—C—OH

(Phenethylamine)
Ephedra alkaloid

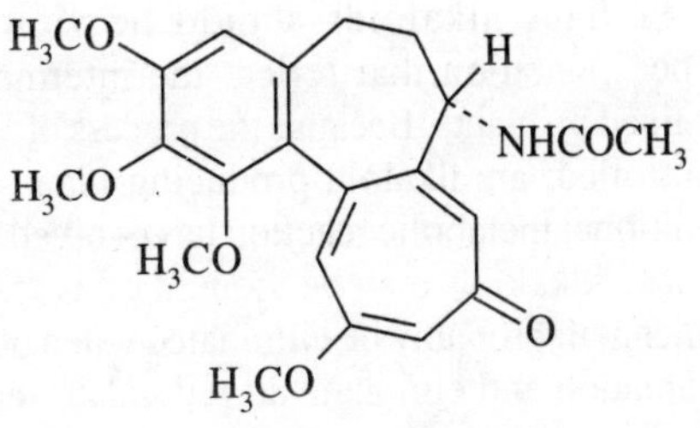

Colchicine alkaloid

Naming of alkaloids

The names of alkaloids are obtained in various ways:

1. From the generic name of the plant yielding them (hydrastine, atropine).
2. From the specific name of the plant yielding them (cocaine, belladonnine).
3. From the common name of the drug yielding them (ergotamine).
4. From their physiological activity (emetine, morphine).
5. Occasionally from their discovery (pelletierine).

Sometimes a prefix or suffix is added to the name of a principal alkaloid to designate another alkaloid from the same source (quinine, quinidine, hydroquinine). By agreement, chemical rules designate that the names of all alkaloids should end in 'ine'.

Role of alkaloids in plants

Much has been written about the possible function of alkaloids in plants and about the reasons why they occur there. Some of the possibilities that have been discussed include their functions as:

1. Poisonous agents protecting the plant against insects and herbivores.
2. End products of detoxification reactions representing a metabolic looking-up of compounds otherwise harmful to the plant.
3. Regulatory growth factors.
4. Reserve substances capable of supplying nitrogen or other elements necessary to the plant's economy.

Although certain exceptions exist because of the diverse nature of alkaloids, the evidence for any result of alkaloid formation useful to the existence of the plant is slight. Perhaps the best example of such a result is found in the wild plants of certain regions where over-grazing by domestic animals has taken place for centuries. An extremely high percentage of these plants contain alkaloids that, because of their bitter taste or toxic properties, apparently confer survival value on the species producing them.

Perhaps alkaloids should be viewed as products of metabolic experimentation that reflect the intermediary evolutionary stages now attained by plants. Because the process of 'alkaloid formation' is genetically controlled, an alkaloid-producing plant is merely a plant in which this additional metabolic reaction has evolved through mutation of one or more genes. Alkaloids may be thought of as resulting from a 'metabolic error', which will probably be eliminated when plants approach a stage of ultimate adaptation and eliminate all redundant features and processes.

They are thus a result of waste product retained within the organism that produces them. It must be emphasized that, unlike many such substances with which we are familiar, the alkaloids are structurally complex and products of energy-requiring reaction sequences.

More details concerning individual alkaloids belonging to different classes of alkaloids will be discussed under the drugs containing them. For studying the groups of alkaloids belonging to particular classes advanced book of pharmacognosy by JSQ may be consulted.

3

Description of Drugs Under Specific Therapeutic Efficacies

This chapter deals with individual drugs and the products derived from them under specific therapeutic efficacies. The drugs under such categories mentioned below are outlined strictly as per the pharmacognosy syllabus and they are to be described as per the requirement of PCI quoted below.

5. Occurrence, distribution, organoleptic evaluation, chemical constituents including tests, wherever applicable, and therapeutic efficacy of following categories of drugs:

(a) **Laxatives** – Aloes, Rhuburb, Castor oil, Ispaghula, Senna.

(b) **Cardiotonics** – Digitalis, Arjuna.

(c) **Carminatives and G.I. regulators** – Urnbelliferous fruits, Coriander, Fennel, Ajowan, Cardamom, Ginger, Black pepper, Asafoetida, Nutmeg, Cinnamon, Clove.

(d) **Astringents** – Catechu.

(e) **Drugs acting on nervous system** – Hyoscyamus, Belladonna, Aconite, Ashwagandha, Ephedra, Opium, Cannabis, Nux vomica.

(f) **Antihypertensives** – Rauwolfia.

(g) **Antitussives** – Vasaka, Tolu balsam, Tulsi.

(h) **Antirheumatics** – Guggul, Colchicum.

(i) **Antitumour** – Vinca.

(j) **Antileprotic** – Chaulmoogra oil.

(k) **Antidiabetics** – Pterocarpus, Gymnema, Sylvestre.

(l) **Diuretics** – Gokhru, Punarmava.

(m) **Antidvsentrics** – Ipecacuanha.

(n) **Antiseptics and disinfectants** – Benzoin, Myrrh, Nim, Curcuma.

(o) **Antimalarials** – Cinchona.

(p) **Oxytocics** – Ergot.

(q) **Vitamins** – Shark liver oil and Amla.

(r) **Enzymes** – Papaya, Diastase, Yeast.

(s) **Perfumes and flavouring agents** – Peppermint oil, Lemon oil, Orange oil, Lemon grass oil, Sandalwood.

(t) **Pharmaceutical aids** – Honey, Arachis oil, Starch, Kaolin, Pectin, Olive oil, Lanolin, Beeswax, Acacia, Tragacanth, Sodium alginate, Agar, Guar gum, Gelatin.

(u) **Miscellaneous** – Liquorice, Garlic, Picrorhiza, Dioscorea, Linseed, Shatavari, Shankhapusphi, Pyrethrum, Tobacco.

LAXATIVES

Laxatives are drugs or products obtained from the drugs which promote bowel movements. They are used to treat constipation. The term constipation may mean infrequent or hard stool. Since normal bowel pattern varies considerably from person to person, constipation is a relative term. Not everyone, for example, has a bowel movement every day.

Constipation can be caused by many factors e.g. by use of low-fibre diet, lack of physical activity, inadequate intake of fluids each day, delay in defecation, stress and travel and other changes contributing the constipation. Constipated persons find it difficult (and even painful) to have bowel movements. They feel bloated, sluggish and uncomfortable. Habitual and recurring constipation needs laxatives. Laxatives come in various forms, but in this chapter we will discuss the plant drugs which are in the syllabus (for the description of other forms of laxatives, pharmacology books may be consulted).

ALOES

Aloe, Ghritkumari, Aliyo (Guj.)

Botanical Source

Aloe is the dried juice collected by incision from the bases of the leaves of various species of Aloe.

Family

Liliaceae.

Geographical Source

There are about 160 species of aloe out of which the following species are important and utilized for the preparation of aloe. They are found in the countries mentioned as under:

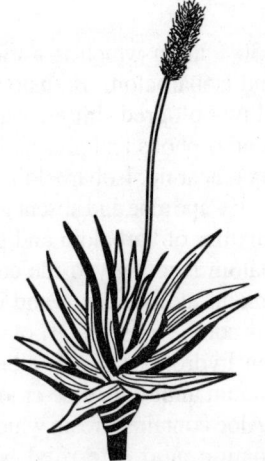

Fig. 3.1. Aloe, Aloe species plant of Aloe vera.

1. *Aloe perryi* Baker: This is found in Socotra and Zanzibar islands and in their neighbouring areas. The aloe obtained from this species is known as Socotrine or Zanzibar aloe.
2. *Aloe vera* Linn: This species is also known as *Aloe vulgaris* Lamarek, *Aloe barbadensis* Mil. or *Aloe officinalis* Forskal. This species is a native of North Africa but now cultivated in Aruba and Bonaire and to a lesser extent in Curacao in West Indies. The aloe obtained from this species is known as Curacao or Barbados aloe.
3. *Aloe ferox* Miller and hybrids of this species with *Aloe africana* and *Aloe spicata*: This species grows in Cape Colony near the Cape of Good Hope in South Africa and aloe obtained is known as Cape aloe.

Cultivation and Collection

The plant is xerophyte and may be herb, shrub or tree and bears a rosette of leaves which are thick, fleshy, sessile and spiny. Flowers are red or yellow. For cultivation in West Indies young offsets are planted in the soil after the rainy season in rows situated at a distance of 60 cm. In the second year leaves are collected by the natives. Because of the spiny nature of leaves the natives protect their hands and feet, cut the leaves near the base, put them into kerosene tins and take them to a central place for the preparation of aloe.

Juice of aloe is present in parenchymatous cells of pericycle surrounding which are mucilage cells. On incision of leaves juice exudes from pericyclic cells and mucilage cells exert pressure on pericycle cells and by single incision juice of the entire leaf is drained out.

Chemical Constituents

Aloe may contain upto 30% aloin which is a mixture of three isomers: barbaloin, b-barbaloin and isobarbaloin. Barbaloin present in all the four varieties is slightly yellow-coloured, bitter, water-soluble, crystalline glycoside. b-barbaloin is amorphous and present in Cape aloe and can be produced from barbaloin on heating. Isobarbaloin is crystalline, present in Curacao aloe and in traces in Cape aloe and absent in Socotrine and Zanzibar aloe and is probably a mixture of barbaloin and polyphenols responsible for its colour tests. Barbaloin is a C-glycoside compared to common O-glycosides. Aloe also contains aloinosides A and B, O-glycosides of aloin in which, a-L-rhamnose is combined with OH of hydroxymethyl group at 11 C atom. Barbaloin on hydrolysis yields aloe-emodin anthrone and glucose. Besides aloe-emodin anthrone, aloe-emodin anthranol and aloe-emodin are also present. Aloe contains a resin which is ester of P-coumaric acid or P-hydroxy cinnamic acid esterified with aloe resinotannol. According to recent work, Cape aloe resin consists of aloe-resin B and aloe-resin A. Aloe-resin B is chromone G-glycoside with glucose and aloe resin A is P-coumaric acid ester of aloe-resin B esterified at one of the OH groups of glucose. Aloe resin does not have any purgative action.

Barbaloin

Aloe-resin B

Uses

Aloe and aloin are strong purgatives and in higher doses may act as abortifacient. If used alone, aloe causes griping and is usually combined with carminatives or antispasmodics like belladonna or hyoscyamus. Ointment of aloe gel is used in sun burns, thermal burns, radiation burns, abrasions and skin irritation and prevents ulceration and malignancy. For bioassay of aloe no suitable animal species has been found.

Indian Aloe

Indian aloe is obtained from *Aloe vera* var. *officinalis*. This is probably the same species as *A. barbadensis* and is found on the coasts of Mumbai, Gujarat and Chennai. Besides in the literature Jafferabad (a port of Saurashtra coast) aloe from *A. abyssinica* is reported. Indian aloe is darker in colour and harder and resembles Socotrine or Cape aloe. Isobarbaloin is absent in Indian aloe and the percentage of aloin in it according to recent work is only about 4%. At present no aloe is exported from Jafferabad.

RHUBARB

Rhizoma Rhei, Rhubarb Rhizome, Rheum,
Rhei Radix, Revandchini (Hindi)

Botanical Source

Rhubarb consists of the peeled dried rhizomes and roots of *Rheum palmatun* Linn, *Rheum officinale* and other species of rhubarb, excepting *Rheum rhaponticum.*

Family

Polygonaceae. Members of this family contain anthracene derivatives and tannins. Some species contain flavonoids including rutin.

Geographical Source

China, Tibet, Germany and other European countries.

Collection

Rhubarb is a very ancient drug. The plant is perennial. Rhizome is large and vertical and roots are thick-branched.

According to recent work, rhubarb is a beet type geophyte and not a real rhizome. Drug is collected from wild plants but is also cultivated to some extent. The plant grows at an altitude of 2500 to 4000 metres. At higher altitude drug of better quality is obtained. Drug is collected in autumn in September or October from 8 to 15 years old plants. Rhizomes are dug out, crown and lateral roots are removed and outer bark separated by peeling. Small rhizomes are kept as such or cut into transverse slices and are known as rounds of commerce. Large rhizomes are cut into longitudinal slices and known as flats. These slices are dried by boring holes and passing thread into them and hanging between shades of trees. Where the climate is not favourable rhubarb is dried on heated stones which are previously heated by wood fire. Drug dried in this way is called high dried and as it is dried more, is usually darker in colour and acquires an empyreumatic odour and is considered inferior.

The above drug is sent to different ports where sometimes the remaining bark is peeled off and graded according to size, shape and quality and then exported to different countries.

Chemical Constituents

Rhubarb contains free anthraquinones, their glycosides reduced derivatives, anthrones or dianthrones and heterodianthrones. The anthraquinones are chrysophanol, aloe-emodin, emodin, physcion and rhein. Anthrones or dianthrones are of chrysophanol, emodin, aloe-emodin or physcion. Hetero-dianthrones contain two different molecules of anthrones and they are from above anthrones. Rhubarb also contains astringent substances such as

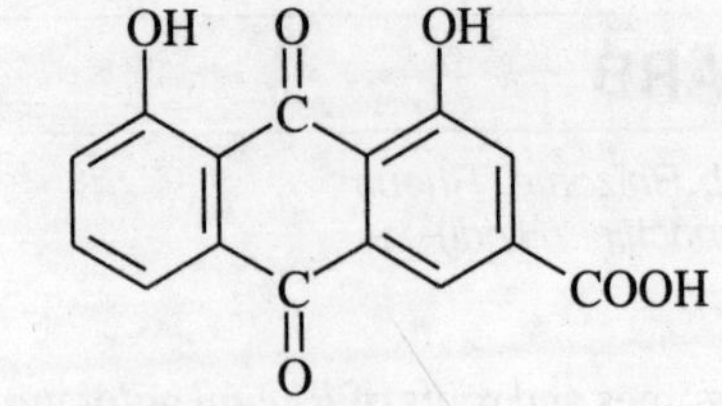

Rhein

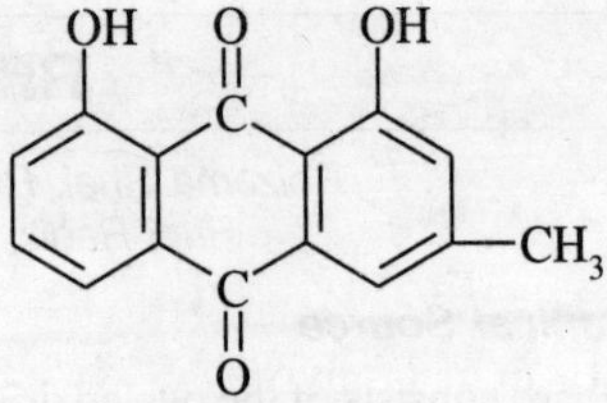

Chrysophanol

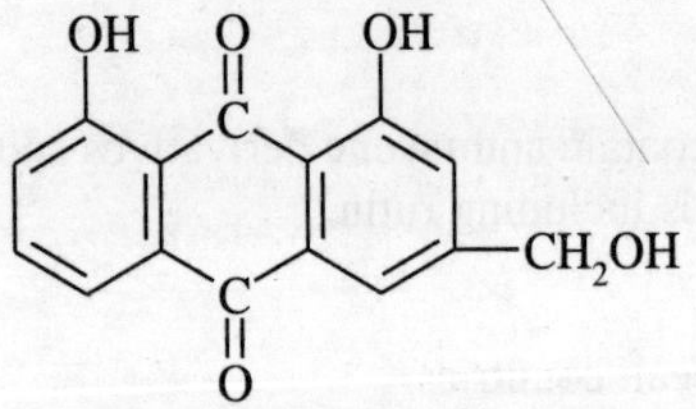

Aloe-emodin

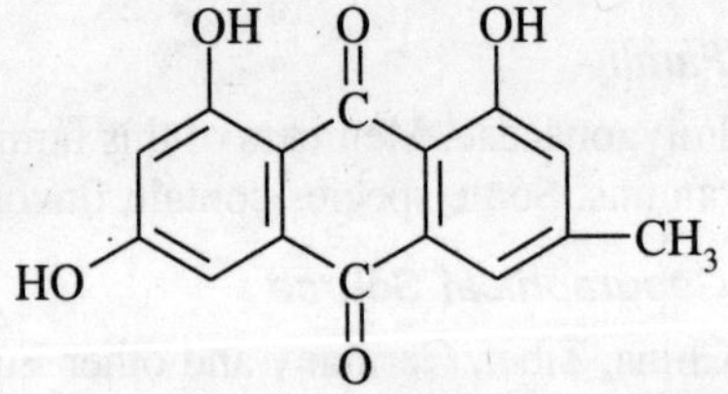

Emodin

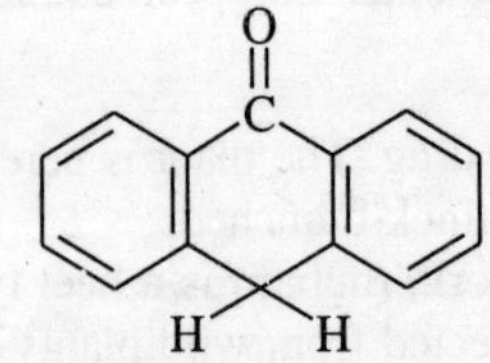

Anthrone

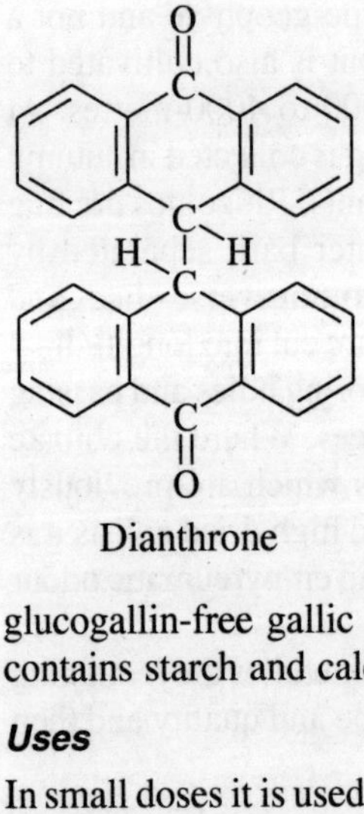

Dianthrone

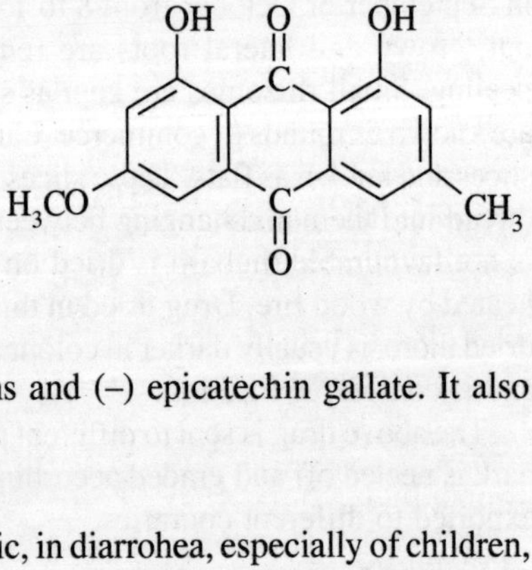

glucogallin-free gallic acid catechins and (–) epicatechin gallate. It also contains starch and calcium oxalate.

Uses

In small doses it is used as a stomachic, in diarrohea, especially of children, and in larger doses as a purgative because of anthracene derivatives.

INDIAN RHUBARB

Indian Rhubarb, Revandchini

Indian Rhubarb consists of the dried rhizome of *Rheum emodi* Wall and *Rheum webbianum* Royle and other species of Rheum. It is collected from

6 to 7 years old plants before the flowenng season and marketed with cortex intact or partially decorticated. Rhubarb I.P. was included in NF 1960.

Chemical Constituents

Indian rhubarb contains free anthraquiones 1.12% while combined anthraquinones as O-glycosides are 4.5%. The anthraquinones both free and in glycosidal combination are chrysophanol, aloe-emodin, emodin and rhein. Sennosides A and B have been isolated by Khorana et al. The tannins present are hydrolysable tannins. Rhaponticin is absent in Indian rhubarb. The greater purgative activity of rhubarb may be attributed to greater peecentage of both free and combined anthraquinones.

It is used in the same way as Chinese rhubarb and is exported and used in the USA.

RHAPONTIC RHUBARB

It is obtained from Rheum rhaponticum. It is 2 to 3 times more active than Chinese rhubarb and in addition to anthracene derivatives it contains rhaponticin, a stilbene derivative, having estrogenic action. Rhaponticin can be identified by the characteristic needle-shaped crystals or blue fluorescence in ultraviolet light. It is not official in the Pharmacopoeias because of rhaponticin.

SENNA LEAVES

Tinnevelley Senna Leaves, Senna Indica, Indian Senna

Botanical Source

Tinnevelley senna consists of dried compound leaflets of *Cassia angustifolia* Vahl.

Family

Leguminosae.

Geographical Source

South India, Tinnevelley district and its adjoining areas.

Collection

Tinnevelley senna plant is cultivated in South India in areas adjoining Tinnevelley and exported from Tuticorin. Cultivation is carried out by planting in moist areas similar to rice. The plant is very sensitive to temperature and if the temperature falls below +10°C, the plant dies. Because of cultivation, this plant has become very luxuriant. The collection of leaves takes place before flowering season. For collection each leaf is carefully picked from the plant by hand and afterwards they are dried in shade with care. Because of drying in shade, their natural green colour is maintained. After drying leaves are packed in bales with pressure. Because of the pressure applied in packing, transverse and oblique impressions are found on the leaves. They are less brittle and hence are more or less entire and in good condition. They were considered better and had good demand and fetched high price but now their price in international market is decreasing because of less percentage of sennosides. Drug collected from dry area is inferior. Every year in India from 5,000 to 7,000 tons of leaves and fruits are obtained by cultivation. Leaves form 67 per cent and fruits form 33 per cent of the drug. However, probably because of improvement of quality, price of senna and quantity of export have increased and in 1978–79, 4782 tons of the drug worth Rs 20 million were exported.

Constituents

Senna leaves contain active constituents 2.5 per cent sennosides A and B. Both sennosides are stereoisomers and sennoside A is dextrorotatory and sennoside B is mesoform. Sennosides A and B are glycosides of rhein-dianthrone or sennidin A and B and glucose. Glycosidation takes place at 8 and 8′ positions. Fairbairn has isloated primary glycosides of sennosides A and B possessing greater physiological activity in which number of sugars may be present upto 10. Senna also contains sennosides C and D which are glycosides of heterodianthrones of rhein-anthrone and aloe-emodin anthrone. Senna also contains free chrysophanol, emodin and their glycosides and free aloe-emodin, rhein, their monoanthrones, dianthrones and their glycosides. Further, in senna, flavones kaempferol and iso-

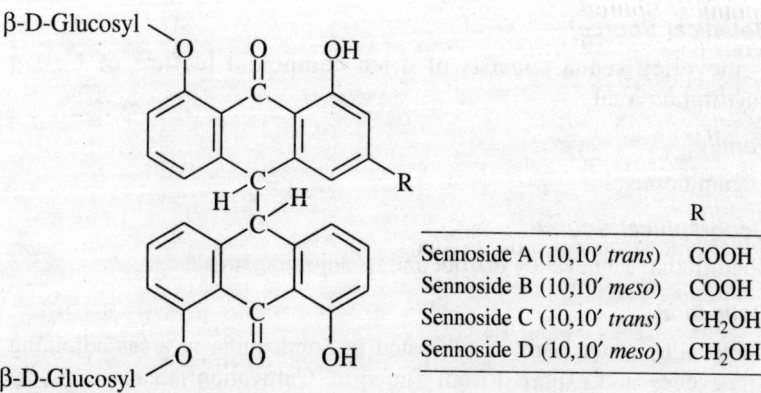

	R
Sennoside A (10,10′ *trans*)	COOH
Sennoside B (10,10′ *meso*)	COOH
Sennoside C (10,10′ *trans*)	CH_2OH
Sennoside D (10,10′ *meso*)	CH_2OH

Fig. 3.2. Sennosides are a group of yellow homo- and heterodimers of anthron glycosides. The aglycones (= sennidins) of the main glycosides are derived from rhein and from aloe emodin (see details under general description of anthraquinone glycosides).

rhamnetin responsible for the colour of the drug, are found. Mucilage is present in the epidermis of the leaf and gives red colour with ruthenium red. Mucilage has no purgative property. Calcium oxalate is also present.

Uses

Senna is used as a purgative drug. Original glycosides of reduced derivatives are more active than free anthraquinones. Anthracene derivatives irritate the large intestine and act as purgatives. If given by injection they are secreted in large intestine and show the purgative property. When the anthracene derivatives containing drugs are used alone they cause griping and thus they are usually combined with carminatives.

Adulterants

• **Dog Senna** consists of leaves of *Cassia obovata*. Leaves have obovate shape and obtuse and tapering apex and quite distinct appearance. They contain about 1% anthraquinone derivatives. They are found in pieces with the broken Alexandrian senna.

• **Arabian, Bombay** or **Mecca senna** consists of leaves from the wild plants of *Cassia angustifolia* growing in Arabia. Leaves resemble Tinnevelley senna and are brownish-green, more elongated and narrower.

• **Palthe senna** consists of leaves of *Cassia auriculata*. It contains leuco-anthocyanidin which gives red colour with 80% sulphuric acid.

SENNA PODS

Sennae Fructus, Senna Legumes, Senna Fruits

Botanical Source

Senna pods are the dried ripe fruits of *Cassia angustifolia* Vahl known as Tinnevelley senna pods.

Family

Leguminosae.

Geographical Source

Upper Nile territories, South India.

Collection

Alexandrian Senna Pods: In the collection of Alexandrian senna leaves, during the coarse sieving, the senna pods remain in the sieve. They are separated and graded according to the quality and condition usually by handpicking. Pods of good quality are entire and do not contain any foreign matter or tissues, while inferior ones are in broken condition and contain foreign matter like pieces of stems, broken leaves, etc. Pods of good quality are used for dispensing while inferior ones are used for manufacturing purposes.

Tinnevelley Senna Pods: Compared to the leaves, less attention is paid in the collection of the pods. Tinnevelley senna pods are inferior to Alexandrian senna pods.

Chemical Constituents

Constituents of senna pods are similar to senna leaves. They contain sennosides A and B. Alexandrian pods have 2.5 to 4.5% while Tinnevelley pods have 1.5 to 2.5% of sennosides. Primary glycosides of sennosides similar to leaves are also present. Other constituents and anthracene derivatives are like those of senna leaves, except that mucilage is absent.

Uses

Senna pods are used as purgative, similar to senna leaves, but cause griping. They are also used for the manufacture of sennosides.

ISPAGHULA

Ispaghula, Ispagol, Ishabgula

Botanical Source

Ispaghula consists of dried seeds of *Plantago ovata* Forskal.

Family

Plantaginaceae.

Geographical Source

The plant was formerly collected by nomadic tribes and grows wild in Punjab, Sind and Persia. At present it is cultivated in North Gujarat around Siddhpur and to some extent in south Rajasthan.

Cultivation

Seeds are sown by broadcasting method in North Gujarat in sandy loamy soil in November. Addition of farmyard manure has favourable effect. Ammonium sulphate is also added as a fertilizer. Water is supplied to the plants at 8 to 10 days interval 7 to 8 times.

Ispaghula is usually not affected by pests or disease but its yield suffers to a great extent if there is any storm or untimely rainfall. Fruits are collected after a period of about 3 months when they are completely mature and ripe. They are dried and seeds are separated. At present about 35,000 ha land is used for ispaghula cultivation and over 29,000 tons of seeds come into the market from which 90 per cent husk and seeds worth about Rs 20 crores are exported.

Chemical Constituents

Ispaghula seeds contain about 10% mucilage which is present in the epidermis of testa. Mucilage consists of pentosan and aldobionic acid. Pentosan on hydrolysis yields xylose and arabinose. Aldobionic acid yields galactouronic acid and rhamnose. Further, protein and fixed oil are present in endosperm and embryo. Fixed oil contains unsaturated fatty acids and β-sitosterol in unsaponifiable matter and may be used for suppressing cholesterol in blood.

Uses

Action of mucilage is purely mechanical. The mucilage is not acted by digestive enzymes and by intestinal bacteria in the gut and passes unchanged. Mucilage is jelly-like and absorbs irritating products of gastrointestinal digestion and bacterial and other toxins. Further, the bacteria get entangled in the gel and mucilage prevents their absorption in the system. Thus, mucilage is used to cure inflammation of the mucous membranes of gastrointestinal and urogenital tracts. Thus, mucilage is used in amoebic and bacillary dysentery, diarrhoea, duodenal ulcer, gonorrhoea and piles. As a result of increase in bulk by swelling of the mucilage, intestinal peristalsis is stimulated by reflex action and drug is used as a bulk laxative especially in habitual constipation. Central Drug Research Institute, Lucknow has developed 'Isaptent' sticks from Isabgul husks. Isaptent is cervix dilator and is used for medical termination of pregnancy. This is quick in action, cheap and safe to use. Other commercial uses of husks are ice-cream stabilizer and as substitute for sodium alginate.

The mucilage neutralises the irritating action and is used as a soothing agent. Thus, it is used in inflammation of skin or mucous membrane of mouth, alimentary system, vagina, bladder and respiratory inflammation.

Gujarat Drugs & Chemicals Ltd. has been promoted by Gujarat Industrial Investment Corporation Ltd. of Gujarat Government involving capital of 1.5 crores at Mehsana (north Gujarat) for manufacturing isabgul formulations mainly for export.

ISPAGHULA HUSK

Ispghulae Testa, Sat Isobgulo

Ispaghula husk consists of the dried seed coats of *Plantago ovata* and is obtained by crushing the seeds and separating by winnowing. It contains not more than 2% of other organic matter.

Uses

In the same way as seed and is preferred as it contains only mucilage.

Allied Drugs

Psyllium, Flea seed. Psyllium consists of the seeds of *Plantago psyllium* and *P. arenaria*.

Family

Plantaginaceae.

Geographical Source

South France, Spain where it is cultivated.

Plantago psyllium seeds are 2–3 mm long, 0.75–1 mm wide, boat-shaped or elongated, ovate, glossy and deep brown in colour. Swelling factor is 12.75.

Plantago arenaria seeds, known as dark psyllium, are 2–2.5 mm, boat-shaped or elliptical, black-brown in colour. Swelling factor is 14.50. Both these seeds contain mucilage and are used in the same way as ispaghula.

Adulterant

Seeds of *Plantago lanceolata*. They are oblong elliptical and yellowish-brown in colour. These seeds contain very little mucilage and the swelling factor is 4.75.

CASTOR OIL

Castor Oil, Oleum Ricini

Botanical Source

Castor oil is the fixed oil obtained by expression of the seeds of *Ricinus communis* Linn.

Family

Euphorbiaceae.

Geographical Source

India and other tropical and sub-tropical countries.

Preparation

Castor oil is obtained from castor seeds. Usually the oil is obtained after removing the seed coat but sometimes it is obtained from seeds as such and it is of inferior quality. For removing seed coats, seeds are placed in grooved rollers and crushed when testa becomes loosened and is removed by blowing in air current. The kernels are placed in oil-expellers and expressed at room temperature with 1–2 tons pressure per square inch till about 30% oil is obtained. Oil is filtered but it contains a poisonous principle ricin a toxalbumin and enzyme lipase. To remove ricin, steam is passed into the oil at a temperature between 80° to 100° when ricin is coagulated and precipitated and lipase becomes inactive. Oil is then filtered. This oil has 1% acidity and only this cold-drawn castor oil is used for medicinal purposes.

Oil cake contains ricin, lipase and about 20% oil. It is crushed and expressed at 40° to 80° with 3 tons pressure per sq. inch. The oil obtained is inferior and not used medicinally but used in industries. The acidity of this oil is 5%.

The residual cake still contains about 8 to 10% oil which can be extracted in soxhlet with lipid solvents. This oil is also used in industry. The residual cake, because of presence of ricin, cannot be used as an animal food but is used as manure and for production of lipase which hydrolyzes fats in glycerine and fatty acids.

Chemical Constituents

Castor oil contains 80% glyceride of ricinoleic acid and other glycerides are of isoricinoleic, stearic and dihydroxy stearic acids. The laxative property is due to ricinoleic acid which forms sodium salt which irritates intestine. Ricinoleic acid is

$$CH_3(CH_2)_5CH(H) . CH_2CH = CH(CH_2)_7COOH$$

and it contains OH group and a double bond. Castor oil also contains vitamin F, a hair growth vitamin.

Uses

Castor oil is mild purgative. Undecylenic acid and its zinc salt obtained from castor oil are used as fungistatic. Castor oil is used as a lubricating agent and in manufacture of Turkish red oil. Hydrogenated castor oil is used as an ointment base. Sulphated hydrogenated castor oil, also known as hydroxystearin sulphate, is used as water-absorbent ointment and cream. Castor oil forms 40% of the total amount of export of natural products from India. Ricinoleic acid 0.5–0.7% is used in vaginal jellies for restoration and maintenance of vaginal acidity. Castor oil is used as plasticizer and in preparation of flexible collodion.

Recently, mechanism of action of castor oil has been explained. Prostaglandin E inhibits reabsorption and increases secretion of water and electrolytes in the intestine and thus acts as a laxative. Ricinoleic acid in the castor oil stimulates endogenous prostaglandin synthesis in the intestine and laxative action takes place. Further, experimentally it was shown that laxative action of castor oil is thus caused to a large extent by the activity of ricinoleic acid. It is indicated in quick treatment of severe constipation.

CARDIOTONICS
CARDIOTONIC AGENTS – CARDIAC TONICS

Heart is perhaps the most important of all the human body organs, which can never rest throughout the lifetime of the living beings. It has to continue to pump the blood throughout the body at a regular and a measured pace. However, under certain pathological and/or abnormal conditions the normal functions tend to become erratic and abnormal. One such and more common condition is congestive heart failure, losing the tonicity of the heart muscle, leading to decrease in cardiac output – pumping loss of blood – and resulting in further decrease in the supply of blood to itself i.e. the heart muscle, which leads to even myocardial infection. The muscle of weak heart tries to overcome this decreased output and in doing so it becomes all the more tired and loses the muscle tone and thus further hampers the cardiac output.

The drugs that increase the tone or force of contraction of heart are called cardiotonics or cardiotonic agents. A good cardiotonic should strengthen the heart, increase the cardiac output and be devoid of any kind of toxic effects.

Cardiac glycosides inhibit Na^+/K^+ ATPase of the cell membrane. Thus, intercellular calcium ions rise inside the cardiac cells. There is, therefore, an increase in the tone of the muscle.

A number of plants have been tried to see if they exerted a slowing and strengthening effect on a weak and failing heart. It was in 1785 that a botanist William Withering found foxglove, *Digitalis purpurea*, a potent plant, which though used first in the treatment of dropsy, proved later on as an important cardiotonic drug. Ever since the finding of digitalis leaves, the species of *Digitalis* have been occupying the important place as the ideal plant product useful as cardiotonics. Their chemical structures are discussed under cardiac glycosides. Also their therapeutic uses with special reference to their structures will be further discussed under each drug.

The drugs included in this category in the syllabus are Digitalis and Arjuna. They are discussed hereunder.

Digitalis, as mentioned in the syllabus, refers to a generalised term for the drug digitalis, under which normally one understands the leaves of the first well-known plant, foxglove, the leaves of *Digitalis purpurea*. *Digitalis* is the generic name of the plant of the family Scrophulariaceae and the genus has quite a few species, which contain similar phytochemical constituents. Of these the species known as lanata has become equally, if not more, important. Hence, we describe these important cardiotaonic drugs here.

DIGITALIS LEAVES

Foxglove Leaves. Folia Digitalis

Botanical Sources

Digitalis consists of dried leaves of *Digitalis purpurea*. After collection leaves are dried immediaely at temperature below 60° and they contain not more than 5% moisture. After drying leaves are stored in moisture-proof containers.

Family

Scrophulariaceae.

Geographical Sources

European countries, England, Germany, France, North America, Kashmir.

Cultivation

Digitalis is a biennial herb growing wild but good quality of the drug is obtained especially from cultivated plants. In the U.S.A., S.B. Penick & Co., by special methods of controlled growth, cultivation, harvest and drying, were obtaining 140 to 160% more potent drug than the standard drug. For cultivation special strains of the seeds are selected which would produce disease-resistant plants with maximum activity. Attention is specially paid to the structure of the soil in seed beds. Soil consists of equal parts of clean sand, garden soil, well-rotted manure and leaf mould. Soil is finely subdivided and mixed well. Before sowing soil is sterilized. Usually, a greater number of seeds are planted than required seedlings. Seedlings are produced which are transplanted by hand or semi-mechanized transplanter which digs the furrow, puts the plant in its place and presses moistened soil on it. Plants are observed periodically to see that they are free from diseases and attack of insects. In dry season sufficient water is supplied to the plant. In the first year, a long stalk with rosette of leaves is produced. Collection of these leaves is carried out from September to November by hand and thus other organic matter and discoloured leaves are avoided. Because of higher percentage of glycosides, leaves of first year are preferred. Leaves are dried in drying chambers with automatic control of temperature and humidity. Collection and capacity of drying chambers are adjusted in such a way that continuous supply of dry leaves is obtained. By quick drying, characteristic green colour of the leaves is maintained. Drying is carried out till moisture is not more than 5%. Leaves are packed under pressure in airtight containers. Leaves are collected in the first year. However, some plants are allowed to grow in the second year when flower stalk and seeds are produced which are utilized for the production of new plants. Leaves of the plants excepting those which are utilized for seed production are harvested and processed as mentioned earlier. Because of F.D.A., S.B. Penick & Co. are not cultivating digitalis at present. At present digitalis leaves used in USA are obtained mostly from England and Germany from selected developed strains of *D. purpurea* and *D. lanata* with maximum drug potency and resistance to plant diseases. The method of cultivation and collection is nearly the same as mentioned above.

Storage

Digitalis leaves are stored in moisture-proof containers with a moisture content not more than 5%. They are protected from light. Usually dessicating agents like calcium oxide or silica gel are used to ensure that drug has no access to moisture.

Chemical Constituents

Digitalis leaves contain monoside (odoroside), bioside (glucoverodoxin), trioside (digitoxin, gitoxin and gitaloxin), tetrasides or primary glycosides (purpurea glycosides A and B). Because of greater stability of secondary glycosides and lesser absorption of primary glycosides a higher content of primary glycosides is not considered ideal and secondary glycosides are used. For isolation of secondary glycosides like digitoxin enzymatic reaction is carried out. The hydrolysis of some important glycosides is as follows:

Purpurea glycoside A → Digitoxin + Glucose
Purpurea glycoside B → Gitoxin + Glucose
Digitoxin → Digitoxigenin + 3 Digitoxose
Gitoxin → Gitoxigenin + 3 Digitoxose
Verodoxin → Gitaloxigenin + Digitalose

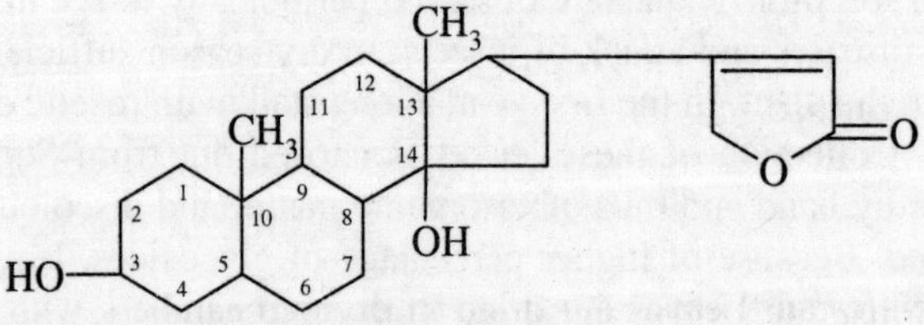

Digitoxigenin

In the above glycosides, the three aglycones are digitoxigenin, gitoxigenin and gitaloxigenin. Gitoxigenin contains an additional OH group at 16 position or is 16 OH digitoxigenin and gitaloxigenin is 16 formyl gitoxigenin. Purpurea glycosides A and B are present in fresh leaves and by their hydrolysis digitoxin and glucose or gitoxin and glucose are obtained, respectively. Hydrolysis of purpurea glycosides can take place by digi-

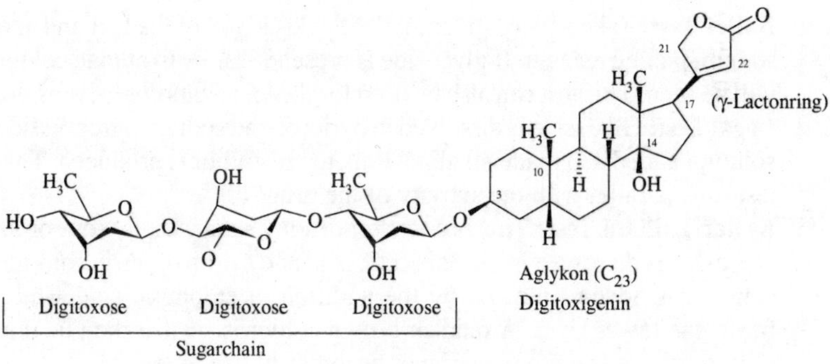

Fig. 3.3. Complete structure of digitoxin showing sugar-sugar linkages with the aglycon digitoxigenin.

puridase present in the leaves. Digitoxin yields on hydrolysis digitoxigenin and three digitoxoses. By hydrolysis of verodoxin, gitaloxigenin and digitalose are obtained. Verodoxin potentiates the activity of digitoxin by synergism and in some pharmacopoeias percentage of verodoxin is indicated along with digitoxin.

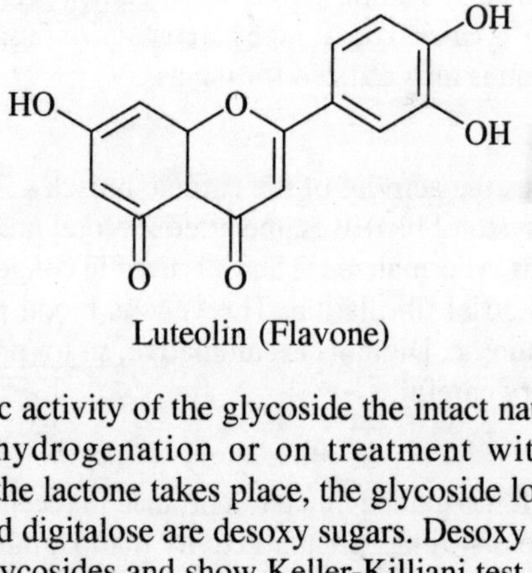

Luteolin (Flavone)

For the cardiac activity of the glycoside the intact nature of lactone is important. On hydrogenation or on treatment with alkali, when isomerization of the lactone takes place, the glycoside loses its activity.

Digitoxose and digitalose are desoxy sugars. Desoxy sugars are found only in cardiac glycosides and show Keller-Killiani test. Digitoxose is 2-desoxy methyl pentose and digitalose is a methoxy 6 desoxy-D-galactose. Digitalis contains steroid saponins digitonin and gitonin and luteolin, a flavone responsible for the colour of the drug.

Chemical Tests

Digitalis glycosides having five-membered lactone ring are C_{23} glycosides. These glycosides show the following tests which are due to the intact lactone (see also Part III).

1. **Baljet Test:** Take a piece of lamina or thick section of the leaf and add sodium picrate reagent. If glycoside is present, yellow to orange colour will be seen. This test can also be used for the localization of glycoside.
2. **Legal Test:** Glycoside is dissolved in pyridine and sodium nitroprusside solution added and made alkaline. Pink to red colour is produced. This test runs parallel with the activity of the drug.
3. **Keller-Killiani Test:** This is a test for desoxy sugar. Digitoxose or its glycoside is dissolved in glacial acetic acid and a drop of ferric chloride solution is added followed by the addition of sulphuric acid which forms the lower layer. A reddish-brown colour is seen at the junction of two liquids and the upper layer becomes bluish green.

If the leaves are used, preliminary extraction is done as follows: 1 gm of the powdered leaves is extracted with 10 ml of 70% alcohol for couple of minutes, filtered and to 5 ml of filtrate 10 ml of water and 0.5 ml of strong solution of lead acetate are added and filtered and the filtrate is shaken with 5 ml of chloroform. Chloroform layer is separated in a porcelain dish and the test is carried out as mentioned above.

Assay

To determine the potency of digitalis and its preparations, bioassay is carried out. In different methods animals like frogs, guinea pigs and cats are used. Sometimes, assay is carried out for the percentage of digitoxose. The colour reaction of lactone is also utilized for the assay.

Uses

Digitalis increases the activity of the cardiac muscles. The contraction of heart ventricle (systole) increases, the arterial blood pressure rises and the frequency of heart is normalized. Thus it is used in congestive heart failure, atrial flutter and atrial fibrillation. The venous blood pressure decreases and it acts as a diuretic. Digitalis is cumulative, so for prolonged treatment one has to be very careful.

Allied Drugs

Digitalis lanata: It has gained much importance in recent years. The leaves of D. lanata have 3–4 times greater activity than D. purpurea.

DIGITALIS LANATA LEAF

Botanical Source

The drug consists of the dried leaves of *Digitalis lanata*.

Family

Scrophulariaceae.

Geographical Source

This species grows in the region adjacent to the Danube in Central Europe. It has been cultivated in England and in the USA. It is also cultivated in India. The plant is biennial.

The leaves are sessile, linear-lanceolate, about 30 cm long and 4 cm broad with entire margin and acuminate apex. The veins leave the mid-rib at an acute angle.

Digitalis lanata contains lanatosides A, B, C and E. Lanatosides A and B are acetyl derivatives of purpurea glycosides A and B respectively. Lanatoside C on hydrolysis yields digoxin, a crystalline active glycoside, acetic acid and glucose. Acetyl group is attached to terminal digitoxose sugar.

Digoxigenin, the aglycone of digoxin, contains an OH group in the 12th position. Lanatoside E yields on hydrolysis gitaloxin, acetic acid and glucose.

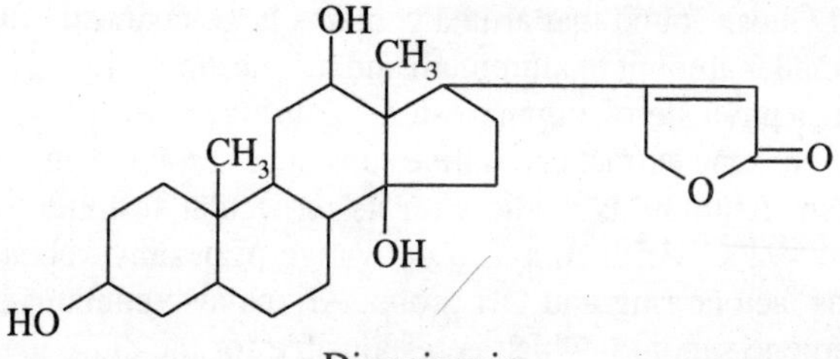

Digoxigenin

The greater activity of *D. lanata* is attributed to the presence of digoxin which is also official in many pharmacopoeias. *D. lanata* is used in the same way as digitalis.

Besides the above, *Digitalis lutea*, so called because of the yellow-coloured flowers, and *Digitalis thapsi*, known as Spanish foxglove, growing in Spain and Italy are considered as allied drugs.

Adulterants

Mullelin leaves are leaves of *Verbascum thapsus*. These leaves are covered with large branched woolly hairs. Other adulterants are primrose leaves (*Primula vulgaris*) and comfrey leaves (*Symphytum officinale*). Many of the adulterants can be identified by shape, margin, venation and nature of trichomes.

ARJUNA BARK

Botanical Source

Arjuna is the dried bark of *Terminalia arjuna*.

Family

Combretaceae.

Members of this family are characterized by the presence of tannins and are used as tanning agents. Myrobalans (Haritaki or Harde) and beleric fruits belong to this family.

Geographical Source

India. Trees are found in north Gujarat at Balaram, a picnic place.

Collection

Arjuna is a large deciduous tree reaching a height of 60' to 80' and trunk is of 10' to 12' in circumference. No information is available about the time of collection of bark. Bark is collected mostly from wild trees by making suitable incisions and dried.

Chemical Constituents

Chopra and Ghosh found that arjuna contains large quantities of calcium salts with smaller amount of aluminum and magnesium salts, 12% tannins, organic acid, a phytosterol, organic ester, colouring matter and sugar. Later on from the benzene extract crystalline substances arjunine and arjunetine were isolated. Arjunine is acidic with its molecular formula $C_{21}H_{32}O_3$, and melts at 192°C. Arjunetine is a derivative of hexahydrobenzoic acid and contains lactone ring and OH group. Arjuna also contains arjunollic acid, a triterpene-saponin, which is responsible for the diuretic property.

Uses

Arjuna is popularly used as a cardiac tonic. Caius, Mhaskar and Isaac found arjuna possessing diuretic property which may be attributed to sapopin. Recently mechanism of cardiovascular action of Arjuna bark is reported. Intravenous administration of the aqueous extract of the dried alcoholic extract of the dried bark produced decrease in blood pressure and heart rate. These extracts also inhibited carotid occlusion response without affecting pressor response induced by intravenous injection of norepinephrine and by electrical stimulation of preganglionic fibres of the abdominal splanchnic nerve. Hypotension and bradycardia were also observed following the injection of extract into the lateral cerebral ventrical and vertebral artery. The results of present study show that the hypotension and bradycardiac effects of *T. arjuna* are mainly of central origin.

Adulterant

Tomentosa bark. Tomentosa bark is obtained from *Terminalia tomentosa* (Family Combretaceae), a plant growing in India. Tomentosa is sometimes used in place of arjuna bark.

CARMINATIVES AND G.I. REGULATORS

This chapter again shows somewhat inconsistency in its heading. This part deals with drugs based on therapeutic efficacy of carminatives and gastrointestinal regulators. Carminatives themselves, in a broader sense, concern with the ailments of gastrointestinal tract (GIT). GIT consists of mainly three regions, the upper one comprising mouth, stomach and upper portion of the duodenum, the middle portion of the lower half of the duodenum to the ileolic sphincter, and the lower portion of the caecum, colon and rectum.

The seat of action is stomach, a part of GIT. The mobility and regulation of digestive secretions are controlled by nervous, biochemical and mechanical factors. These processes are well coordinated to ensure the necessary secretion of digestive juices in order to accomplish the digestion of food materials. It is, however, a common fact that the secretions and/or mortality get altered as per the need. This leads to disturbances and calls for symptomatic treatment.

The GI regulators may regulate the increase in secretion, causing gastric hyperacidity and peptic ulcers and decrease in mobility of GIT leading to constipation. Other direct or indirect symptoms of GI tract are gastric distension, eructation (noisy oral expulsion of gas from stomach) and heart burn.

There are a number of ailments which are connected with GIT, especially to its upper and lower portions, which are more susceptible to different kinds of disorders, which require a number of drugs for their treatment. Such drugs, to name a few of their categories, are: carminatives, bitters, emetics, antiulcer agents, demulcents, laxatives, purgatives, antidiarrhoeal drugs, etc.

As pointed out above, the syllabus could have preferably included all those drugs together which are required to treat different categories of diseases of GIT. This would make the syllabus more consistent and rational.

CARMINATIVES

Carminatives are substances obtained from drugs or drugs chewed as such or used in other kinds of preparations which help in ejecting gases from the stomach and provide relief from discomfort and distension after (heavy) meals. The action is through irritation of the gastric mucosa which would stimulate the gastric movements and also relax the sphincters to cause expulsion of the gas from stomach.

Carminatives are thus aromatic substances which assist eructation reflex. Their mode of action is, however, not clearly understood. Many volatile oils and volatile oils containing drugs included in the syllabus are described here.

The drugs included in this category of therapeutic efficacy are: Umbelliferous fruits, Coriander, Fennel, Ajowan, Cardamom, Ginger, Black pepper, Asafoetida, Nutmeg, Cinnamon and Clove.

Since there are quite a few drugs belonging to the family Umbelliferae, it is considered worthwhile to describe briefly the common structural characteristics of umbelliferae fruits in Part III.

CORIANDER

Fructus Coriandri, Coriander Fruits, Dhaniya (Hindi),
Dhana (Guj.), Kazbara (Arabic)

Botanical Source

Coriander consists of dried ripe fruits of *Coriandrum sativum* Linn.

Family

Umbelliferae.

Geographical Source

Cultivated in many countries of Central and Eastern Europe, especially Russia and Thuringia, Mediterranean countries, Morocco and India.

Collection

The plant is an annual herb, upto 1 metre in height. All the parts of the green plant have unpleasant bug-like smell, hence the name coriander. The green leaves of the plant, kothmir (Guj.) are used as spice. Fruits are collected when mature and ripe and dried. During drying fruits develop aromatic smell and unpleasant bug-like odour disappears.

Chemical Constituents

Volatile oil is 0.5–1.0%. Main constituent is the pleasant smelling d-linalool upto 90%. Other constituents are terpene hydrocarbons like pinene, cymene, terpinene and small quantities of borneol and geraniol. (see also general account on volatile oils).

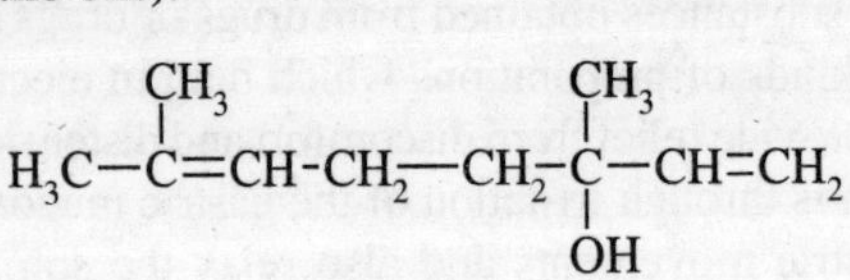

$$H_3C-\underset{\underset{CH_3}{|}}{C}=CH-CH_2-CH_2-\underset{\underset{OH}{|}}{\overset{\overset{CH_3}{|}}{C}}-CH=CH_2$$

Linalool

Recently, in addition to above, geranyl acetate, decanal and a nev compound trans-tridecene-(2)-al-(1) have been isolated. Trans-tridecene-(2)-al-(1) (tridecenal) is responsible for the bug-like smell of the green plant.

$$H_3C-(CH_2)_{\overline{9}}-CH=CH-CHO$$

Tridecenal/Trans-tridecene-(2)-al-(1)

In some Indian samples thymol has also been found. The fruit also contains fixed oil and protein.

Uses

Coriander is used as an aromatic, carminative and flavouring agent. Oil of coriander is one of the constituents in aromatic elixir preparation. The volatile oil separated by steam distillation also shows antibacterial and antifungal activity.

FENNEL

Fructus foeniculii. Fennel fruit, Badi saunph (Hindi), Variyali (Guj.)

Botanical Source

Fennel consists of the dried ripe fruits of *Foeniculum vulgar* Miller obtained by cultivation.

Family

Umbelliferae.

Geographical Source

Indigenous to Mediterranean countries and Asia. Cultivated in many countries of Central and Eastern Europe, India and Japan. Commercial varieties are Saxon (Germany) and from Galicia and Russia.

Cultivation

Fennel is a perennial herb and is cultivated by planting fresh seeds in spring in the usual ways. Stems with fruits are colleted next September, dried, thrashed and fruits separated.

Chemical Constituents

3–7% volatile oil which contains 50–60% anethole, 5–8% methyl chavicol (estragole) and 18–20% fenchone. Anethole is p-propenyl anisole and is aromatic and has sweet odour and taste. Fenchone is a colourless pungent liquid and has camphoraceous taste and smell. Fenchone is bicyclical monoterpene, and is optically active. It is responsible for bitter burning taste of oil. Father fennel contains about 20% fixed oil and 20% proteins.

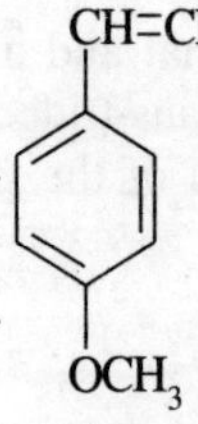

CH=CH-CH₃   CH₂-CH=CH₂

Anethole 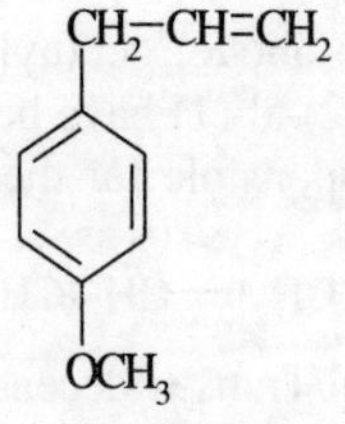   Methyl chavicol (estragole) 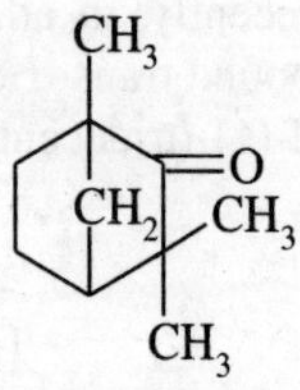   Fenchone

Uses

It is respiratory stimulant and is used as an expectorant. It is an aromatic, carminative and flavouring agent and is popularly added in cough and stomach mixtures. Because of sweet taste, anethole is used in mouth and dental preparations. Recently, a variety of fennel growing in Ooti (South India) has been found to contain methyl chavicol as the chief constituent and is free from anethole.

Adulterant

Fennel is adulterated with exhausted fennel in which part of volatile oil is removed either by extraction with alcohol or steam-distillation.

- **Alcohol-exhausted Fennel:** These fruits do not change much in appearance and have fusel oil odour. Percentage of volatile oil is 1–2%.
- **Steam-exhausted Fennel:** They are darker in appearance. They contain less volatile oil and sink in water.

AJOWAN

Ajwan Fruits, Ajowain (Hindi), Ajwain (Urdu)

Botanical Source

Ajowan consists of the dried ripe fruits of *Trachyspermum ammi* (L.) Sprague (Syn. *Carum copticum*; *Ptychotis ajowan*).

Family

Umbelliferae.

Geographical Source

Cultivated mainly in India.

Chemical Constituents

Volatile oil is 3.5–5.0%. Main constituent is the pleasant smelling thymol from 30 to 50%. Also contains carvacrol, limonene, camphene, etc.

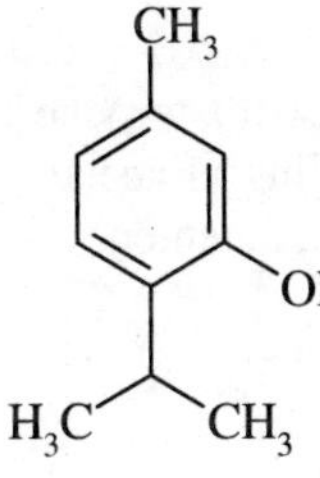

Thymol

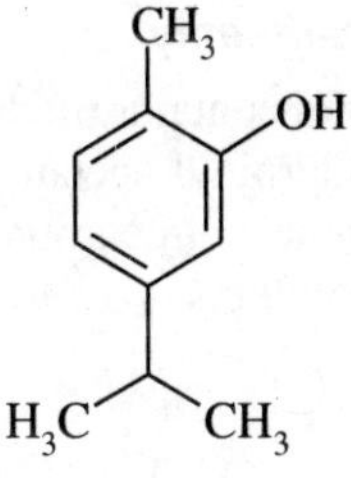

Carvacrol

Uses

It is used as a spice and is highly esteemed as a spice in India. It is an important source for thymol. Ajowan is used in the treatment of colds, coughs, asthma, rheumatism and indigestion.

CARDAMOM

Cardamom fruit, Cardamom seed, Ilayachi (Hindi and Guj.)

Botanical Source

Cardamom consists of the dried ripe seeds of *Elettaria cardamomum* var. *minuscula*. Seeds are removed from fruits when required for use.

Family

Zingiberaceae.

Geographical Source

Cultivated in Karnataka and Kerala States in South India and Guatemala and Sri Lanka.

Even though seeds are used as drug, in many pharmacopoeias fruits are official. If seeds are separated, there is loss of volatile oil by volatization and in some cases by rupturing of the seeds and pericarp has protective property. According to Clevenger, the loss of volatile oil may be upto 30%. Fruits of different varieties can be easily identified as they have different shapes and sizes and the presence of foreign organic matter is easily determined. There are four official varieties of cardamom:

1. Mysore or Ceylon-Mysore
2. Malabar or Ceylon-Malabar
3. Mangalore
4. Aleppy cardamom

(Diagrams and morphology in Part III).

Chemical Constituents

Volatile oil 3–6%, contains oxide cineole (50%), terpene alcohols borneol, terpineol, ester terpinyl acetate, linalool, linolyl acetate, linalool, linolyl acetate and terpene hydrocarbons limonene, dipentene and terpinene, fixed oil, starch and proteins.

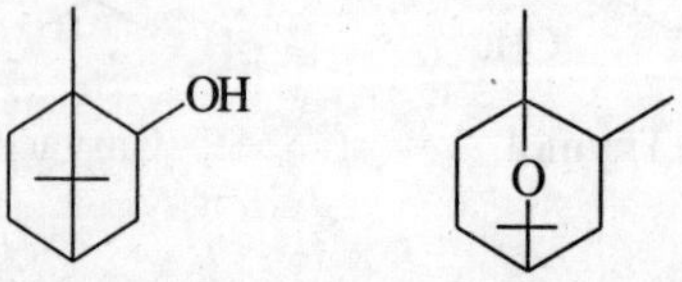

Borneol   Cineole

Uses

Cardamom is used as an aromatic, carminative, stimulant and flavouring agent. It is popularly used as a spice.

Adulterant

- **Long Wild Native Cardamom:** This is obtained in Ceylon from wild plants of *Elettaria cardamomum* var. *major*. This variety is not cultivated and cardamom fruits are more elongated upto 4 cm in length, 1 cm in diameter, dark brown and coarsely striated. The seeds are about 4 mm long, less aromatic and bitter. The volatile oil has different composition.
- **Amomum Species:** Several species of Amomum yield fruits which are usually much larger in size but less aromatic. *Amomum aromaticum* and *A. kepulaga* yield Bengal cardamoms (Bari Ilayachi) and round or cluster cardamoms, respectively. Their seeds are adulterated with the authentic drug.

CLOVE

Caryophylli, Clove buds, Clove flowers, Lovang (Hindi), Laving (Guj.)

Botanical Source

Clove consists of the dried flower buds of *Eugenia caryophyllus* Spreng and contains not more than 5% of its stalks and not more than 1% other organic matter.

Family

Myrtaceae.

Members of this family are evergreen shrubs or trees. Schizolysigenous oil glands are present in young stems, leaves and flowers in many species of this family. Some species contain tannins. Vascular bundles are bicollateral. Eucalyptus and Jambool belong to this family.

Geographical Source

Clove tree is native of Molucca Islands (present Indonesia). At present clove is cultivated mainly in Islands of Zanzibar, Pemba, Amboiana and Sumatra. It is also found in Madagascar, Penang, Mauritius, West Indies and Sri Lanka.

Cultivation

Clove tree is evergreen and 15 to 20 metres in height. For cultivation seeds are sown in well-drained suitable soil at a distance of about 25 cm. Clove plant requires moist, warm and equable climate with well distributed rainfall. During cultivation plants should be protected against pests and diseases. In the beginning seeds cannot bear full sunlight, so protection is given by constructing frames about 1 metre high and covering them with banana leaves. Banana leaves gradually decay and more sunlight falls on the young seedlings. When seedlings are about 9 months old they are able to bear full sunlight. Then the frames are removed and when seedlings are about 1 metre high they are transplanted at a distance of 6 metres in the beginning of rainy season. For the first two to three years young clove trees are shaded by planting banana trees in between. Clove can be collected every year from trees of 6 years old till they are 70 years old. Every year 3–4 kg clove can be collected from each tree. For continuous and regular supply every year new plantations are added.

Collection

Inflorescence of clove is panicle or compound receme and branches are opposite and decussate. Clove buds are at first white, then green and finally become crimson-red in colour. Collection of crimson-red coloured buds is carried out in dry weather from August to December. For collection of buds, natives climb the trees or put ladders and pick the buds, with the stalk. Mobile platforms are also used for collection. Trees are also beaten by means of bamboo sticks, clove buds fall on the ground and are collected. After collection stalks are separated and then they are put on coconut mats or concrete floors and dried in the sun. During night they are covered. Drying takes about three days. As a result of drying clove buds become dark reddish-brown and lose about 70% of the weight. Clove is then graded according to size, condition and quality, packed into bales and exported.

At present Zanzibar and Pemba islands produce each year about 8000 tons, which meets 4/5th of world's supply.

Chemical Constituents

Clove contains volatile oil about 14–21% and pyrogallol tannins. Volatile oil contains about 85–90% eugenol, 3% acetyl eugenol and sesquiterpenes and caryophyllenes. The characteristic aroma of clove is due to the presence of methyl amyl ketone, a minor constituent of volatile oil. Other substances are methyl furfural and dimethyl furfural. Eugenol is a colourless liquid and is chemically allyl guaicol. Eugenol is used for the synthesis of vanillin.

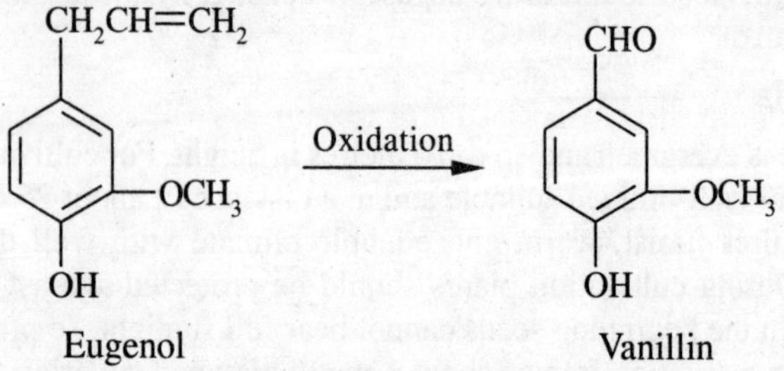

$$CH_2CH=CH_2 \qquad\qquad CHO$$

Eugenol →(Oxidation)→ Vanillin

Uses

Clove is used as an antiseptic, aromatic stimulant, carminative and as flavouring agent. Clove and clove oil are popularly used in toothache, dental preparations and in mouthwashes. Clove oil and zinc oxide are used in temporary filling of dental cavities. Eugenol also has local anaesthetic action. Large doses are poisonous because of irritating action on striated muscles. Clove is mainly used as spice and clove oil in perfumery.

Adulterants

1. **Exhausted Clove:** In this drug, volatile oil is partially or entirely removed by distillation and thus they contain less volatile oil. Exhausted cloves are darker in colour, more shrunken, do not yield oil when indented with fingernail and float in freshly boiled and cooled water.
2. **Clove Stalks:** During collection, buds are collected along with stalks and subsequently separated. Stalks are, however, not completely removed. Pharmacopoeial limit of clove stalks is 5%. The percentage of volatile oil in clove stalks is only 5%.
3. **Clove Fruits:** Mother Clove, Anthophylli. Some clove buds ripen to fruits and are found in the drug. The ripened fruits are 2–2.5 cm long, ovate and tapering below. At the upper part calyx teeth intrun towards style. Clove fruits are dark brown and their outer surface is rough. Each fruit contains a single firm seed. Seeds contain starch and by its presence adulteration of clove fruits can be determined. Clove fruits also contain less percentage of volatile oil and that is why it is considered an adulterant.
4. **Blown Clove:** They are fully developed clove flowers from which usually corolla and stamens get detached. Mixture of detached corolla and stamens is known as clove dust.

NUTMEG

Semen myristicae, Myristica, Jayfal (Guj.)

Botanical Source

Nutmeg is the kernel of the dried ripe seed of *Myristica fragrans* Houtten, deprived of its arillus and seed coat and with or without a thin coating of lime.

Family

Myristicaceae.

Geographical Source

A native of Mollucca islands in Indonesia and at present cultivated in West Indies and other tropical countries.

Collection

Plant is a dioecious tree bearing male and female flowers separately. Only female plant supplies the drug. Fruits are light yellow, drupaceous ovoid berries. They are 5–7 cm long and 4–5 cm wide and dehisce longitudinally. The fleshy pericarp splits and exposes dark brown seed coat and crimson reticulate arillus. Fruits are collected from November to December or from April to June from 8 years old plants in the morning. Collection is done by hand or with a stick and hook device. In West Indies they are allowed to fall and collected. The arillus is stripped off and forms a separate article of commerce called mace. Seeds are dried with charcoal fire keeping them in trays at a height of about 3 metres. The testa is removed by cracking the seeds with wooden mallet and kernels separated. The immature, wormy and broken kernels are removed and graded according to size and condition. Nutmeg is derived from anatropous ovule and the markings like raphe, hilum, micropyle are present on the seed coat. Since the seed coat is separated no true raphe, hilum and micropyle are present on the kernels but only their impressions. Sometimes kernels are coated with lime which protects them. It was considered by Dutch that coating with lime destroys the germinating capacity. According to Wallis, germinating capacity is completely lost by drying and above precaution was superfluous.

Chemical Constituents

Nutmeg contains, as the active constituent, volatile oil 5–15%, which is secreted in large bubble-like cells in the inner perisperm. Volatile oil contains 4–8% myristicin, elemicin, terpene alcohols like borneol, geraniol and hydrocarbons pinene, camphene and dipentene. Further, volatile oil contains safrol, eugenol and isoeugenol. Mainly myristicin and to a lesser extent safrol, eugenol and isoeugenol are considered responsible for the activity of the drug. Elemicine is related to amphetamine.

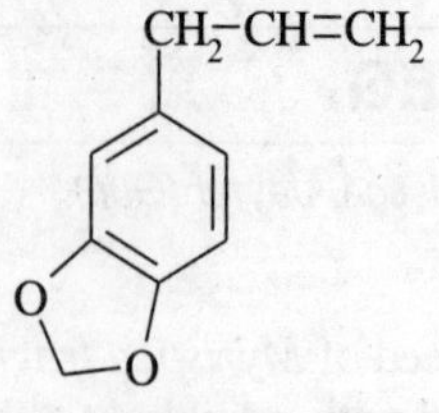

CH₂–CH=CH₂ (Safrol structure)

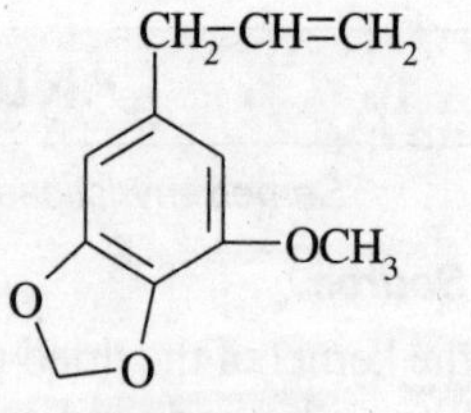

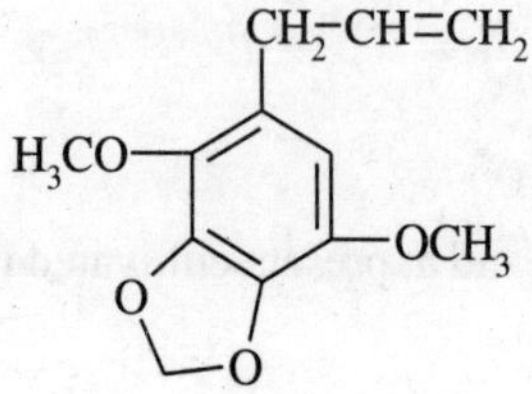

Safrol

CH₂–CH=CH₂ (Myristicin structure with OCH₃)

Myristicin

CH₂–CH=CH₂ (Apiole structure with H₃CO and OCH₃)

Apiole

CH₂–CH=CH₂ (Elemicin structure with H₃CO, OCH₃, OCH₃)

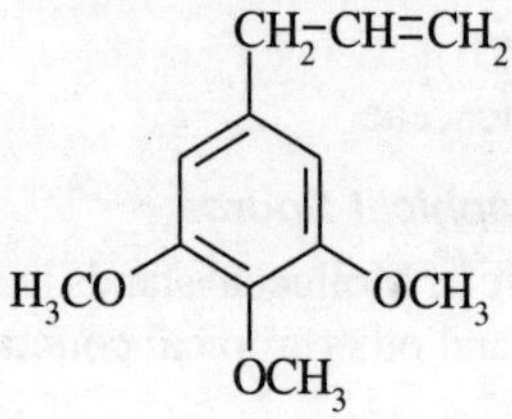

Elemicin

Nutmeg also contains fat or fixed oil, 25% to 30%, and is known as nutmeg butter. Nutmeg butter is aromatic because of the presence of volatile oil and is an orange-coloured mass. Starch, amylodextrin and saponin are also present.

Uses

Nutmeg is aromatic carminative and flavouring agent. In higher doses it is toxic because of myristicin. On central nervous system it has narcotic and anaesthetic action and peripherally has irritant action and irritates intestine and uterus and is considered as an abortificient. Recently nutmeg has been found as a useful remedy in controlling diarrhoea associated with certain carcinomas.

Allied Drugs

1. **Bombay Nutmeg:** Indian nutmeg is known as Bombay nutmeg because it is exported from Mumbai. It is obtained from *Myristica malabarica* and is obtained from South India. Kernels are long and narrow. Volatile oil is less and the drug has very little aromatic odour.
2. **Papua Nutmeg:** They are obtained from *M. argentea*. Seeds are larger, narrower and less aromatic.

MACE

Banda mace, Javantri, Jaypatri

Mace is the arillus of the seed of *M. fragrans*. As mentioned under the collection of nutmeg, mace gets exposed during dehiscence of the fruit and completely encloses the seed. If it is removed entirely it is called double blade and if cut into two pieces and removed it is called single blade. After collection it is flattened by treading under feet or pressing between the boards. It is then dried by exposure to sun for 2 to 4 days. When fresh, it has crimson red colour but during drying it turns golden yellow.

Mace contains volatile oil similar to nutmeg, fixed oil about 20% and amylodextrin which gives red colour with iodine. Mace is used similar to nutmeg.

Mace gives yellow colour with alkali or concentrated sulphuric acid, while Bombay mace and Papua mace give dark red and cherry red colour, respectively.

CINNAMON BARK

Cortex cinnamonni, Ceylon cinnamon,
Ceylon Taj (Guj), Dalchini (Hindi)

Botanical Source
Cinnamon is the dried inner bark of the coppiced shoots of *Cinnamomum zeylanicum* Nees.

Family
Lauraceae.

Geographical Source
Sri Lanka, Java, Sumatra, West Indies, Seychelles, Jamaica, Brazil.

Preparation
The pieces of the barks are graded according to thickness and then they are dried in the shade. During drying, they roll into quills. Then compound quills are made by packing small quills into large ones. They are then cut into pieces of 1 metre length. The remains of cuttings are known as quillings or featherings. During drying, the original pale colour of the bark is changed to brown as some of the phlobaphenes are formed.

The quality of the bark is determined according to thickness. The thinner the bark, the better it is. The compound quills are then graded and packed into bales and exported. The outer peeled portions are known as cinnamon chips. Chips yield volatile oil of low specific gravity and low aldehyde content. Quillings and featherings are used for distillation of volatile oil. The outer layers contain very little volatile oil so by peeling, bark of a good quality is obtained.

Constituents
Cinnamon contains volatile oil 0.5 to 1.4%. Volatile oil is present in numerous unicellular oil cells in secondary phloem. Volatile oil contains

50 to 75% cinnamic aldehyde $C_6H_5CH=CHCHO$, about 5 to 10% eugenol and terpene hydrocarbons, phellandrene, pinene and caryophyllenes and other terpenes. Further, mucilage, phlobatannins, calcium oxalate and starch are present in the bark.

Chemical Tests

1. One drop of volatile oil is dissolved in 5 ml of alcohol and a drop of ferric chloride solution is added. A pale green colour is produced. With ferric chloride cinnamic aldehyde gives brown colour and eugenol, because of phenolic OH, gives blue colour and an intermediary green colour is obtained.
2. In cassia bark oil, brown colour is obtained as it contains only cinnamic aldehyde.
3. Prepare a chloroform extract by extracting few milligrams with 1 ml chloroform on slide and to 2 drops of chloroform extract or of volatile oil, add 2 drops of 10% aqueous solution of phenylhydrazin hydrochloride and cover with cover slip. Small rod-shaped crystals of the phenyl hydrazone of cinnamic aldehyde are seen.

Uses

It is used as an aromatic carminative, flavouring agent, stomachic and antiseptic and mild astringent.

CASSIA BARK

Chinese cinnamon, Cassia lignea

Botanical Source

Cassia bark is obtained from *Cinnamomum cassia* Blume.

Family

Lauraceae.

Geographical Source

South-eastern provinces of China and Cochin.

Cultivation

Cassia bark is collected from cultivated plants. They are grown in terraces by planting the seeds. Collection is done from trees 6 to 10 years old. Branches about 3 cm thick and 40 cm long are cut above the soil. Twigs and leaves are removed. Then two longitudinal cuts and transverse ring cuts are made and bark is stripped off. Then cork and some parts of outer cortex are peeled off and the product is dried and packed into bales and exported. In cassia bark compared to Ceylon cinnamon bark, less attention is paid to cultivation. As plants are not coppiced and bark is not completely peeled, it is considered inferior to Ceylon cinnamon bark.

Chemical Constituents

Volatile oil is 1–2% and contains 75–90% cinnamic aldehyde, 13-methoxy cinnamic aldehyde, caryophyllene and methyl O-cumin aldehyde and coumarin. Methyl O-cumin aldehyde is responsible for the inferior smell of the volatile oil. Eugenol is absent.

Both cinnamon and cassia can be distinguished by TLC and fluorescence. Cassia oil contains coumarin which gives strong green-blue fluorescence on addition of alkali not seen in cinnamon oil.

Uses

It is used similar to cinnamon.

GINGER

Rhizome zingiberis, Zingiber, Ginger, Soonth (Guj.), Saunth (Hindi)

Botanical Source

Ginger consists of the rhizome of *Zingiber officinale* Roscoe, scraped and dried in the sun.

Family

Zingiberaceae.

Geographical Source

Jamaica, South India (Cochin), Africa, Japan.

Cultivation

The plant of ginger is a perennial herb about 1 metre high with sympodial branching rhizome. For cultivation the rhizome is cut into pieces and each piece containing a bud is planted into trenches in well-drained and loamy soil in March or April.

Ginger cultivated and collected in January as above is called plantation ginger and is of high quality. Jamaica exports to all parts of world more than 2 million pounds of ginger every year.

- **Cochin Ginger:** Cultivated in South India in the same way as described above. This ginger is only partially peeled and bleached by dipping into milk of lime. Cochin ginger is thus coated and bleached. Pungency of this ginger is the same as that of Jamaica ginger but it is less aromatic.
- **African Ginger:** This is darker and smaller than Cochin ginger. It is imperfectly washed and coated. In recent years quality of this ginger has improved. This ginger is more pungent but lacks the aroma of Jamaica ginger.

Chemical Constituents

Ginger contains 1–2% volatile oil, 5–8% pungent principle, resinous mass and starch. Volatile oil is responsible for the aromatic smell and consists of zingiberene 6%, a sesquiterpene hydrocarbon zingiberol, a sesquiterpene alcohol and bisabolene. Gingerol is a yellow pungent oily liquid and yields gingerone, a ketone, and aliphatic aldehydes. Shogaol is formed by loss of water from gingerol. Shogaol and gingerone are less pungent. The pungency of gingerol and ginger is destroyed when boiled with 5% potassium hydroxide or other alkalies.

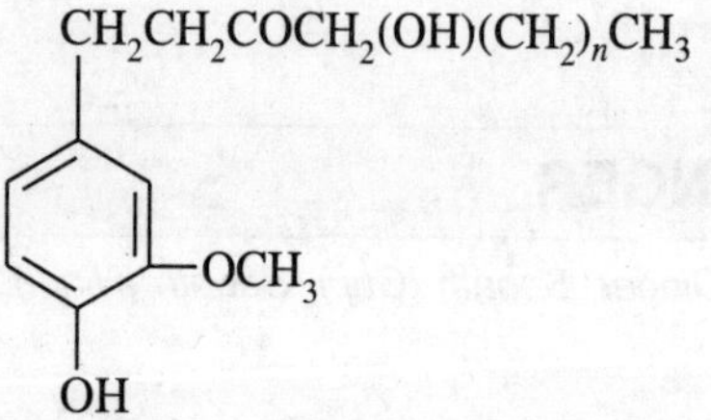

$$CH_2CH_2COCH_2(OH)(CH_2)_nCH_3$$

OCH$_3$

OH

Gingerol

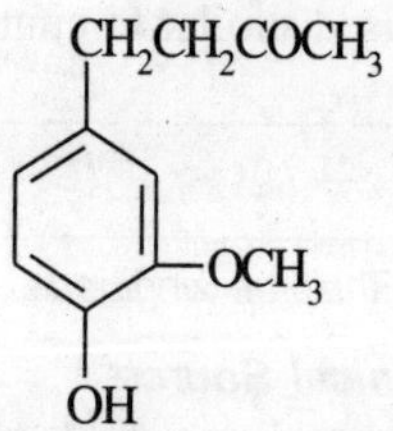

$$CH_2CH_2COCH_3$$

OCH$_3$

OH

Gingerone

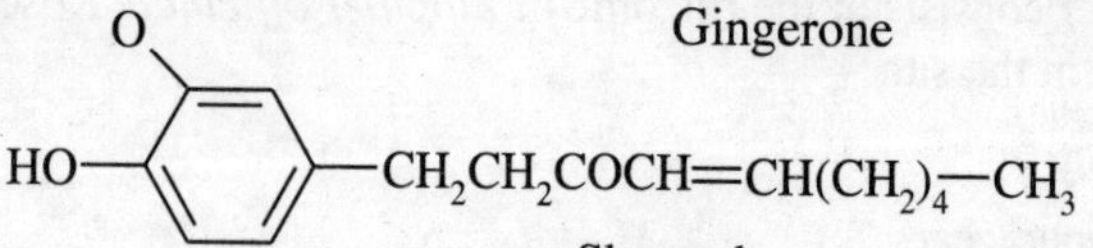

$$HO--CH_2CH_2COCH=CH(CH_2)_4-CH_3$$

Shogaol

Uses

Ginger is stomachic, stimulant and aromatic carminative. It is used more as a spice. Much of the ginger at present is used in manufacture of gingerale.

Pharmacopoeial Standards

1. *90% alcohol-soluble extractive is not less than 4.5%.*
   - Ginger exhausted with alcohol has 1.5% extractive. Water-exhausted ginger cannot be evaluated in this way.
2. *Water-soluble extractive is not less than 10%.*
   - Water-exhausted ginger has 6% extractive. Alcohol-exhausted ginger passes this standard.
3. *Total ash is not more than 6%.*
   - In ginger, not well-washed or limed, total ash is more.
4. *Water-soluble ash is not less than 1.7%.*
   - In water-extracted drug this ash is 0.5% and water-exhausted drug can be identified by this standard.

Adulteration

Adulteration of ginger by exhausted or not well prepared or limed drug can be determined by the above standards.

Sometimes in exhausted ginger, capsicum or paradise grains are added to increase pungency. Paradise grains are the seeds of Alframomum melegueta (Zingiberaceae). Pungency of capsicum and paradise grains is not destroyed by boiling with alkali while it is destroyed in case of ginger. Adulteration of ginger by capsicum and paradise grains can be determined in this way.

BLACK PEPPER

Kali Mirch, Golmirch

Botanical Sources

Pepper or Black pepper consists of the dried unripe or nearly ripe fruits of *Piper nigrum*, family Piperaceae.

Geographical Source

Malaysia, Indonesia, India, South America and the West Indies.

Pepper is perhaps the oldest known spice and as such it was known to Theophrastus and other ancient medical men and philosophers. As early as A.D. 1000 it became an important imported article in England. This and many other eastern spices are said to have become so competitive that these led to the discovery of the sea route to India, which in turn motivated European nations to colonise countries.

Pepper crop is systematically looked after and the spikes of 20–30 sessile flowers develop sessile fruits. The fruits are collected when their lower part turns red. They are dried in open and/or by artificial heat, the latter being preferred.

White pepper, used in the East, is also prepared from the black pepper. But in this case the *Piper nigrum* fruits are allowed to fully mature and ripe. After a few days of storage and soaking in water, their outer part of the pericarp is removed by rubbing. The white fruits so obtained are then washed and dried.

Chemical Constituents

Black pepper contains volatile oil, alkaloids and resin. The volatile oil, 1–2.5%, is responsible for the aroma of pepper and comprises of terpenes, like α- and β-pinene, dipentene, phellandrene and sesquiterpenes. The

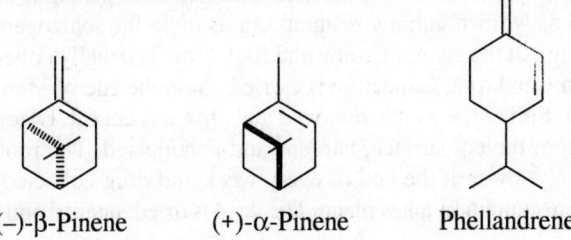

(–)-β-Pinene   (+)-α-Pinene   Phellandrene

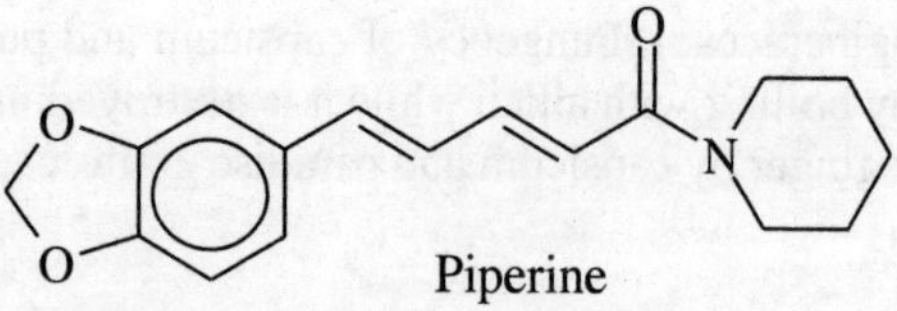

Piperine

alkaloids, 5–9%, consist of crystalline alkaloids, piperine and piperettine and impart the drug its pungency. The resinous content also contributes to the pungency of the drug.

Uses

Black pepper is used as a condiment and spice. It has been used earlier to treat gonorrhoea and chronic bronchitis.

The syllabus based on the therapeutic use of black papper does justify its inclusion in this chapter here. However, since the drug also contains, and that too 5–9% alkaloids, it is described along with drugs containing alkaloids under the now commonly used phytochemical classification. It will, therefore, be found included under alkaloids in my advanced book, "Pharmacognosy".

ASAFOETIDA

Asofoetida, Devil's dung, Hing (Hindi & Guj.)

Botanical Source

Asafoetida is an oleogum resin obtained from the rhizome and root of *Ferula foetida* Regal, *F. rubricaulis* Boiss, *F. asafoetida* L. and other species of *Ferula*.

Family

Umbelliferae.

Geographical Source

Eastern Iran, Western Afghanistan.

Collection

The plant is a perennial branching herb about 3 metres in height. Asafoetida is present as whitish gummy resinous emulsion in the schizogenous ducts of the cortex of the stem, rhizome and root. Drug is usually collected from the rhizome and root. Collection is carried out in the end of March, before flowering. Soil of the root is removed and crown is cut off. Oleogum resin exudes from the cut surface, hardens and is collected. The root is sliced successively lower at the end of every week and drug collected as above till no more exudation takes place. The drug is dried, packed and exported.

Chemical Constituents

Asafoetida contains 4–9% volatile oil, 65% resin, 20% gum and about 10% ash. Volatile oil contains pinene and organic disulphides including isobutyl propenyl disulphide $C_7H_{14}S_2$ responsible for the alliaceous odour. Resin consists of asaresinol ferulate, an ester of asaresinol and ferulic acid, free ferulic acid and a resene asaresene. Because of the presence of free ferulic acid asafoetida shows combined umbelliferone test. Ferulic acid when treated with concentrated hydrochloric acid is converted into umbellic acid which loses water and forms lactone, 7-OH coumarin or umbelliferone. Umbelliferone shows blue fluorescence with ammonia. In galbanum free umbelliferone is present and when ammonia is added it shows directly blue fluorescence. In asafoetida, umbelliferone is only produced by its reaction with hydrochloric acid, and so it contains combined umbelliferone.

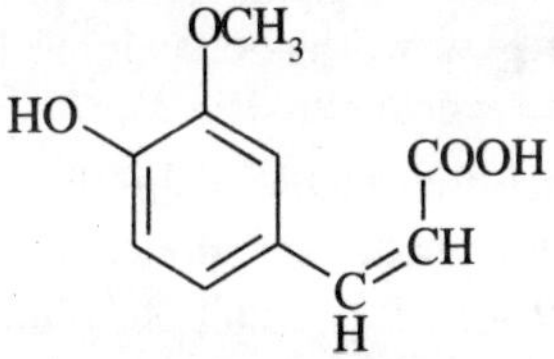

Ferulic acid
(Hydroxy-methoxy
cinnamic acid)

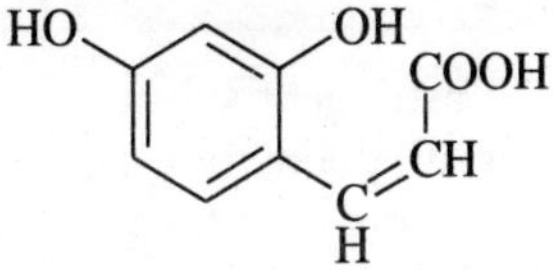

Umbellic acid
(Dihydroxy
cinnamic acid)

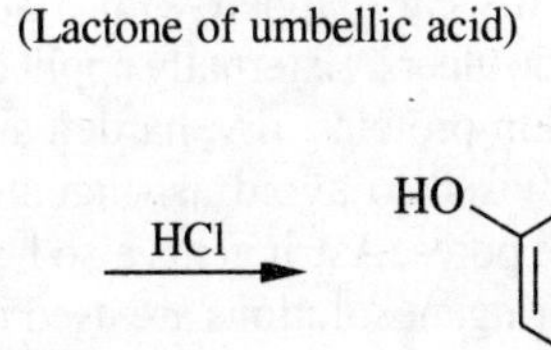

Umbelliferone
(Lactone of umbellic acid)

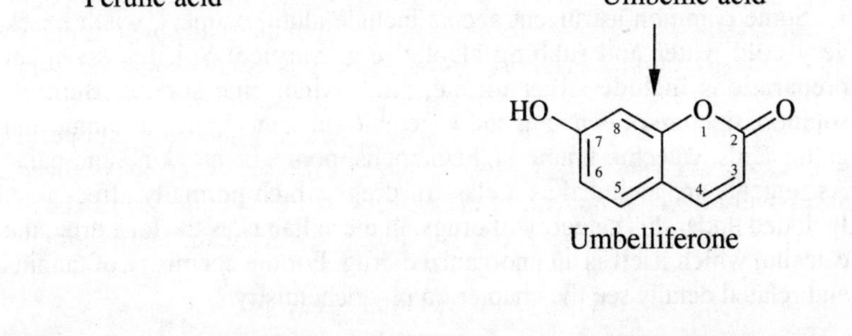

Ferulic acid

Umbellic acid

Umbelliferone

Chemical Tests

1. When triturated with water it forms yellowish-orange emulsion.
2. To the fractured surface add sulphuric acid, a red or reddish-brown colour is produced. When washed with water, the colour changes to violet.
3. Add to the fractured surface 50% nitric acid. Green colour is produced.
4. **Combined umbelliferone test:** Boil 0.5 gm of the drug triturated with sand with 3 ml of hydrochloric acid and 3 ml of water for several minutes. Filter and to the filtrate add equal volume of alcohol and excess of strong solution of ammonia. A blue fluorescence is produced.

   The above test performed without hydrochloric acid does not show blue fluorescence.

ASTRINGENTS

An astringent substance is a chemical substance that tends to shrink or constrict body tissues, usually locally after topical medicinal application. The word "astringent" derives from Latin *astringere* meaning "to bind fast". Few common examples are calamine lotion, witch hazel and catechu.

Astringency is also the dry, mouth-puckering sensation caused by tannins found in many barks, leaves and fruits such as ashoka tea leaf, galls and triphala fruits. The tannins denature the salivary proteins, causing a rough "sandpapery" sensation in the mouth. Astringency tastes unpleasant to many mammals, including humans.

Astringent medicines cause shrinkage of mucous membranes or exposed tissues and are often used internally to check discharge of blood serum or mucous secretions. This can happen with a sore throat, hemorrhages, diarrhoea, or with peptic ulcers. Externally applied astringents, which cause mild coagulation of skin proteins, dry, harden and protect the skin. Acne sufferers are often advised to avoid astringents, which are believed to worsen the clogging of pores. Astringents also help heal stretch marks and other scars. Mildly astringent solutions are used in the relief of such minor skin irritations as those resulting from superficial cuts, allergies, insect bites, or fungal infections such as athlete's foot.

Some common astringent agents include alum, oatmeal, witch hazel, very cold water and rubbing alcohol e.g. Surgical Spirit. Astringent preparations include silver nitrate, zinc oxide, zinc sulfate, Burow's solution, tincture of benzoin, and vegetable substances such as tannic and gallic acids, catechu. krameria, hemamelis, pomegranate, kino and galls. Astringents are included as a class of drugs which normally affect skin. Included under this category of drugs, in the syllabus, is the lone drug, the catechu, which itself is an unorganized drug. For the chemistry of tannins and related details see the chapter on phytochemistry.

CATECHU

The syllabus mentions just catechu as a drug under the class of astringents. There are, however, two types of catechus which are of equal importance, though they just differ in the colours of final product. Interestingly though they belong to totally different botanical and geographical resources. Other differences relate to method of preparation, chemical constituents, analytical test, etc.

There are Pale Catechu and Black Catechu. They are discussed separately as follows.

PALE CATECHU

Gambir, Catechu

Botanical Source

Gambir or pale catechu is the dried aqueous extract prepared from the leaves and shoots of *Uncaria gambier* Roxb.

Family

Rubiaceae.

Geographical Source

Malaya (Johore, Penang), Indonesia (Java, Sumatra), Borneo.

Collection

Plant is a climbing shrub and cultivated by planting the seeds in nurseries and seedlings transplanted when about 9 months old. Plant grows better in direct light at an elevation of not more than 170 metres and by copicing. When plant is about 2 years old and about 2 metres in height, leafy twigs upto 50 cm in length are cut at an interval of 4 to 6 months till the plants are 10 years old. The leaves and twigs are put into a large wooden pan with iron bottom about 1½ metres in diameter which is full of boiling water. The material is further boiled for 3 hours and stirred well. Leaves and twigs are taken out and extract is decanted. The mark is pressed and washed and liquid transferred to the vessel and combined liquids concentrated till it becomes yellowish-green pasty mass. It is cooled in shallow wooden tubes and stirred continuously till it gets cooled. As a result of stirring during cooling, crystallization of catechin takes place. This cooled semi-solid mass is allowed to solidify in trays or tin containers and cut into cubes of uniform size stamped with the name of manufacturer, dried in the sun, packed and exported.

Sometimes 60 lb semi-solid mass without cutting and drying is packed into bales and sold. This catechu is called bale-gambir and contains more water, less tannin and is inferior in quality.

Characters

Pale catechu occurs in cubes each side of which is about 2.5 cm. Sometimes cubes are broken or attached to one another. Colour is reddish-brown. Inner surface is porous and its colour is pale brown to buff. It has no odour and taste is astringent, but sometimes bitter and later sweet. When mounted in lactophenol and seen in the microscope needle-shaped crystals of catechin are seen which are sometimes interlacing.

Chemical Constituents

Pale catechu contains 7–33% catechin which is the structural unit of catechol tennins or phlobatannins. It occurs in white needle-shaped crystals and is soluble in hot water and alcohol. It is not real tannin, but pseudotannin and does not give precipitate with antipyrine. Catechu tannic acid is 22–25%; it is non-crystalline phlobatannin. Catechu tannic acid on decomposition yields insoluble, dark-coloured phlobaphene catechu red, which is also present as an independent constituent. Quercetin, a flavone, and gambir-fluorescein, fluorescent substance are also present.

(+)-Catechin

Chemical Tests

1. **Gambir-fluorescein Test:** Boil a little powdered drug with alcohol, filter and add sodium hydroxide solution to the filtrate, stir and add few ml of light petroleum. Petroleum layer shows green fluorescence. Black catechu does not show this test.

2. Heat about 0.5 gm powder with 5 ml chloroform on water-bath and filter in white porcelain dish and evaporate on water-bath. A greenish-yellow residue, because of chlorophyll present in the drug, is seen. In black catechu, as chlorophyll is absent, this test is negative.

3. Dip a matchstick in decoction of pale catechu, dry in the air and dip it in concentrated hydrochloric acid and warm it near the burner. Magenta or purple colour is produced. In this test, by the action of hydrochloric acid on catechins, or catechol tannins, phloroglucinol is produced which with lignin of the matchstick shows the above test.

4. **Vanillin-hydrochloric acid Test:** (Vanillin 1 : alcohol 10 : dil. hydrochloric acid 10) Catechu shows pink or red colour. In this test also phloroglucinol is produced which with vanillin shows the above colour.

Tests Nos. 3 and 4 are also positive in case of black catechu.

Uses

Catechu has local astringent action and is used in diarrhoea and in lozenges. It is mainly used in dye and tanning industries. In the countries of its origin it is added to betel leaves.

BLACK CATECHU

Catechu Nigrum, Cutch, Khadir (Sans.) Katha (Hindi) Katha (Guj.)

Botanical Source

Black catechu is the dried aqueous extract, prepared from the heartwood of *Acacia catechu* Wild.

Family

Leguminosae.

Geographical Source

India, Burma.

Collection

For preparation of the drug, the tree is felled and bark and sapwood separated from the stem. Small chips of the heartwood are made and boiled with water in earthenware vessels, decoction is filtered and concentrated in iron vessels till it acquires a syrup consistency. It is cooled and allowed to solidify in wooden frames covered with paper or leaves. It is then cut into pieces, packed and exported. Since it is concentrated in iron vessles colour of the catechu becomes darker because of tannins. If during cooling it is stirred, crystals of catechin are produced and as a result black catechu becomes translucent. At present stainless steel vessels are used for the manufacture and catechu is thus lighter in colour.

Characters

Black catechu occurs in irregular black or brownish black mass. Outer surface is firm and brittle and shows covering of leaves. When broken, fractured surface appears glassy and porous and sometimes it is soft.

Chemical Constituents

Black catechu contains 4–12% aca-catechin or acacia catechin, 25–30% catechu tannic acid, catechu red, quercetin and 20–30% gum. It does not contain chlorophyll and gambir fluorescein as in pale catechu.

Test

Black catechu gives positive tests Nos. 3 and 4 given by pale catechu.

Uses

Both catechus are astringent and are used in diarrhoea and in lozenges (see Part II).

DRUGS ACTING ON NERVOUS SYSTEM

Drugs and medicines which act and influence central nervous system (CNS) distinguish themselves as the important products of clinical and therapeutic values. It is estimated that one out of seven drugs prescribed is acting on this system, and this ratio is much higher (1 : 3) in elderly patients. One should understand the fundamentals of the anatomy and physiology of brain and its parts for understanding the pathophysiology of CNS disorders and the action of drugs.

In the following paragraphs an account on general organization of CNS is given, before the drugs included in the syllabus under this heading are described individually.

The CNS consists of cerebrum, cerebellum, medulla oblongata and spinal cord. Some other major or minor parts which regulate their own and each other's activities need mention here are thalamus, hypothalamus, midbrain, pons, etc.

Cerebral cortex is the largest part of the brain and is involved in higher functions like fine voluntary movements, pain, temperation regulation, vision, smell, hearing, etc. Disturbance in cerebral cortex may lead to many disorders, like motor defects, epilepsy, dementia, etc.

Cerebellum, the second largest part, is concerned with reflex regulation of muscle tone, posture and integration and coordination of skeletal muscle contractions. It is acting as a link between the cerebral cortex and peripheral motor activities.

Medulla oblongata and pons are the parts of hindbrain. They control vital functions like blood pressure, heart rate and respiration. Spinal cord is concerned with reflex movements, control of muscle tone and the upper and the lower motor neurons.

Drugs connected with CNS are classified according to their general stimulatory or depressant action, keeping in mind their sub-division as to their specific action such as anticonvulsant and psychopharmacological activites.

From the natural drugs and their products there are groups of drugs belonging to narcotic (opioid) analgesics, hallucinogenic drugs, which are now misused and have negative implications for the society at large.

Some classes of the drugs acting on CNS are:

1. Drugs affecting mental activity.
2. Analeptic drugs (CNS stimulants), e.g. Nux vomica, Ephedra.
3. Central depressant of motor function (CNS depressants), e.g. Opium, Hyoscyamus, Belladonna, Ashwagandha.
4. Drugs used in psychiatric disorders, e.g. Cannabis.

5. Drugs used to relieve pain, e.g. Opium.
6. Drugs used for parkinsonism and other motor disorders, e.g. Levodopa.

The readers are advised to consult general physiology and pharmacology books to acquire knowledge about CNS, its organization, mechanism of action of CNS drugs and classification of CNS drugs.

Drugs acting on nervous system, included in the syllabus, are described below.

HYOSCYAMUS

Folia hyoscyamus, Hyoscyamus herb, Hyoscyamus leaf, Henbane, Khorsani Ajma (Hindi)

Botanical Source

Hyoscyamus consists of the dried leaves and floweing tops of *Hyoscyamus niger* Linn. It contains not less than 0.05% alkaloids, calculated as hyoscyamine.

Family

Solanaceae.

Geographical Source

Native of Europe and west and north Asia. Biennial plant is cultivated and obtained from England, Germany, Balkan countries. Poland, Russia and Kashmir.

Plant Habit

Hyoscyamus occurs as an annual and biennial herb and drug is collected from cultivated plants. In England biennial herb is cultivated, while annual plant is cultivated in continent.

1. **Biennial Plant:** In the first year it produces a small stem and a rosette of periolate leaves near the soil. Flowers ars not formed in the first year. In the second year stem is branched up to 1.5 metres in height and leaves are sessile. Flowers are produced in May-June. Corolla is yellow-coloured with deep purple veins.
2. **Annual Plant:** Stem is simple unbranched and about 0.5 metre in height. Leaves are sessile and smaller than biennial plant. The plant bears flowers in July or August. Flowers are paler than those of biennial plant and veins are less deep.

Cultivation

Drug is usually obtained from cultivated biennial herb. Seeds are sown in June or July. In the first year a rosette of leaves is produced. Leaves are collected and used as drug. In the second year the plant bears leaves and flowering tops which are collected in August and September in dry weather and in the morning. They are dried at 40°C to 50°C in drying sheds heated from outside. The dried drug it stored in air-tight containers at low temperature, protected from light and moisture.

Chemical Constituents

Hyoscyamus contains 0.045–0.15% alkaloids, mainly hyoscyamine and traces of hyoscine. Hoscyamine or atropine is an ester of tropic acid and tropine.

$$\text{Hyoscyamine or Atropine} + H_2O = \text{Tropic acid} + \text{Tropine}$$

Hyoscine or scopolamine is related to hyoscyamine and is ester of scopine and tropic acid.

$$\text{Hyoscine} + H_2O = \text{Tropic acid} + \text{Scopine}$$

Alkaloids* are present mainly in the mid-rib and petiole but absent in stems. Hyoscyamus originally contains optically active laevorotatory alkaloid l-hyoscyamine. Optically active alkaloids possess greater medicinal activity than their corresponding optically inactive isomers. During extraction from the plant, because of the action of heat or chemical agents like acid or alkali, optical activity of hyoscyamine is lost and the corresponding optically inactive racemic atropine is obtained. Atropine is an isomer of hyoscyamine and consists of equal parts of l-hyoscyamine and d-hyoscyamine. Atropine possesses lesser activity than hyoscyamine.

Hyoscyamine or Atropine   Hyoscine or scopolamine

Stoll found the method of isolation of optically active l-hyoscyamine from hyoscyamus at low temperature without the use of acid or alkali. l-Hyoscyamine is available in several commercial pharmaceutical preparations.

Uses

Tropine alkaloids hyoscyamine, hyoscine and atropine block cholinergic reactions by competitive displacement of acetylcholine at the receptor sites and are anticholinergic and are thus parasympatholytics and various secretions like salivary secretion, secretion of the alimentary system and perspiration are checked or reduced. Belladonna is used to check profuse

---

* For detailed account on tropane (solanaceous) alkaloids consult Pharmacognosy, 16th ed. by the same author.

perspiration of patients suffering from tuberculosis. Alkaloids are relaxant to bronchial muscle and are antispasmodic and are used in asthma, bronchitis and whooping cough. Hyoscyamine has also depressant action on the gastrointestinal tract and decreases its peristalsis and secretion and is used in gastroenteritis, hyperacidity and ulcer. Atropine dilates the pupil, but is now replaced by homatropine, which is used by ophthalmologists. Atropine has antiemetic action and is used to suppress parasympathomimetic side reactions like vomiting of morphine injection. It is used in poisoning caused by cholinesterase inhibitors like physostigmine and organophosphorus esters as insecticides. Hyoscyamine has local anaesthetic and anodyne action and so liniment and plaster of belladonna are used to remove peripheral pains. Hyoscine or scopolamine has especially sedative action on central nervous system and is used in excitability, in shocks including those of aerial bombardments, in air and sea sickness and as truth serum for getting the information from war prisoners. As drug, mainly hyoscine hydrobromide is used. Hyoscine is found in *Duboisia* species found in Australia, leaves and rhizomes of *Scopolia carniolica* and *Datura* species found in India all belonging to Solanaceae.

Standards

Total ash not more than 8–12%. In hyoscyamus, because of the glandular trichomes, clay sticks to the clammy leaves and total ash may be up to 22%. Higher quantity of clay can be determined by acid-insoluble ash.

BELLADONNA

Folia belladonnae, Belladonna herb, Belladonna leaves,
Deadly nightshade leaves, Sag-angur Patti (Hindi)

Botanical Source

Belladonna consists of dried leaves and other aerial parts of *Atropa belladonna* Linn. (known as European belladonna) or *Atropa acuminata* Royle ex Lindley (known as Indian belladonna). It contains not less than 0.3% of the alkaloids, calculated as hyoscyamine.

Family

Solanaceae.

Geographical Source

Plant is a native of Central and Southern Europe. It is cultivated in England, Germany, Balkan countries. America and India.

Plant Habit

Plant is perennial herb about 1.5 metres in height. Root is fleshy, tapering and bears numerous rootlets. Stem is straight, herbaceous, branched, glabrous or slightly hairy. Leaves are alternate. Because of adnation, leaves in the upper part are in pairs of two, of which one leaf is larger and the other smaller.

Cultivation

For sowing, the seeds are selected which would produce strong sturdy plants, rich in leaves and containing high percentage of alkaloids. Seeds are sown in nurseries and seedlings are transplanted deep in well-drained, moist, calcareous and loamy soil in April. Water clogging is harmful to the plants. Addition of farmyard manure has favourable effect on the growth of plants. Weeds are removed.

Collection

The leaves are collected in dry weather in late summer. Next year plant reaches a height of 4 ft and during the flowering season, from 15th June to 15th July, plants are cut few inches above the ground and leaves and flowering tops are separated. From the cut plants second harvest is made in August and September and sometimes again a third harvest in October. In the second and third year, two to three harvests similar to first year are made. In the fourth year after harvesting, roots are dug out, which form separate article.

Chemical Constituents*

Belladonna herb contains 0.3–1%, average 0.4%, alkaloids. l-Hyoscyamine should be 3/4 of the total alkaloids. The remaining alkaloids are atropine, apoatropine and traces of hyoscine. Belladonna also contains non-alkaloidal volatile bases, pyridine N-methyl pyrrolidine and a diamine having no medicinal property. Belladonna contains a flourescent coumarin derivative, scopoletin or β-methyl aesculetin also. If ammonia is added to alcoholic solution of scopoletin it shows blue fluorescence. This test is useful in identification of belladonna poisoning. It also contains calcium oxalate.

Standard

Total ash not more than 14%, acid-insoluble ash not more than 3%.

Uses

Belladonna has action similar to hyoscyamus which is also used in purgatives to prevent griping but has milder action.

Indian Belladonna

Indian belladonna was official in B.P. and I.P. This species is found in Western Himalayan regions from Kashmir to Simla and also to a lesser extent in Himachal territory of Kangra and Kulu.

---

* See structures under hyoscyamus.

BELLADONNA ROOT

Radix belladonnae

Botanical Source

Belladonna root consists of dried root and rootstocks of *Atropa belladonna*. It contains not less than 0.4% alkaloids calculated as hyoscyamine.

Family

Solanaceae.

Geographical Source

England, Germany and Balkan countries, U.S.A., Kashmir.

Collection

The plant is a perennial herb, about 1.5 metres high. Drug is collected from 3 to 4 years old cultivated plants.

Chemical Constituents

Belladonna roots contain 0.4–0.8% alkaloids. The main alkaloid present is hyoscyamine. Atropine and scopolamine are present in small quantities. Belladonna root contains apoatropine and belladonna not found in leaves. Apoatropine is the ester of atropic acid with tropine, and belladonna is dimeric alkaloid of apoatropine. Belladonna roots, because of belladonna, were considered useful in the treatment of parkinsonism. In addition, roots contain β-methyl aesculetin, calcium oxalate and starch.

Uses

Belladonna roots are parasympatholytic and used as local anaesthetic, anodyne, in cough and bronchitis and checking secretions especially perspiration of tuberculosis.

Indian Belladonna Roots I.P.

Botanical Source

Indian belladonna root consists of dried root and rootstock of *Atropa acuminata*.

Family

Solanaceae.

Geographical Source

India, Himalaya, Kashmir.

Collection

As mentioned earlier *Atropa acuminata* is not considered as a separate species but is a variety of *Atropa belladonna* var. *acuminata*.

In Indian belladonna root, besides root and rootstock, stem bases are present up to 50%.

Chemical Constituents and Uses

Similar to European belladonna root.

At present in Kashmir (India) cultivation of *A. belladonna* is carried out instead of *A. acuminata*.

Although the syllabus does not include the drug stramonium, yet the importance of solanaceous alkaloid drugs collectively gives enough reason to describe in brief stramonium here.

STRAMONIUM

Folia Stramonii, Stramonium leaves, Stramonium herb, Thornapple leaves, Jamson or Jamestown weed

Botanical Source

Stramonium consists of the dried leaves and flowering tops of *Datura stramonium* Linn. and *Datura tatula* Linn.

Family

Solanaceae.

Geographical Source

Stramonium probably originated in Caspian Sea territories and from there spread to Europe in the first century. At present it grows wild in waste places besides Europe, in Asia, America and South Africa. Stramonium is cultivated in Germany, France, Hungary and South America.

Plant Habit

D. stramonium and *D. tatula* both are annual plants and resemble each other. Their stem is herbaceous, branched and glabrous or only lightly hairy. By cultivation the plant reaches a height of about one metre. The flowers of *D. stramonium* are white and stem green-coloured while in case of *D. tatula*, flowers are purple-coloured and stem and veins of leaves have purplish tint. *D. tatula* is now considered a variety of *D. stramonium* and not a separate species.

Cultivation

For cultivation, seeds are sown in calcareous soil 63 cm apart in rows at a distance of 1 metre. Farmyard manure is applied to the soil. In August the plant reaches a height of 1 metre and bears flowers and fruits. In the end of August stems with leaves and flowering tops are collected and dried as soon as possible at 45°C to 50°C. Leaves get shrivelled because of contraction.

Chemical Constituents*

It is mentioned that the drug from European countries contains more hyoscyamine and less hyoscine while *Datura* species from India contain more hyoscine or scopolamine and less hyoscyamine. Stramonium contains 0.2–0.6% alkaloids, mainly hyoscyamine. Hyoscine is present in traces. Sometimes atropine is present which is believed to have been formed by racemization of hyoscyamine.

Uses

Stramonium is used similar to belladonna as an antispasmodic in respiratory affections and used as powder which is burnt and inhaled or used in asthma as cigarettes which are smoked.

DATURA HERB I.P.

Botanical Sources

Datura herb consists of the dried leaves and flowering tops of *Datura metel* Linn. and *Datura metel* var. *fastuosa*.

Family

Solanaceae.

Geographical Source

India.

Plant Habit

Datura metel known as white datura is dichotomously branched and spreading. Usually this plant is herbaceous but sometimes becomes like a shrub. Lower branches and base of the plant are woody. In *Datura metel* var. *fastuosa*, stem, flowers and main veins of leaves are purple-coloured. Corolla is bilobed or sometimes trilobed. Other characters of *D. metel* var. *fastuosa* are similar to *D. metel*.

Chemical Constituents

Drug contains 0.5% alkaloids. It is reported that Indian daturas contain mainly hyoscine with small quantity of hyoscyamine and atropine. Shah

---

* See structures under hyoscyamus.

and Khanna have shown that *D. metel* and *D. metel* var. *fastuosa* both contain hyoscine and hyoscyamine, nearly in equal proportions. The percentage of alkaloids in *D. metel* var. *fastuosa* is 1½ times more than of *D. metel*.

In Ayurveda black datura is considered more efficacious or more toxic and this has been confirmed as stated above.

Uses

D. metel is used in the manufacture of hyoscine or scopolamine. Its uses are mentioned on page dealing with hyoscyamus and belladonna.

Adulterant

Datura innoxia: It is found throughout India. It is a perennial herb with a thick fleshy and hairy stem. Leaves are thick and pubescent. Corolla is single, white, 10-toothed and calyx inflated.

Fruit is a capsule with prominent spines. Leaves contain both hyoscine iand hyoscyamine.

WITHANIA

Withania root, Ashwagandha

Botanical Source

Withania consists of the dried roots and stem bases of *Withania somnifera*.

Family

Solanaceae.

Withania is widely distributed from southern Europe to India and Africa. In India it is cultivated in Neemuch near Ajmer and Manasa in M.P. There are five varieties of Withania found in different parts and at different elevations in India and have shown variations in plant habit and morphological characters of stem, root, leaves, flowers and fruits. The plant is a perennial, branched, erect, undershrub. For the drug tuberous roots are used.

Chemical Constituents

Withania contains alkaloids and steroid lactones. Recently Schwarting and co-workers isolated from withania biochemically heterogenous alkaloids, like tropine and pseudotropine, hygrine (pyrrolidine derivative)3-α-tigloyloxytropine (3-α-tropyl tiglate), cuscohygrine (two pyrrolidine moieties), d-l-isopelletierine and two new alkaloids anaferine and anahygrine. Recently a new alkaloid withasomnine has been isolated. Withasomnine is phenyl 1,5-trimethylene pyrazole.

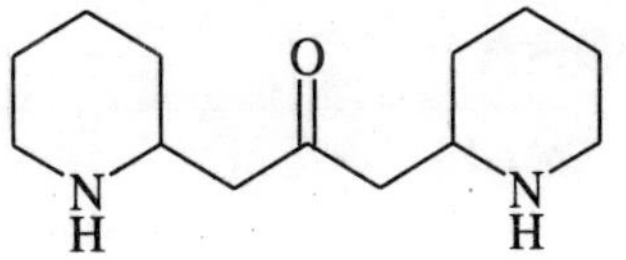

Anaferine

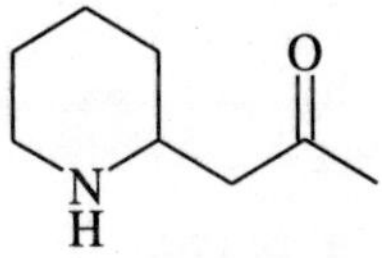

Isopelletierine

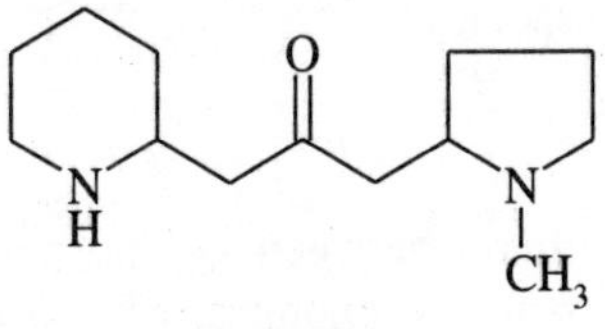

Anahygrine

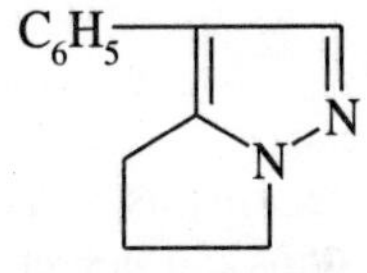

Withasomnine

Recently steroid lactones have been isolated from leaves. Three different chemotypes were discovered from 24 populations by Israeli workers collected in different parts of the country.

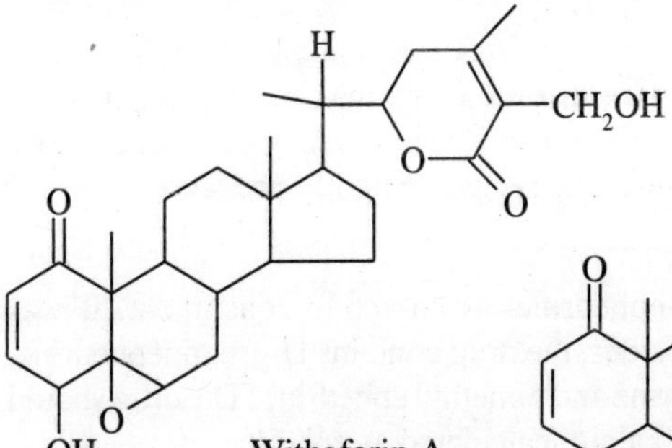

Withaferin A

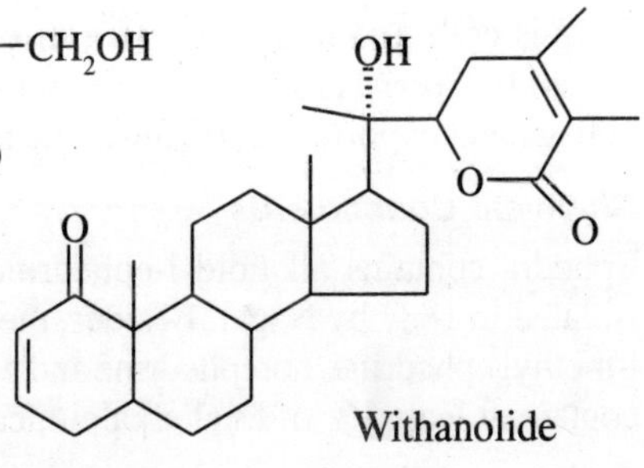

Withanolide

Steroid lactones

Chemotype A contains predominantly withaferin A (0.2%) responsible for the bacteriostatic and antitumour properties. Chemotype II contains a compound similar in structure to withaferin and chemotype III contains a mixture of related compounds containing a new group of steroid lactones withanolides.

Uses

Withania has a great reputation as tonic and aphrodisiac. It is used as sedative in insomnia. It is used in asthma, bronchitis, tuberculosis, leucorrhoea, rheumatoid arthritis and as antiinflammatory drug. Recently anticancer activity has been found in the drug in India. During earlier plague epidemic withania root was applied externally in tumors; it is likely that steroid lactones may be responsible for the activity. It has been reported that cultivated roots have no narcotic property. Withania is considered as an adaptogen and so is used in number of diseases. The antistress activity is mentioned along with tulsi (*Ocimum sanctum*).

EPHEDRA

Ma-Huang, Ephedra

Botanical Source

Ephedra consists of the dried aerial parts of *Ephedra sinica* Stapf, *Ephedra equisetina* Bunge and other *Ephedra* species.

Family

Gnetaceae.

This family is considered transitional between gymnosperms and angiosperms and as such is very important to taxonomists. *Ephedra* species are grouped into Ephedraceae according to some authors.

Geographical Source

China, Pakistan and North-West India.

Collection

Ephedra plant is a small woody dioecious shrub about 60–90 cm high. Drug is collected in autumn as it then contains maximum percentage of alkaloids. Green slender twigs are collected in autumn, dried, packed loose in bags and exported. Sometimes the twigs are tightly pressed.

Chemical Constituents

Ephedra contains alkaloid l-ephedrine, as an active constituent. It was isolated in 1887 by Nagai. Besides, the drug contains D-pseudoephedrine, l-methyl ephedrine, norephedrine and dimethyl ephedrine. The drug should contain at least 1% of total alkaloid, calculated as epherine.

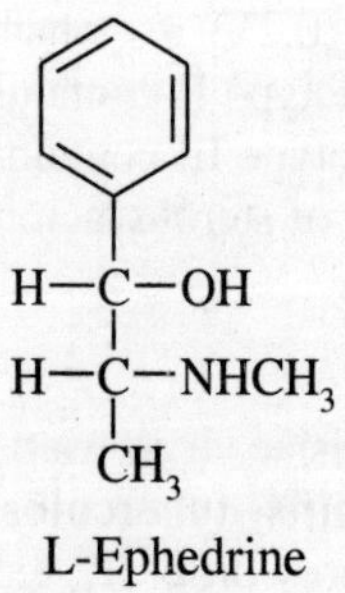

L-Ephedrine 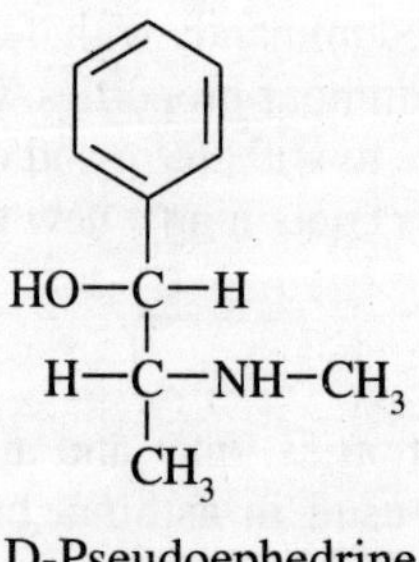   D-Pseudoephedrine 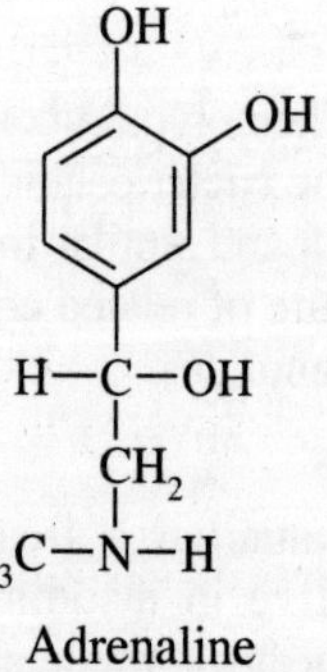   Adrenaline

Uses

Ephedrine is sympathomimetic and is used in asthma, hay fever, rhinitis, bronchitis and also whooping cough. It has the same action as adrenaline, but its action is slower and more prolonged and can be given orally.

Ephedrine is bronchodilator and CNS stimulant. It causes cardiac stimulation and vasoconstriction and also causes rise in blood pressure. Ephedra species are difficult to identify correctly, so action would be uncertain. It is therefore desirable to use the alkaloid ephedrine instead of the herb.

ACONITE

Radix aconite, Aconite root, Monkshood, Wolf's bane, Vachhnag (Guj.)

Botanical Source

Aconite consists of the dried tubercles or tuberous roots of *Aconitum napellus* Linn. collected from wild or cultivated plants.

Family

Ranunculaceae.

Geographical Source

The plant is a native of mountainous, temperate regions of Europe and is found in Alps and Carpathian mountains, mountains of Germany and Himalaya. Aconite is cultivated in England but is obtained from wild plants in countries of Europe and Asia.

Chemical Constituents*

Aconite contains 0.5–1.5% alkaloids. The alkaloids are derivatives of amino-alcohols and are pentacyclic diterpene C_{19} alkaloids and may be considered derived from phyllocladene. They are usually diesters and by

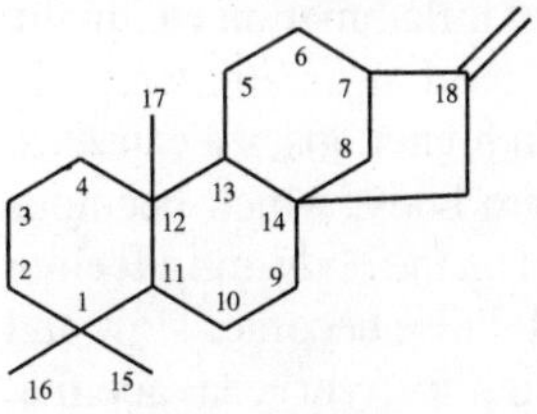

Phyllocladene

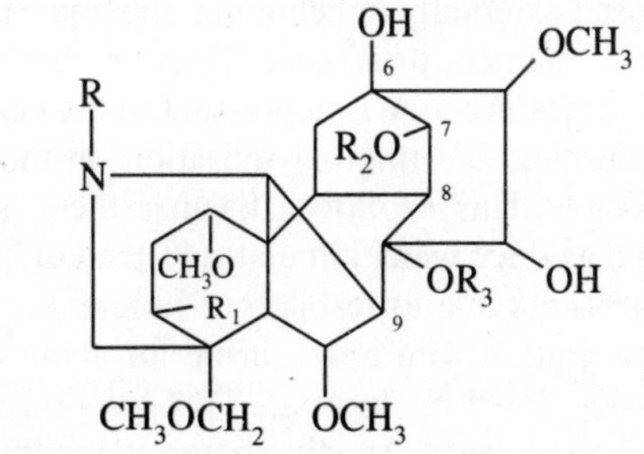

	R	R_1	R_2	R_3
Aconine	C_2H_5	OH	H	H
Benzoylaconine	C_2H_5	OH	$CO.C_4H_5$	H
Aconitine	C_2H_5	OH	$CO.C_6H_5$	$CO.CH_3$

---

* Diploma students are not expected to know detailed chemical structures.

their hydrolysis two acids are obtained. The main alkaloid is aconitine and by its hydrolysis acetic acid, benzoic acid and aconine are obtained. In the structure of aconitine C_{16} and C_{17} are joined with the nitrogen of methyl amine or ethyl amine. Further C_{17} and C_9 are joined by exocyclic ring.

Hypoaconitine and mesaconitine resemble each other but have with nitrogen CH_3 group instead of C_2H_5 and at a C_2 position there is H instead of OH group. Hypoaconitine and mesaconitine are found in asiatic species of aconite.

By partial hydrolysis of aconitine first acetic acid and benzoyl aconine are obtained. Benzoyl aconine on hydrolysis yields aconine and benzoic acid.

$$\text{Aconitine} \xrightarrow{\text{Hydrolysis}} \text{Benzoyl aconine} + \text{Acetic acid}$$

$$\text{Benzoyl aconine} \xrightarrow{\text{Hydrolysis}} \text{Aconine} + \text{Benzoic acid}$$

The toxicity of alkaloids decreases with hydrolysis. Thus aconitine is maximum toxic, benzoyl aconine is intermediary and aconine is least toxic. Benzoyl aconine and aconine possess 1/400 and 1/4000 toxicity of aconitine respectively. *A. napellus* further contains hypoaconitine, mesaconitine, napelline, neopelline and slight sparteine and ephedrine. Aconite also contains tricarboxylic acid, aconitic acid and plenty of starch.

Uses

Aconitine is one of our strong plant poisons and 2% to 3 mg can lead to respiratory failure, heart failure and ultimately death. Aconite and its preparations are poisonous and rarely used internally except in homeopathy. It is used externally in neuralgia, rheumatism and inflammation etc. in the form of liniment of aconite. Tincture aconite is used as an antipyretic in small doses. Aconite is depressant to the heart. In higher doses it causes at first burning and tingling sensation on the entire body, which becomes intolerable. This is followed by anaesthetic action on the body and a feeling of cold as if ice water circulates instead of blood. Pulse becomes slow and death occurs due to respiratory failure. According to Ayurveda, aconite, by maceration with cow's urine for about a week changing cow's urine everyday, loses its depressant property on the heart and instead acquires stimulant property. Aconite so treated is administered in much higher doses apparently without any toxic effect. Pharmacological experiments in Dr. K.C. Bose's laboratory support the above belief.

Indian Aconites

In the I.P., 2nd edition, 1966, *A. napellus*, the European species, is official. In India *A. chasmanthum* (official in I.P., 1956), *A. deinorhizum*, *A. spicata*, *A. balfourii* and *A. lacinatum* are found and exported.

- **A. chasmanthum:** Roots are dried and tuberous resembling *A. napellus* but smaller upto 3.5 cm long, less wrinkled and darker in colour. Starch is gelatinized. The drug contains indaconitine resembling aconitine in chemical structure and medicinal use.
- **A. deinorhizum:** It is one of the main Indian Aconite species exported to foreign countries. Roots are larger, yellow to brown in colour and coarsely wrinkled. Fracture is horny because of gelatinization of starch. It contains pseudoindaconitine. It is nearly two times more toxic than aconitine.
- **Atis root:** (Ativish – Guj.) Atis consists of roots of *Aconitum heterophyllum*. Roots are small, ovate and greyish. Taste is bitter but does not produce numbness. It contains atisine and heteratisine, alkaloids which are phenanthrene derivatives. These alkaloids are comparatively very little toxic. Atis is popularly used in Ayurveda as febrifuge, bitter tonic and in intestinal diseases.

OPIUM

Afim (Hindi), Afin (Guj.)

Botanical Source

Opium is the dried latex obtained by incision from capsular fruits of *Papaver somniferum* Linn.

Family

Papaveraceae.

The plants of this family contain latex. *Argemone mexicana* plant found wild especially in dry regions of India belongs to this family.

Geographical Source

Turkey, Yugoslavia (Macedonia), India, Pakistan, Iran, U.S.S.R. Illicit opium is obtained from Turkey, China and border areas of Burma, Thailand and Laos known as 'Golden Triangle', India and Pakistan. Lately Afghanistan is producing lot of opium for misuse.

Plant Habit

Opium is obtained from poppy plant. Poppy plant is an annual herb, about 1 metre in height and bears about 5–8 capsules. Laticiferous vessels are present in all the parts of the plant except the roots but they are maximum in the phloem of the capsule. There are different varieties of the plant like album, nigrum, glabrum or violet-grey, usually known according to colour of flowers, and seeds. Different countires adopt different methods for cultivation, collection and production. We deseribe here the production of opium in India.

Papaver somniferum var. *album*, which bears white flowers, is more widely cultivated in India in Uttar Pradesh, Rajasthan and Madhya Pradesh.

Cultivation

The opium poppy is a very delicate plant and requires extreme care in its cultivation. It requires a well ploughed and pulverised soil. It is grown in India as winter (Rabi) crop from November to March. The land is enriched with farmyard manure, sheep penning, green manure and compost. After irrigation and final ploughing, the seeds are sown by broadcast method. About 3–4 kg of seeds per hectare are used. When the plants are about 10 cm tall at the rosette stage, weeding and thinning are carried out. Irrigation is done once in 20 days. Poppy takes about 100 days from the time of sowing to the time of flowering. The petals fall off in four days and capsules become ready for collection of opium in about 15 days from the time of flowering.

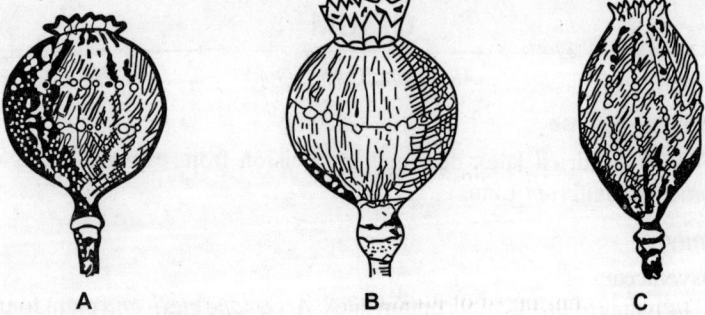

Fig. 3.4. Opium, *Papaver somniferum*. **A:** Poppy capsule cut transversely in Turkish opium. **B:** Capsule with one transverse incision in Macedonian opium. **C:** Capsule cut longitudinally in Indian opium.

Collection

In India collection of opium starts in the middle of February and extends upto April, depending on climatic conditions and time of sowing of the seeds. The unripe capsules which have attained maturity are incised in the afternoon with an implant consisting of four blades tied together with cotton in between at a distance of about 1 mm, the incision being made only at a certain depth of outer wall cutting the phloem tissue. The incisions are made longitudinally from top to bottom of the capsule. The latex which is white to pinkish in colour gradually solidifies and turns brown in contact with air. This remains as pellicles on the surface of the capsules and is collected next morning with the help of a scoop. Each capsule is lanced three to five times on alternate days till no more latex oozes out. The lancing of the capsules of the whole field takes about three weeks. Opium of the first lancing has the highest morphine content and morphine goes on decreasing in opium of subsequent lancings. The air dry latex thus collected is raw opium which is stored by cultivators in plastic buckets. The opium collected is mixed and turned over two to three times a day for about 12 days to make a uniform product. The raw opium is then submitted to the Government agencies and has consistency of 60' to 70'.

Storage and utilization of opium

In India the raw opium collected in the field by the cultivators is brought to the weightment centres and from there transferred to the factories at Ghazipur (U.P.) and Neemuch (M.P.). When opium is received in these factories every consignment is tested for dry solids (consistency), morphine content and adulterants like starch, sugar, gums, tannins and other foreign materials. The raw good opium is stored in separate vats. It is disposed of as: (1) Export opium, (2) Medicinal opium, (3) Excise opium, and (4) Raw material for production of alkaloid. In 1978–79 India produced 1300 tons of opium at 90°C which is about 81% world's production.

Characters

- **Turkish Government opium:** It is available in cylindrical cakes which are about 9 cm high and 14 cm in diameter and about 2 kg in weight. These cakes are externally coated with powdered poppy leaves and as a result they appear mottled and are greenish-grey. Colour is chocolate-brown, texture uniform and slight granular.
- **Yugoslavian opium:** It resembles the cakes of Turkish opium and contains 10–17% morphine. Because of high percentage of morphine this opium is considered of good quality.
- **Indian opium:** It occurs in masses of various sizes, which are often soft and shiny and become hard and brittle after drying, usually moulded in masses of uniform size and shape, blackish brown in colour and with strong characteristic odour.

Medicinal opium

Opium is used as an ingredient in many pharmaceutical preparations like tinctures, pills, powders, tablets, etc. Medicinal opium is prepared as (a) Opium I.P. and (b) Opium Powder I.P. Opium I.P. contains not less than 9.5% anhydrous morphine and opium powder I.P. not less than 9.5–10.5% morphine. Medicinal opium is sold to pharmaceutical firms having valid licences.

Chemical Constituents

Opium contains more than 30 alkaloids. These alkaloids are either of phenanthrene ring system or of benzyl isoquinoline ring system. Morphine (8–20%), codeine (1–4%) and thebaine (0.2–2%) belonging to phenanthrene system are strong bases showing litmus test and are toxic.

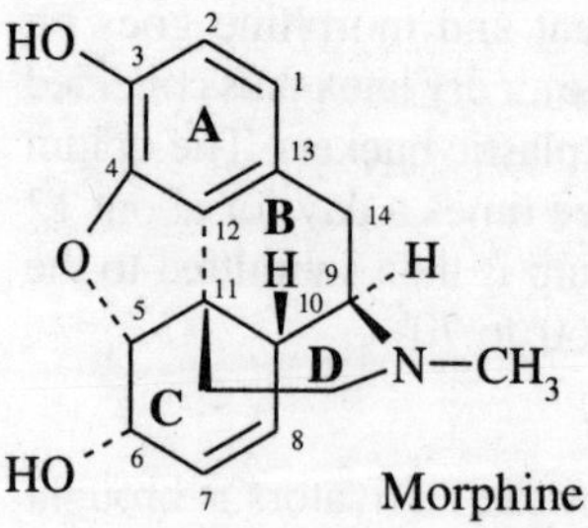

Morphine

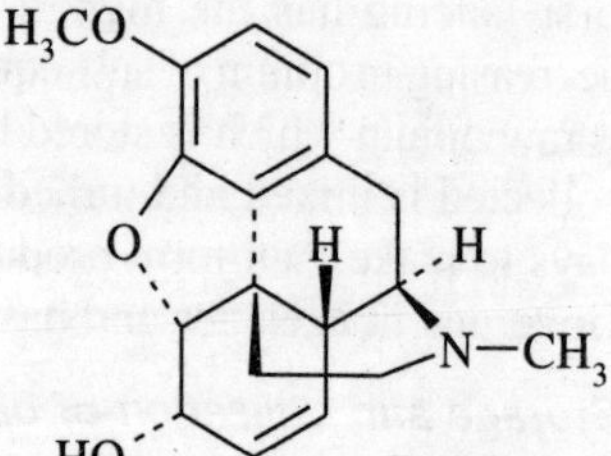

Codeine

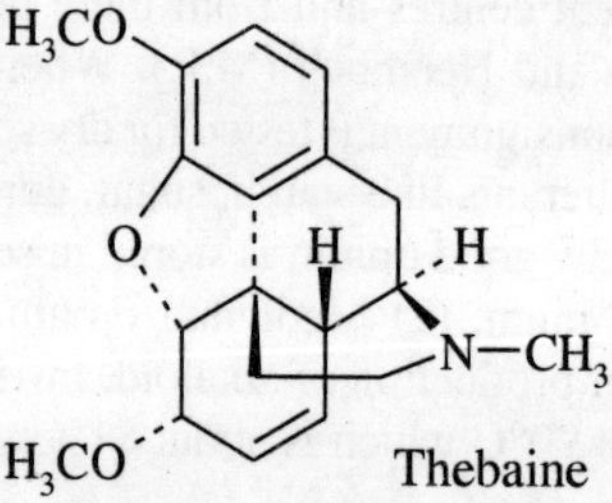

Thebaine

Papaverine, narcotine and narceine belonging to isoquinoline ring system are weak bases and show only very little toxicity.

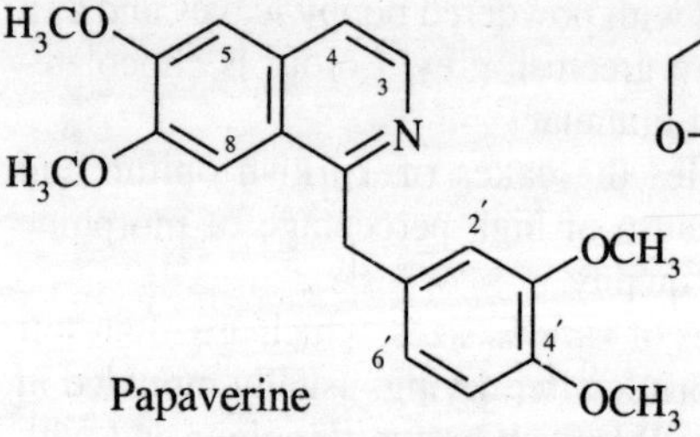

Papaverine

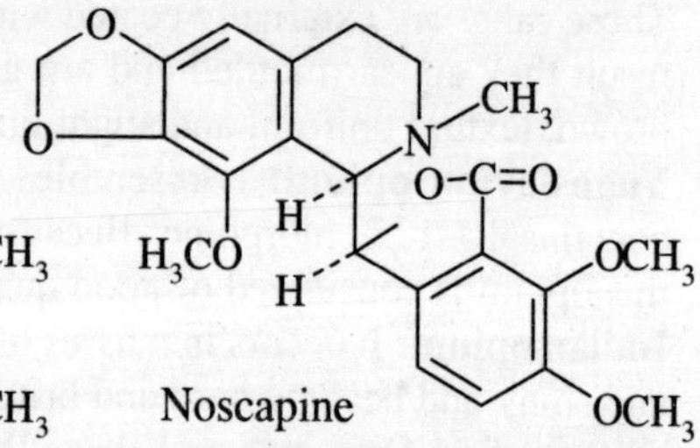

Noscapine

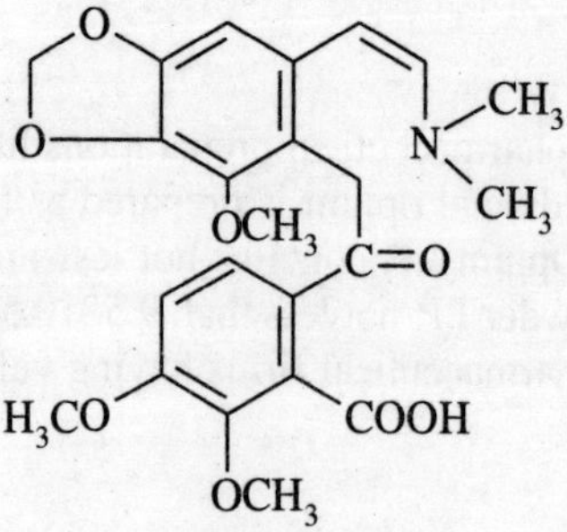

Narceine

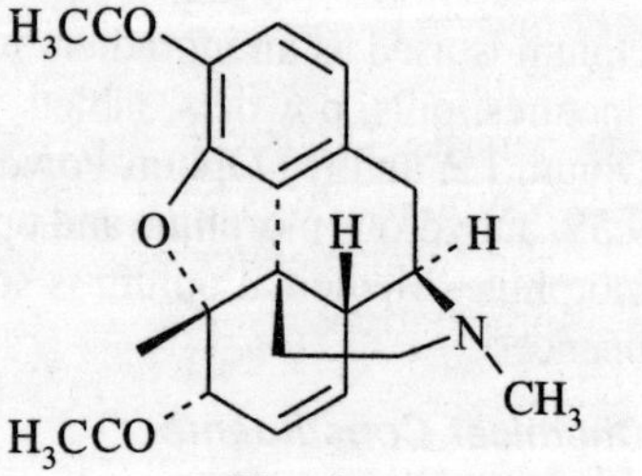

Heroin

Other alkaloids are **narceine, protopine, laudanine, codamine, cryptopine, anthopine** and **maconidine**.

Some opium alkaloids like protopine and hydrocotarnine do not have any of the above ring systems.

The molecule of morphine has both a phenolic and an alcoholic hydroxyl group and on acetylation forms diacetyl morphine or heroin.

Codeine is an ether of morphine, which is used medicinally also.

The alkaloids of opium are in combination with meconic acid and sulphuric acid. Meconic acid is present to the extent of 3–5%. It can also exist free and is said to be present only in opium.

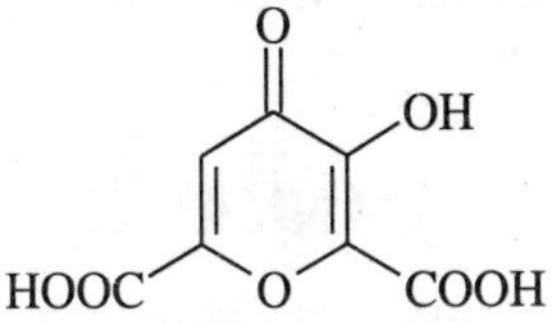

Meconic acid

It is a dibasic acid and can be easily detected in free or in combined state, as a meconate, and thus it helps in identifying/detecting the presence of opium by the formation of a deep red colour with a solution of ferric chloride.

Recently it has been reported that certain species of *Papaver*, which do not show the presence of morphine, may also contain meconic acid. It may, therefore, be of considerable interest to the chemotaxonomists as a chemotaxonomic marker for the family Papaveraceae. Also a related acid, namely chelidonic acid, has been found in some species of Papaveraceae, e.g. in the roots of Greater Celandine.

Opium contains sugar, salts, albumins, colouring matter and moisture. Opium does not contain starch, calcium oxalate and tannins, which are potential adulterants of opium and their presence helps in detecting the adulterants.

Chemical Tests

1. Boil 0.1 gm of opium with 5 ml of water, filter and add to the filtrate few drops of ferric chloride solution. Deep reddish-purple colour is obtained. Add few drops of dilute hydrochloric acid. The colour persists. This test is due to meconic acid.
2. Morphine gives dark violet colour with concentrated sulphuric acid and formaldehyde and this test is used for identification of opium preparations.

Uses

Morphine has both analgesic and sedative or hypnotic action on central nervous system and where both these actions are required as in severe injury, burns, pains, it is used with great success. It is used in diarrhoea, dysentery and cough. Codeine is methyl morphine and checks cough whatever the cause. Syrup codeine phosphate is popular in cough and bronchitis. Codeine increases analgesic action of other analgesics and is combined with aspirin, antipyrine, quinine, etc. Papaverine has spasmolytic action. Narcotine has non-narcotic property and so it is called noscapine. It is central antitussive and is found useful in respiratory disesses. Opium and morphine cause euphoria and are habit-forming and gradually higher and higher doses are required and cause addiction. Several synthetic derivatives have been prepared. Heroin or diacetylmorphine is even more dangerous than morphine.

CANNABIS

Indian hemp, Hashish, Bhang, Ganja,
Charas, Cannabis indica, Marihuana

Botanical Source

Cannabis consists of dried flowering and fruiting tops of the pistillate plants of *Cannabis sativa* Linn.

Family

Cannabinaceae.

Some authors put cannabis into the Moraceae family. The members of this family are aromatic dioecious herbs, have leaves with persistent stipules and unicellular hairs with cystoliths.

Geographical Source

Tropical parts of India such as Maharashtra, North India, Bengal, also Africa and America.

Plant and Habit

Cannabis is an annual dioecious herb and only female plants supply the drug. In temperate countries the plant produces in its stem pericyclic fibres which are separated and washed and known as hemp fibres and are used in surgical dressings. The seeds contain about 20% fixed oil known as hempseed oil used in the manufacture of paints and soap and its cake as cattle food. In temperate countries narcotic resin is not produced in flowers and fruits. In India and other tropical countries narcotic resin is produced in large quantity in the glandular trichomes, found in flowering and fruiting tops of the plant. In tropical countries the plant produces practically no pericyclic fibres. According to recent work production of fibres or resin is not due to climate but according to genetic factors. Cannabis is obtained from cultivated plants and there are several preparations known as flat and round ganja, charas and bhang. Collection is made in February and March.

- **Flat Ganja:** Stems are cut about 15 cm above the ground and kept for few hours in sunlight. They are then cut into pieces of 30 cm length and flower and fruit free portions of the stems removed. Pieces are made into bundles and pressed usually by treading. Because of the resin, pieces stick together and form a flat mass. The flat ganja is thus resinous mass of flowering tops. Flat ganja is prepared in Nasik, and also in Ahmednagar district of Maharashtra State.
- **Round Ganja:** It is prepared in Bengal, similar to flat ganja but with greater care. More resin-free parts are removed and each twig is rolled individually and resinous mass becomes cylindrical. Round ganja is considered of better quality.
- **Charas:** Charas is the crude resin obtained by crushing the flowering tops in the hand and collecting it in a piece of cloth placed below. Charas is purified by passing though cloth. Sometimes people with leather aprons walk through the plants, charas sticks on the leather. It is scraped and collected. Charas is smoked by many *sanyasis* or by criminals.
- **Bhang:** It consists of leaves of male or female plants obtained from cultivated or wild plants. Because of less percentage of resin, bhang is not suitable as a drug. It is used as mild narcotic especially by worshippers of Shiva on Shivratri.

Chemical Constituents

The percentage of resin and its constituents are different according to climate, method of preparation and genetic structure. The percentage of resin varies from 2.5–20%.

Indian cannabis is carefully prepared and it contains 15–20% resin. Resin is semi-solid, brown-coloured and amorphous. Resin contains many constituents and these constituents have psychotropic, narcotic, sedative, analgesic or antibiotic properties.

Cannabis resin contains cannabidiol (antibacterial against Gram-positive bacteria), cannabidiolic acid (sedative and antibiotic), cannabinol (inactive), cannabigerol (antibiotic), cannabichromene (sedative) and most important active constituent Δ^1-*trans*-tetrahydrocannabinol (Δ^1-THC) (psychotropic and analgesic) and other constituents. In the formulae numbering is mentioned according to Mechoulam and Gaoani.

For Δ^9-THC, besides monoterpene structure dibenzopyran structure (–)Δ^1-THC is mentioned. The same componnd was isolated by two research teams and one team called this substance monoterpene derivative as mentioned above, while the other team called it dibenzopyran derivative. Both the structures are mentioned in the literature; however, dibenzopyran structure is more widely accepted. Besides, Δ^9-tetrahydrocannabinol and Δ^8-tetrahydrocannabinol possess euphoric and hallucinogenic activity. Δ^9-THC is biosynthesized via acetate-mevolonate pathway and the precursors are cannabidiolic acid and cannabidiol (CBD).

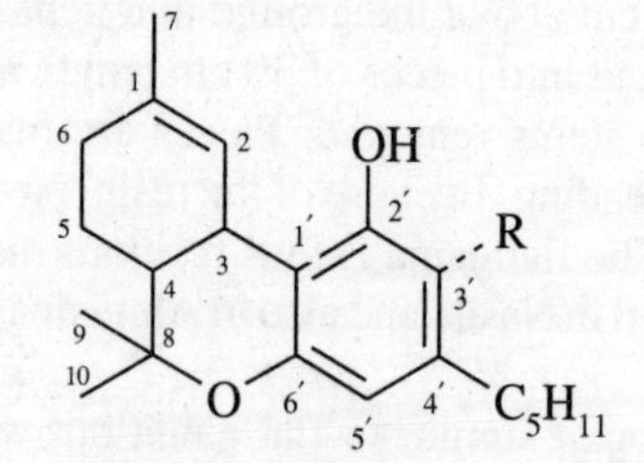

Δ^1-Tetrahydrocannabinol (R=H)
Monoterpene structure

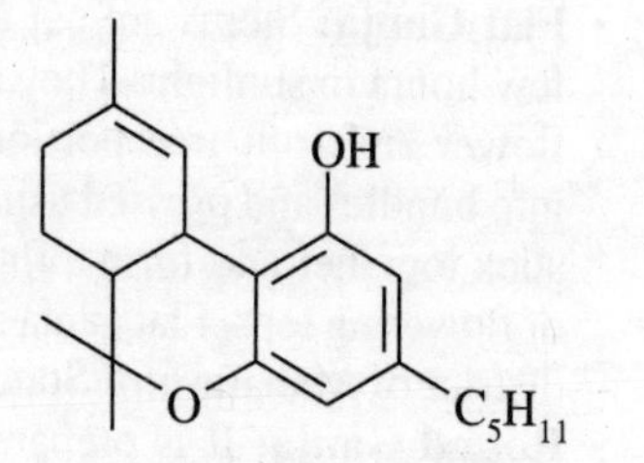

Tetrahydrocannabinol

Mevalonate | Acetate
derived | derived

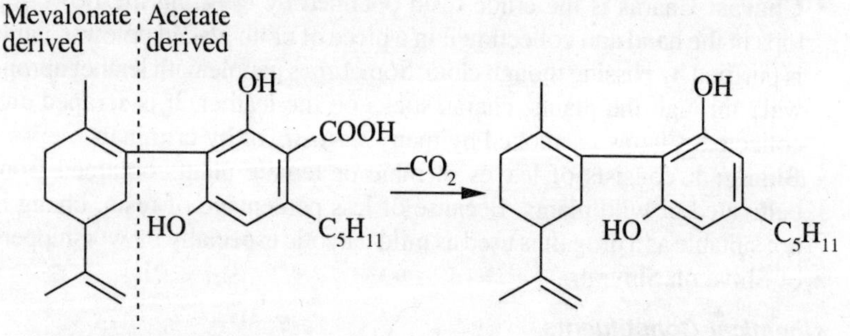

Cannabidiol–carboxylic acid   Cannabidiol

Cannabidiolic acid, cannabidiol Δ^9-tetrahydrocannabinol cannabinol Δ^9-THC is the active constituent and other constituents show mild action as antibacterial and sedative action as mentioned above. The constituents of cannabis are unstable and are transformed into one another. Cannabis also contains volatile oil, trigonelline and cholene.

Storage

The drug must be dried thoroughly and is stored in well-closed containers. If this precaution is not observed and the drug is kept under ordinary conditions the drug deteriorates. The deterioration of the drug is brought about by the oxidative action of oxidase upon the resin.

Uses

Cannabis resin is sedative, analgesic and narcotic. It has psychotropic properties similar to L.S.D. and mescaline. In the beginning it causes intoxication, euphoria and later mental disturbances and along with it personality disturbance, hallucinations and sometimes depression. The above actions are more by smoking and inhalation than by taking it orally. The psychotropic action is explained by increase of noradrenaline and dopamine in brain. Cannabis causes only psychic dependence. The person is fully conscious during intoxication.

At present it is very little used as a drug, but because of its psychotropic property, it causes addiction and at present problem is more socioeconomic.

Marihuana (Mexican cannabis)

It contains 15% resin. It contains resin in all aerial parts of the stem. Cigarettes prepared from marihuana were imported into the U.S.A. and this cigarette smoking addiction took place in school children and government took strict measures against import and sales of marihuana. As a result of government measures, marihuana is now not used as a drug in the U.S.A.

NUX VOMICA

Semen strychni, Nux vomica seed, Kuchla (Hindi), Zer kachuro (Guj.)

Botanical Source

Nux vomica consists of the dried ripe seeds of *Strychnos nux-vomica* containing not less than 1.2% strychnine.

Family

Loganiaceae.

Members of this family are found in tropics and are characterized by the presence of indole alkaloids. Besides strychnine, strychnos alkaloids having curare-like action are important.

Geographical Source

South India, Malabar coast (Kerala), Eastern Ghats, Bengal, Sri Lanka and North Australia.

Collection

The plant is a small tree, 10–13 metres in height. The fruits are 3–5 cm in diameter and are subspherical yellowish-brown orange-like berries. The epicarp is leathery and the pulp is bitter, whitish and mucilaginous in which 2–5 seeds are embedded. Ripe and mature fruits are collected in November to February by the natives. Epicarp is separated and seeds are removed and washed to remove adherent pulp. They are dried on mats in the sun and graded according to size and exported. In India, nux vomica is collected from wild plants as the cost of collection is less because of cheap labour.

Chemical Constituents

Nux vomica contains about 2.5–3.5% bitter indole alkaloids. **Strychnine** ($C_{21}H_{22}O_2N_2$), average 1.25%, is therapeutically active and a toxic alkaloid and is located in central portion of endosperm. Strychnine is crystalline and gives violet colour with ammonium vanadate and conc. sulphuric acid.

Brucine, about 1.5%, is chemically dimethoxystrychnine. It is much less toxic and has very little physiological action. It is intensely bitter and is used as a standard for determining the **bitter value** of many bitter drugs. With concentrated nitric acid brucine gives yellow to orange colour. Brucine is more in the outer part. **Vomicine** and **pseudostrychnine** are minor alkaloids. Alkaloids are combined with chlorgenic acid or caffeotannic acid. Chlorogenic acid with ammonia in the presence of oxygen of air becomes green and plays a role as respiratory agent in the plant. **Loganin**, a glycoside, is present in the seeds which on hydrolysis yields **loganetin**. Cell walls of endosperm of nux vomica are thick-walled and contain reserve material hemicellulose consisting of **mannan** and galactan, which on hydrolysis yield **mannose** and **galactose**. Fixed oil is 3%, and aleurone grains are present in the endosperm of the seed.

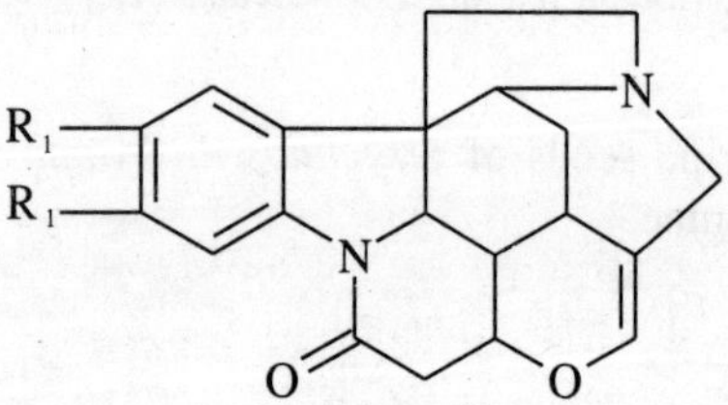

Strychnine

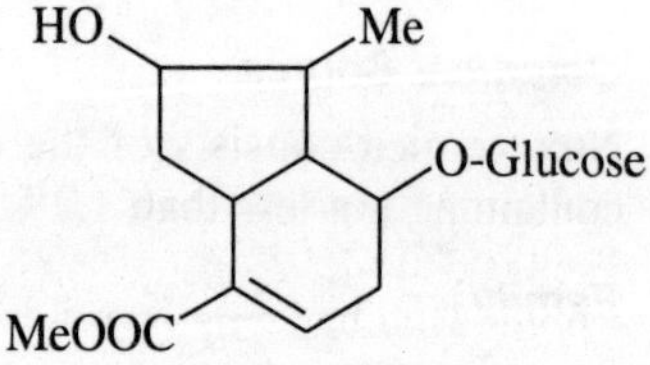

Loganin

	R_1	R_2
Strychnine	H	H
Brucine	OCH_3	OCH_3

Strychnine and brucine belong to a group of dihydroindole alkaloids and were among the first alkaloids to be discovered in the plant kingdom. Strychnine and brucine are **monoacidic bases**.

Strychnine is found abundantly in *Strychnos nux-vomica* and *S. ignatii* and has also been reported to be in *Strychnos cinnamifolia*, *S. colubrina*, *S. ligustrina*, *S. lucida*. and *S. tieute*.

Chemical Tests

1. **Strychnos Test:** To a thick section of endosperm add ammonium vanadate and sulphuric acid. Middle portion of endosperm is stained purple because of strychnine.
2. Strychnine also gives violet colour with potassium dichromate and conc. sulphuric acid.
3. **Brucine Test:** To a thick section add concentrated nitric acid. Outer part of endosperm is stained yellow to orange because of brucine.

The above tests can be used as localization tests.

4. **Hemicellulose Test:** To a thick section add iodine and sulphuric acid. The cell walls are stained blue.
5. **Organoleptic Test:** Put a little drug at the tip of the tongue. It tastes bitter.
6. **Biological Test:** 2 μg (2/1000 mg) of strychnine if injected into the tail of a two-week old mouse will cause palpitation of the tail.

Uses

Strychnine has a stimulant action on spinal cord and reflex movements are better. Nux vomica is a bitter stomachic and increases the tone of intestine and it is used in atonic dyspepsia. It is used in tropical neurasthenia. It is considered nerve and sex tonic. It is used as circulatory stimulant in surgical shock and is useful in certain cases of poisoning like alcohol. In toxic doses strychnine causes violent tetanus-like convulsions and death takes place due to asyphxia and respiratory failure. Brucine acts similar to strychnine but has 1/50th of its activity. At present strychnine is seldom used in modern medicine, but is used as vermine killer. Brucine, because of its bitter taste, is used as alcohol denaturant. Nux vomica (vomiting nut) contrary to its name has no vomiting properties. However, *Strychnos potatorum* has emetic action.

Adulterants

1. Dried ripe seeds of *Strychnos potatorum*. These seeds are smaller in size and thicker than nux vomica. They are bitter in taste and have emetic property. In India, they are used for clearing the turbid water and are known as clearing nuts.

   The seeds contain diaboline, an indole alkaloid, and other alkaloids. Strychnine is, however, absent.

   The total alkaloids produce convulsions in different species of animals when administered parentally. The alkaloids decrease barbiturate sleeping time in mice. The alkaloids increase amphetamine toxicity in aggregated mice. The LD_{50} is 50 mg/kg. In India, they are used in chronic diarrhoea, irritation of urinary organs, gonorrhoea and diabetes.
2. Dried ripe seeds of *Strychnos nux blanda*. They are brighter and have yellowish-buff colour. They do not contain any alkaloid and are free from bitter taste.

Allied Drug

Ignatius Beans.

Ignatius Beans

Botanical Source

These are dried ripe seeds of *Strychnos ignatii*.

Family

Loganiaceae.

Geographical Source

Native of South Philippines Islands.

Characters

Seeds are about 1.5 cm long, dark grey and ovoid. Trichomes are not lignified and easily rubbed off and so in commercial drug trichornes are absent.

Chemical Constituents

2.5–3% alkaloids of which strychnine is 45–60%.

Uses

Similar to nux vomica and for the manufacture of strychnine and brucine.

ANTIHYPERTENSIVES
ANTIHYPERTENSIVE AGENTS

Antihypertensives are drugs which are responsible for the reduction and/ or lowering of abnormal high blood pressure caused by hypertension, a common cardiovascular disorder of the present modern age. According to WHO definition one-third of men and two-fifths of women over 40 years of age are hypertensive. This is due to the fact that with the advancement of age there is pari-pasu increase in blood pressure (BP). Generally a person with diastolic pressure above 100 mm Hg is considered to be a hypertensive and requires treatment by use of an antihypertensive (agent). Systolic BP on the other hand is often fluctuating, but if it persists very high, it is also fraught with danger.

With a view to understand the use of antihypertensive, it is necessary to know the disease hypertension, its causes and also perhaps its etiology briefly.

Hypertension is identified into primary hypertension and secondary hypertension.

Primary hypertension is characterized by the elevation of diastolic BP, a normal cardiac output (in most of the cases) and an increase in peripheral resistance with a documented etiology. The etiology of primary hypertension is not quite clear, though several factors are implicated in its genesis. These factors are stated as under:

1. Genetic i.e. family history of vascular disease.
2. Obesity and glucose intolerance.

3. High salt intake.
4. Cigarette smoking.
5. Hyperlipidaemia.
6. Increased serum renin levels.
7. Hypersensitivity of sympathetic system.

Some 80–90% cases of hypertension belong to primary hypertension.

Secondary hypertension is the kind of hypertension of which the etiology is known. It is secondary to other disorders, which can be one of the following disorders:

1. Acute or chronic renal disease (particularly glomerulonephritis).
2. Renal artery stenosis.
3. Hyperaldosteronism.
4. Cushing's syndrome.
5. Acromegaly.
6. Pheochromocytoma.
7. Drugs like oral contraceptives, estrogens, steroid carbenoxolone and sympathomimetics.

Hypertension is one of the major risk factors of various diseases like myocardial ischaemia, cardiac failure, renal failure and stroke.

RAUWOLFIA

Sarpagandha, Chhotachand,
Pagla ki Jadibutti (Dawa), Rauwolfia Roots

Botanical Source

Rauwolfia consists of dried roots and rhizomes of 3–4 years old plants of *Rauwolfia serpentina* collected in autumn and with bark intact and contains not less than 0.15% reserpine-rescinnamine groups of alkaloids.

Family

Apocynaceae.

Geographical Source

The plant is a small shrub, about 1 metre in height and occurs mainly in India, Pakistan, Burma, Thailand and Java. Rauwolfia is found abundant in tropical deciduous forests of Himalayas and in bamboo forests. Commercial supplies are obtained from India and Thailand. In India, there are three varieties, Bihar, Dehradun and Assam.

Cultivation

Cultivation of Rauwolfia is usually carried out by seed propagation. Sterile seeds are eliminated by immersing them in saline. Sterile seeds are light, float and are separated. Fertile seeds sink and are utilized. Fresh seeds germinate more and preferably fresh seeds are used. In vegetative propagation, especially in root-cuttings, development of roots is better if growth hormones are used.

Rauwolfia plants should be protected from nematodes of *Heterodora*, from fungus *Fusaria* and *Alternaria* and from Mosaic virus.

Collection

Roots and rhizomes of Rauwolfia are collected in October–November after hot and dry period. In Indian Phannacopoeia collection of roots of 3–4 years old plants is mentioned, but in culture it is found that roots of two years old plants are equally good. For collection of roots, plants are dug out, aerial parts are removed and roots are separated. Roots are washed and dried in air till moisture is about 10–12%. Roots should be stored protected from light.

At present, drug is collected both from wild and cultivated plants.

Chemical Constituents*

Rauwolfia contains 1.5–3% alkaloids. Alkaloids are mainly present in the cortex. Medicinally important alkaloids are: (1) Weakly basic tertiary indole alkaloids, reserpine, rescinnamine and deserpidine. They are derivatites of yohimbine. Reserpine is 0.1% in the roots and contains at the 18 position trimethoxy benzoic acid while rescinnamine contains trimethoxy cinnamic acid. Deserpidine is 11-demethoxy reserpine. (2) The second group of alkaloids are medium basic tertiary indoline or of dihydroindole series as ajmaline. (3) The third series are strongly basic quaternary anhydronium bases as serpentine and tetrahydroserpentine or ajmalicine. The ring E of serpentine group is pyran ring and so exhibits heterocyclic structure.

Uses

Rauwolfia is used as hypothesive and tranquilizer. Reserpine, being the main alkaloid, is responsible for the activity and is used in anxiety conditions and other neuropsychiatric diseases. Reserpine reduces or diminishes noradrenaline and serotonin in the brain and thus possesses neurotropic properties and is used in anxiety conditions, fear, tension, aggressiveness and chronic schizophrenia. Reserpine also antagonises LSD at CNS level and sedates the patient. Serpentine supplements hypotensive action of reserpine and is often combined with it. Ajmaline, because of action similar to quinidine, is used in angina pectoris and cardiac arrhythmia. Ajmalicine has property of increasing blood supply to the brain.

---

* Diploma students are normally not expected to know and draw exact chemical structures. Suffice it to know the basic ring structures in different kinds of alkaloids, here and elsewhere.

Structures of the Chemical Constituents of Rauwolfia

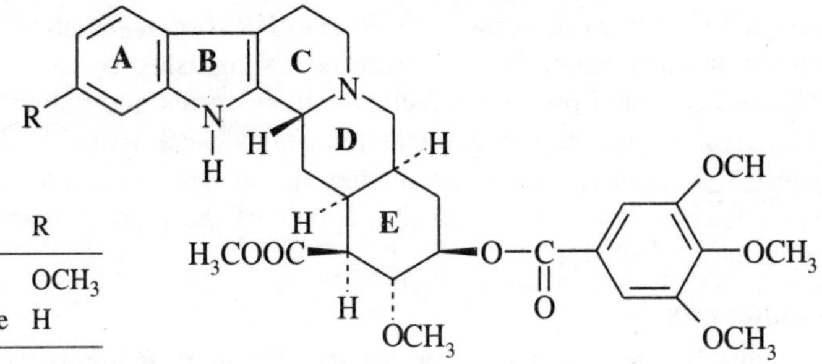

R
Reserpine OCH₃
Deserpidine H

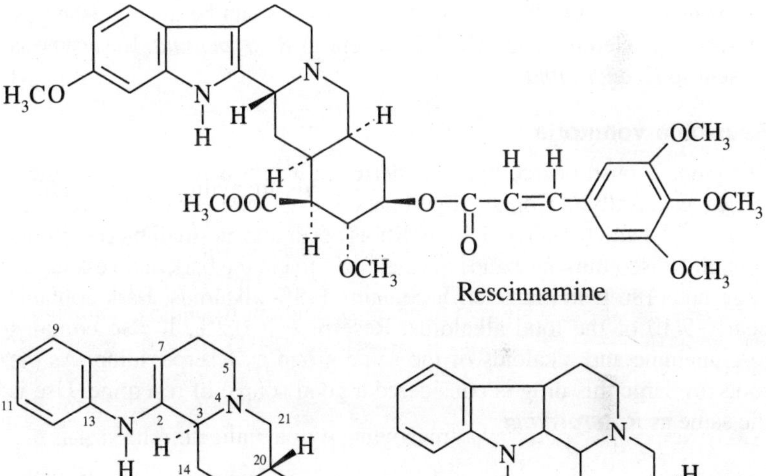

Rescinnamine

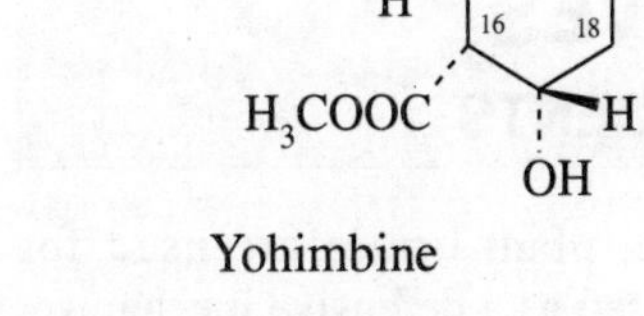

Yohimbine

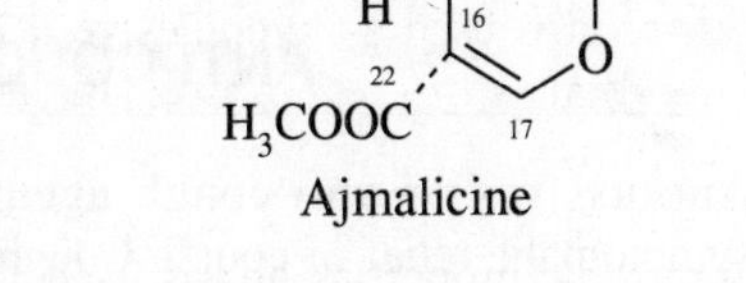

Ajmalicine

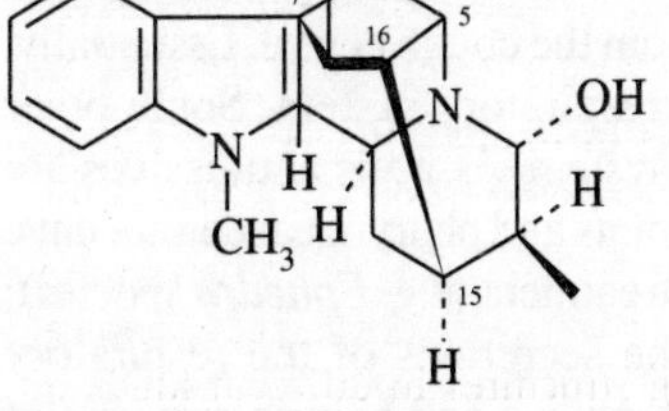

Ajmaline

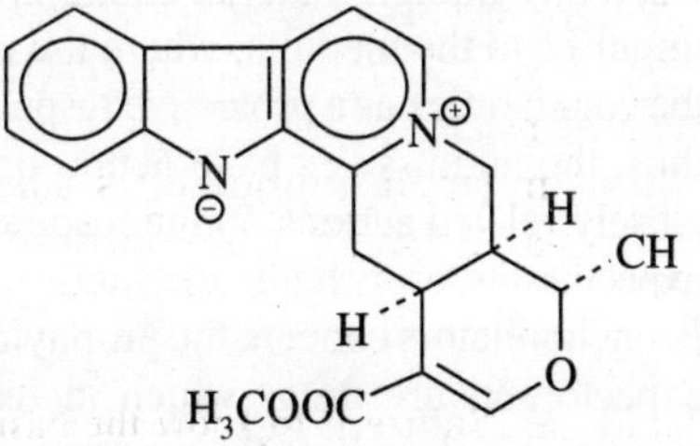

Serpentine

Allied Species

There are several species of *Rauwolfia* found in India. Roots of *R. canescens* are used similar to *R. serpentina*. Roots of *R. canescens* are bigger and known as Badachand. This drug can be distinguished by the absence of stratified cork and presence of stone cells in cortex and phloem, and by large vessels up to 90 μ in diameter. It contains 1–2% alkaloids. Reserpine is less, 0.5%, but rescinnamine and deserpidine are more. It also contains Rauwolscine. It is interesting that leaves of the plant contain highest percentage of alkaloids.

Adulterants

In India, besides the above species *R. micrantha*, *R. densiflora* and *R. perakensis* are found. The roots of these species can be distinguished by presence of sclerenchyma which is absent in *R. serpentina*. Reserpine is present in *R. micrantha*.

Rauwolfia vomitoria

The plant is bush or tree upto 10 metres in height and found in tropical Africa, especially in Congo, Nigeria and Ivory Coast. The roots are large in size and diameter is 0.1–1.5 cm. Roots occur also in small pieces. Roots contain 5 discontinuous bands of sclerenchyma in the bark and vessels are large upto 180 μ in diameter. It contains 1–3% alkaloids. Bark contains nearly 9/10 of the total alkaloids. Reserpine is 0.2%. It also contains rescinnamine and alkaloids of the same group as reserpoxidine. As the roots are large this drug is considered a good source of reserpine. Use is the same as *R. serpentina*.

ANTITUSSIVES
ANTI-COUGH AGENTS

Antitussives or anti-cough agents from plant origin are used for symptomatic relief of cough. Cough is caused as a defensive mechanism when any foreign material enters the respiratory tract conveying sensory impulses to the medulla, where the cough centre is situated. This leads to the cough reflex as a protective response from the cough centre. Essentially, thus, the antitussives have action on the respiratory system. Some other closely related actions on the respiratory system vis-a-vis antitussives are expectorants, bronchodilators, antiexpectorants and pharyngeal demulcents. Bronchodilators concern the prophylactic treatment (e.g. *Ephedra* species); expectorants are drugs which increase the secretions of the respiratory system, which induce the viscosity of the mucus and help in removal of the content from the respiratory tract. With dry cough, especially, the patients experience irritation and pain, reflexly stimulating secretion of mucus from the bronchial glands.

Anti-expectorants reduce bronchial secretions. Pharyngeal demulcents are used locally in the throat to remove irritating cough. They increase salivary secretion.

Cough is a protective function, but constant coughing particularly in old age and convalescent persons may be discomforting and damaging to the respiratory muscles. It may also disturb the circulatory system in hypertensive individuals. Thus, the use of a cough drepressant provides a great relief to the patient.

In this category of antitussives there are three drugs vasaka, tolu balsam and **Tulsi** included in the syllabus, which are described below one by one.

VASAKA LEAVES

Adhatoda, Vasaka folium, Adulasa, Ardushi, Sinhmukhi

Botanical Source

Vasaka consists of the fresh or dried leaves of *Adhatoda vasica* Nees.

Family

Acanthaceae.

Geographical Source

Plains of India, the Ranges of Himalayas up to 4000 ft, Sri Lanka, Burma and Malaya.

Cultivation

Plant is evergreen shrub, reaching a height of 3–8 ft. Flowers have open bilabiate corolla and have the appearance of lion's mouth and hence the Sanskrit name – Sinhmukhi. The plant is gregarious and used as hedge and is easily cultivated by stem cuttings. Leaves are collected throughout the year and used both in fresh and dry condition.

Chemical Constituents

Vasaka leaves contain crystalline bitter alkaloids vasicine, vasicinone and 6-hydroxy vasicine. They are quinazoline derivatives.

Vasicine is identical with peganin isolated from *Peganum harmala* (Rutaceae). Vasicine is auto-oxidizable and forms vasicinone, a ketone at 8 position. According to Amin and Mehta, vasicinone is present in leaves and, formed from vasicine, is responsible for the activity. Alkaloids have bronchodilator and antihistaminic action. Vasaka leaves contain volatile oil. Volatile oil is expectorant and is considered to have antitubercular property. Vasaka contains betain and vasakin, a non-nitrogenous crystalline substance having atropine-like action.

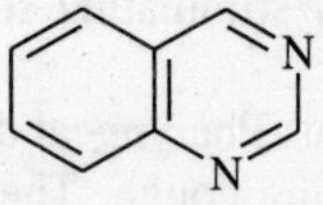

Quinazoline

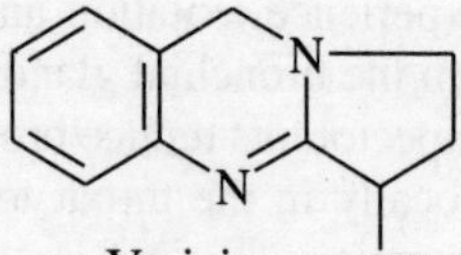

Vasicine OH

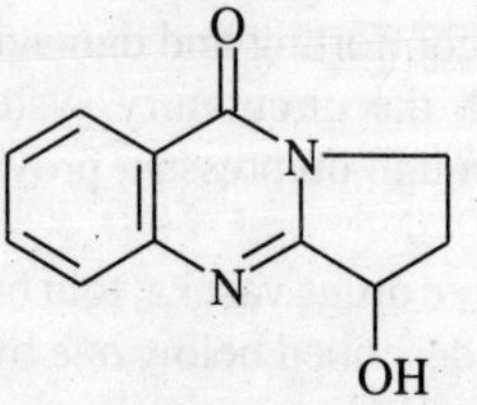

Vasicinone

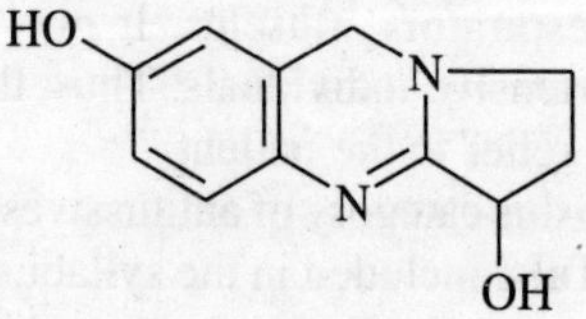

6-Hydroxy vasicine

Uses

Vasaka is expectorant and bronchodilator, used in cough and acute and chronic bronchitis. Its claim in Ayurveda as an antitubercular drug has not been proved. Vasicine has also oxytocic action similar to ergometrine or oxytocine. Investigation in the West resulted in an extract of this plant being marketed as bromhexine, which is used mainly as an antitussive and mucokinetic drug.

BALSAM TOLU

Balsamum tolutanum, Balsam of Tolu, Tolu balsam

Botanical Source

Tolu balsam is obtained by incision on the stem of *Myroxylon balsamum* (*Myroxylon toluifera*).

Family

Leguminosae.

Geographical Source

Along the lower Magdalena river in Columbia, West Indies, Cuba and Venezuela. The name Tolu is derived from the name of the place Tolu near Cartagena on the north coast of Columbia.

Collection

Tolu balsam is a pathological product and resin is present in the cortex of young twigs only. As the twigs become older, because of secondary growth, cortex is cut off and resin is not present normally in the bark of the stem. As a result of injury a large number of resin ducts are produced in secondary wood and new bark. For collection, V-shaped cavities sloping inwards and downwards are made and suitable receptacle is placed below the cavities. Resin exudes and is collected in calabash cups and transferred to tin containers.

Chemical Constituents

Tolu balsam contains 75–80% resin. Resin contains resin ester of tolu-resinotannol esterified with benzoic acid and cinnamic acid and 7–8% cinnamein which is a mixture of benzyl benzoate and benzyl cinnamate. About 20% free balsamic acids are found. It also contains vanillin and styrol. Total balsamic acids in the drug, both free and combined, are 35–50%. Recently the drug has been shown to contain other esters, eugenol, styrene and ferulic acid.

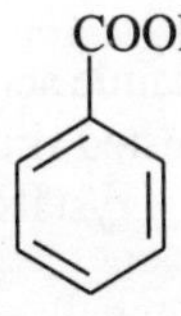

COOH

Benzoic acid

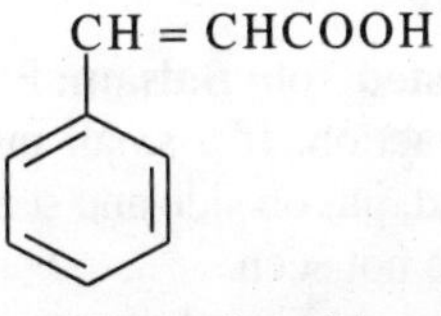

CH = CHCOOH

Cinnamic acid

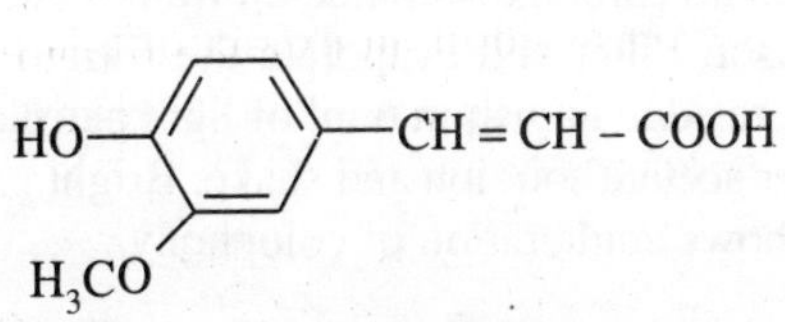

HO—⟨⟩—CH = CH – COOH
H₃CO

Ferulic acid

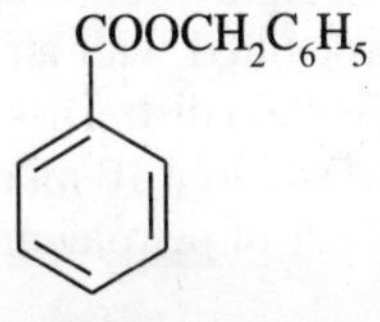

COOCH₂C₆H₅

Benzyl benzoate

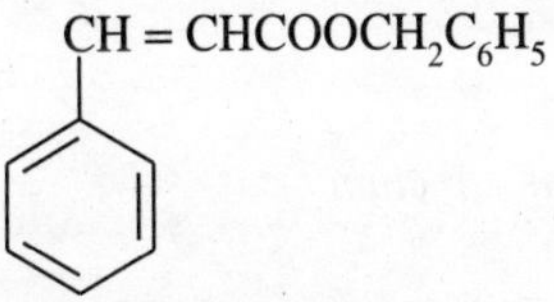

CH = CHCOOCH₂C₆H₅

Benzyl cinnamate (Cinnamein)

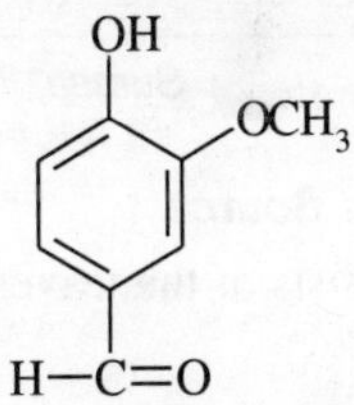

OH
OCH₃
H—C=O

Vanillin

Tests

1. Dissolve 1 gm of tolu balsam in 10 ml of alcohol by heating. The solution shows acidic reaction with litmus and the insoluble residue is not more than 4%.

2. Boil 1 gm balsam with 5 ml water, filter and note the smell of filtrate. To the filtrate add 3 ml of 1% aqueous potassium permanganate solution and heat and smell. Cinnamic acid present in the balsam is oxidized to benzaldehyde giving bitter almond-like smell.

3. Add few drops of ferric chloride to alcoholic solution of tolu balsam. Green colour is seen because of toluresinotannol.

Uses

Balsam of Tolu was included in the US Pharmacopeia in 1820 as well and has been used as an antitussive, in the form of lozenges for coughs and sore throats, in cough syrups and as a vapour inhalant for respiratory ailments with documented antiseptic and expectorant properties. The internal dosage is reported to be ½ to 1 gram taken three times daily.

Today it is used extensively in topical preparations for the treatment of wounds, ulcers and scabies, and can be found in hair tonics, anti-dandruff preparations, feminine hygiene sprays and as a natural fragrance in soaps, detergents, creams, lotions and perfumes.

Adulterants

1. **Exhausted Tolu Balsam:** From tolu balsam cinnamic acid is removed by extraction. If a small quantity of this exhausted drug is heated, softened, put on side and seen under microscope, crystals of cinnamic acid are not seen.
2. **Colophony:** The adulteration of colophony can be detected as follows: Boil 5 gm of the drug with 25 ml carbon disulphide on water-bath in a flask fitted with air condensor. Filter and evaporate the filtrate in a porcelain dish. Dissolve the residue in dish in 6 ml of light petroleum and add to it 10 ml of copper acetate solution and shake. Bright green colour of petroleum layer shows adulteration of colophony.

TULSI

Surasa, Tulasi, Tulsi, Holy basil, Raihan

Botanical Source

Tulsi consists of the leaves of *Ocimum sanctum*.

Family

Labiatae. The plant is found throughout India and is considered sacred and worshipped and is grown near Hindu houses and temples.

Chemical Constituents

Leaves contain 0.7% volatile oil. Volatile oil contains about 71% eugenol and 20% methyl eugenol. The oil contains also carvacrol and sesquiterpene hydrocarbon caryophyllene. The oil from plants in Phillipines possesses sweet anise-like odour. It contains methyl chavicol, cineole and linalool (see structures under volatile oils).

Uses

Leaves are anti-catarrhal, expectorant and spasmolytic and are used in cold, cough, fever and gastric disorders. They are used as aromatic carminative, stimulant and flavouring agent. The drug is antiseptic and is used also externally in skin diseases. Recently anti-stress activity of Tulsi (*Ocimum sanctum*) and Ashwagandha (*Withania somnifera*) was determined by estimation of succinic dehydrogenase (SDH) in mice brain and liver. Studies on cell-mediated immunity and some other clinical assessments of these drugs were made in human beings.

ANTIRHEUMATICS
ANTIRHEUMATIC AGENTS

Antirheumatics are used to manage symptoms of rheumatoid arthritis (pain, swelling) and in more severe cases to slow down joint destruction and preserve joint function. Before describing the drugs it is considered necessary to know first, in short, the disease, Rheumatism itself.

Rheumatism

Rheumatism is the term used to describe any pain or inflammation in or around the bones, muscles or joints. Rheumatism includes arthritis which specifically means inflammation of the joints. Rheumatism is a medical term once frequently used to describe disorders associated with many different parts of the body. Most often, people associate rheumatism with arthritis or with rheumatic fever, a complication of strep throat that can result in damage to the heart. However, the term rheumatism might apply to the symptoms of numerous conditions that can cause pain and/or weakness.

Rheumatism is not a single disease. It pertains to a whole range of conditions, all of which cause pain. These conditions affect the joints, the muscles and the ligaments. Rheumatism is more common among the middle-aged and elderly people. The exact cause of most forms of rheumatism is not known. Exposure to wet and cold may aggravate the pain. There are many types of rheumatism, and some of the most common ones are rheumatoid arthritis, osteoarthritis, gout, ankylosing spondylitis, tennis elbow, frozen shoulder, cervical spondylitis and fibrositis. The common causes of rheumatism are infections, genetic factors and hormonal imbalance.

Fig. 3.5 shows how the rheumatic disorders are classified.

More discussion on the topic in question i.e. antirheumatics is beyond the scope of this book.

The antirheumatic drugs in the syllabus, namely Guggal and Colchicum are described below.

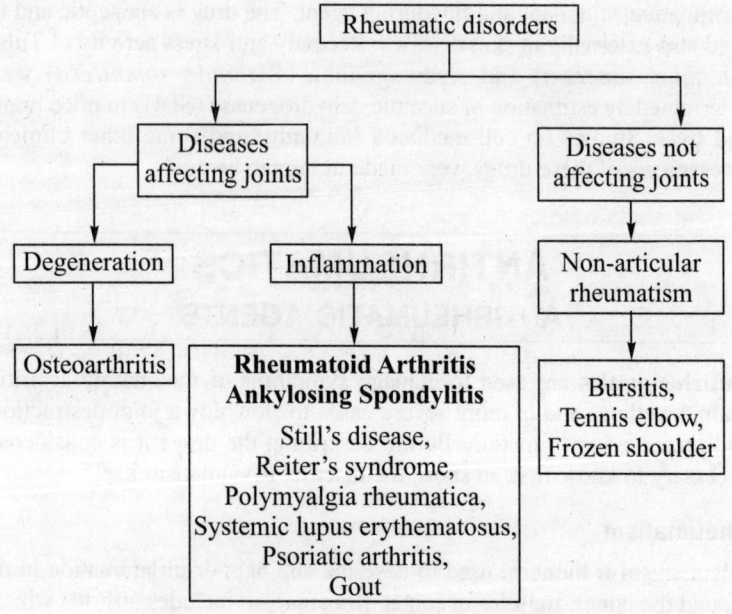

Fig. 3.5. Classification of rheumatic disorders.

GUGGUL

Gum Gugul, Indian Bdellium (Eng.), Guggula, Gugal,
Guggul (Sansk., Hindi & Guj.), Muqil (Urdu)

Botanical Source
Guggul consists of exudate of *Commiphora wightii* (Syn. *Commiphora mukul*; *Balsamodendron mukul*).

Family
Burseraceae.

Geographical Source
It is a small perennial tree or shrub upto 1.2–1.8 m high, occurring in rocky tracts of Rajasthan and Gujarat.

Collection
The exudate is collected in winter season by marking the incision in the bark or in summer, the exudate falling from the bark itself.

Characters
The drug occurs in vermicular or stalactitic pieces of pale yellow or brown to dark brown mass or conglomerate of tears. It makes milky emulsion in

water and readily burns. When fresh it is viscid and golden-coloured. It has faintly balsamic aromatic odour and bitter and astringent taste.

Chemical Constituents

It is an oleo-gum-resin and contains essential oil gum resin and steroids. The sterols are named as guggulsterols I, II and III, with guggulsterone, sugar and amino acids, camphorene, cambrene and allylumbrol. Also present are flavonoids and ellagic acid.

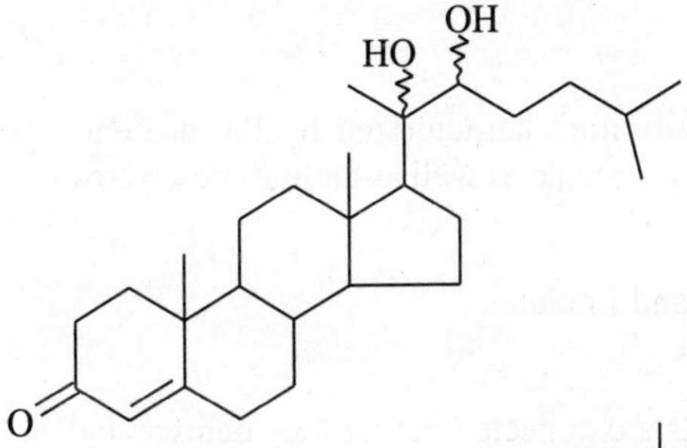

Guggulsterol I

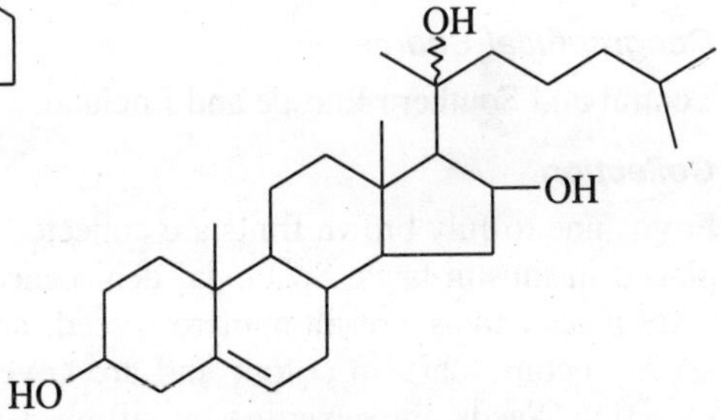

Guggulsterol II

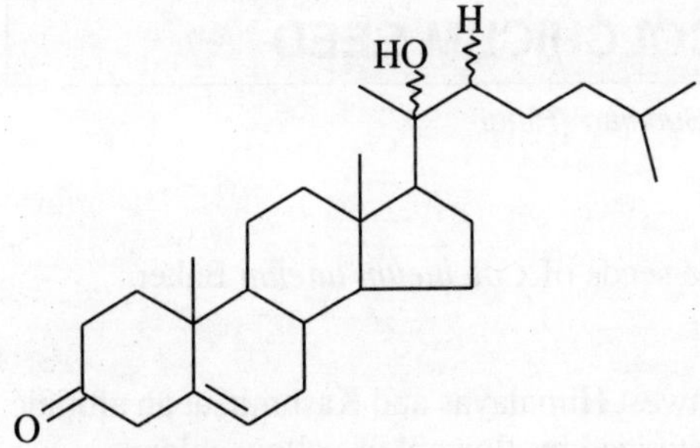

Guggulsterol III

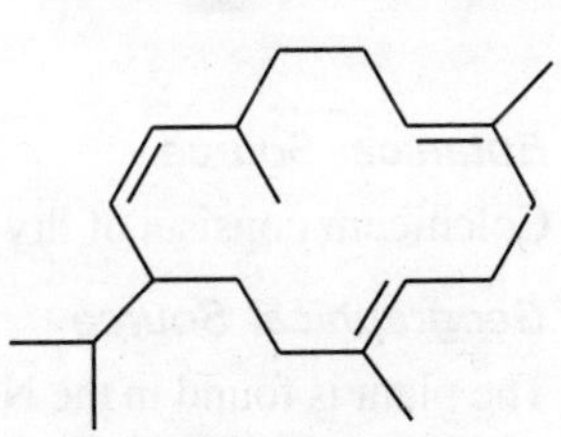

Cambrene

Uses

The drug is used as an antirheumatic, expectorant, antiseptic, astringent and demulcent. It is also said to be an aphrodisiac and emmenogogue. It is one of the latest drugs and is now famous for its well-known use as hypolipidaemic. A large number of preparations are now in the market for its hitherto acquired importance as an Ayurvedic, Unani and alternative medicine.

COLCHICUM SEED

Semen colchici, Autumn Crocus Seed,
Meadow Saffron Seed, European Colchicum Seed

Botanical Source

Colchicum consists of dried ripe seeds of *Colchicum autumnale* Linn. containing not less than 0.3% alkaloids calculated as colchicine.

Family

Liliaceae.

The members of this family are characterized by the presence of alkaloids, steroidal saponins and cardiac as well as anthracene glycosides.

Geographical Source

Central and Southern Europe and England.

Collection

From June to July brown fruits are collected before they dehisce and are placed in muslin bags. Septicidal dehiscence of fruits into three valves takes place and as a result numerous seeds are liberated. During ripening seeds become dark in colour and are covered by a sweet saccharine secretion. Seeds are separated by sifting. Colchicum seeds are derived from amphitrophous ovules and have a short raphe.

INDIAN COLCHICUM SEED

Surinjan (Hindi)

Botanical Source

Colchicum consists of dry ripe seeds of *Colchicum luteum* Baker.

Geographical Source

The plant is found in the Northwest Himalayas and Kashmir, at an altitude of 4000 to 7000 ft. It is characterized by flowers of yellow colour.

Characters

Seeds are 2–5 mm long and are oval but may become angular due to shrinkage. Testa is dark brown and finely pitted. There are two beaks – one at the hilar end, which is better developed, and another at the micropylar end. The two beaks are connected by a wavy somewhat feeble ridge. Endosperm forms the major portion of seed and contains fixed oil and aleurone grains. Near the micropylar end is a small spindle-shaped embryo.

COLCHICUM CORM

Radix colchici, Cormus colchici,
Autumn Crocus Corm, Meadow Saffron Corm

Botanical Source

Colchicum corm is the fresh or dried corm of *Colchicum autumnale* Linn.

Family

Liliaceae.

Geographical Source

Central and Southern Europe, England.

Cultivation

For cultivation, old corms are planted in the month of August and September in deep rich soil. New corms develop and next year in June-July, before flowering, corms are dug out, their outer membraneous scales removed and cut into thin transverse slices. Sometimes longitudinal slices are prepared. These slices are put into trays and dried completely at temperature not exceeding 65°C.

INDIAN COLCHICUM CORM

Surinjan

Botanical Source

Indian colchicum corm is the dried corm of *Colchicum luteum* Baker. The outer membraneous scales of the corm are removed after collection and the corm is dried.

Family

Liliaceae.

Geographical Source

India, North-Western Himalayas 1300 to 2600 metres, Kashmir.

Collection

Indian colchicum plant has yellow-coloured flowers. In other respects it resembles *C. autumnale*. Corm is dug out in May to July and remains of flowering stem and clay attached to it are removed. In India, these corms are tied in cloth, dipped into boiling water and taken out. By this process colchicine decreases but starch of the corm gets hardened and gelatinized and insects and other organisms do not deteriorate the drug. It is suggested that if the drug is brought into contact with steam instead of boiling water, colchicine content would not decrease and starch would be gelatinized.

Chemical Constituents

Colchicum contains colchicine and other alkaloids, 0.2–1.0% (average 0.5%). Alkaloids are located in the inner part of the seed-coat. Colchicine does not have basic properties as its nitrogen in the side chain has acetyl group.

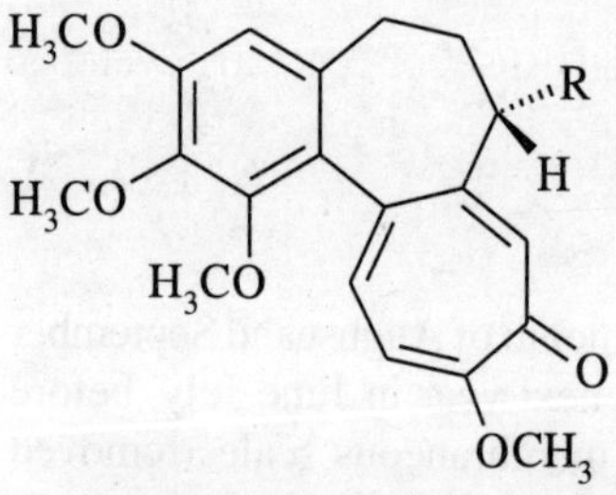

	R
Colchicine	NH—C—CH$_3$ with =O
Demecolcine	NHCH$_3$

It is yellowish-white amorphous substance and turns darker on exposure to air.

Besides colchicine, demecolcine and other alkaloids are also present.

Colchicine gives yellow colour with strong mineral acids. Colchicum seeds contain resin, called colchicoresin, fixed oil, glucose and starch. Corm also contains resin and starch.

Colchicine is also reported to have been isolated from *Colchicum vernum* Ker-Gawl, *Gloriosa superba* Linn., *Merendera attica* Boiss & Spun, *M. sabolifera* C.M.A. and *Androcymbium gramineum* McBr. The related alkaloid androcymbine has been isolated from *Androcymbium melanthioides* Linn.

Chemical Tests

The drug with 70% sulphuric acid or concentrated hydrochloric acid gives yellow colour because of colchicine.

Uses

Colchicum seed and colchicine are used to relieve pain and inflammation of gout and rheumatism. Colchicine is mitotic inhibitor and is used in malignant tumours but is toxic. Demecolcine is less toxic, its toxicity being 1/30 to 1/40 of colchicine and is recommended in myeloid leukaemia. In higher doses colchicine is toxic, causes diarrhoea, vomiting and death due to respiratory failure. Colchicine is used for causing polyploidy. It increases the number of chromosomes, from 2N to 4N or more, and is employed in horticulture and drug cultivation to increase the constituents.

ANTITUMOURS
ANTITUMOUR AGENTS

Cancer is a class of diseases or disorders characterized by uncontrolled division of cells and the ability of these to spread, either by direct growth into adjacent tissue through invasion, or by implantation into distant sites by metastasis (where cancer cells are transported through the blood stream or lymphatic system). Cancer may affect people at all ages, but risk tends to increase with age. It is one of the principal causes of death in developed countries. The term antitumour refers to malignant disease at and in any part of the body. The disease is characterized by the formation of tumours due to cell proliferation of tissues of organs in any part of the body, resulting in abnormal growth at concerned site. Death of the organism ensues if the uncontrolled formation of abnormal cells and/or tumours is not arrested. There are various kinds of treatment undertaken to provide relief temporarily or cure the symptoms to prolong the life of the patient. These treatments are surgery, radiation and drugs, commonly called the therapeutic agents.

There are many types of cancer. Severity of symptoms depends on the site and character of the malignancy and whether there is metastasis. A definitive diagnosis usually requires the histologic examination of tissue by a pathologist. This tissue is obtained by biopsy or surgery. Most cancers can be treated and some cured, depending on the specific type, location, and stage. Once diagnosed, cancer is usually treated with a combination of surgery, chemotherapy and radiotherapy. As research develops, treatments are becoming more specific for the type of cancer pathology. Drugs that target specific cancers already exist for several types of cancer. If untreated, cancers may eventually cause illness and death, though this is not always the case.

The unregulated growth that characterizes cancer is caused by damage to DNA resulting in mutations to genes that encode for proteins controlling cell division. Many mutation events may be required to transform a normal cell into a malignant cell. These mutations can be caused by radiation, chemicals or physical agents that cause cancer, which are called carcinogens, or by certain viruses that can insert their DNA into the human genome. Mutations occur spontaneously and may be passed down from one cell generation to the next as a result of mutations within germ lines. However, some carcinogens also appear to work through non-mutagenic pathways that affect the level of transcription of certain genes without causing genetic mutation. Many forms of cancer are associated with exposure to environmental factors such as tobacco, smoke, radiation, alcohol and certain viruses. Some risk factors can be avoided or reduced.

Plants have long been shown to contain phytochemicals which have been successfully used for their antitumour activity. To mention a few important plants, out of the many, having such antitumour activity are Podophyllum (*Podophyllum hexandrum, P. peltatum*), Mistletoe (*Viscum album*), Mezereon (*Daphne mezereon*), (*Taxcus brevifolia*) and Catharanthus (*Catharanthus roseus*).

Natural drugs and phytochemicals which have shown tumour-inhibitory properties are called antitumours or antitumour agents. These tumour-inhibitory phytochemicals represent a wide variety of structures. Amongst them are terpenes, lignans, alkaloids, triterpenoids, steroids, non-heterocyclic peptides, etc.

As an antitumour drug the syllabus has only one drug, the most important and well-known drug, the Vinca, which is described below.

CATHARANTHUS

Catharanthus, Vinca, Madagascar perivinkle, Barmasi (Guj., Hindi)

Botanical Source

Catharanthus is the dried entire plant of *Catharanthus roseus* (*Vinca rosea*).

Family

Apocyanceae.

Geographical Source

The plant is a native of Madagascar and is found in many tropical and subtropical countries, specially in India, Australia, South Africa and North and South America. The plant is cultivated as garden plant in Europe and India.

Characters

Vinca plant is an erect, ever-blooming, hairy herb or undershrub, which is woody at the base. It is 40–80 cm in height. The flowers in cultivated varieties are violet, pink or white. The leaves are opposite, oblong and petiolate with entire margin (Fig. 3.6). Fruits are divergent follicles*.

The drug is obtained both from wild and cultivated sources in many parts of the world.

Chemical Constituents

About 90 alkaloids have been isolated from Catharanthus. Alkaloids are present in the entire shrub, but leaves and roots contain more alkaloids, some alkaloids such as ajmalicine, serpentine, lochnerine and tetrahydro-

---

* Teachers may see the detailed description, including photos of the plants and anatomic brief in *Pharmacognosy*, 16th ed. by the same author.

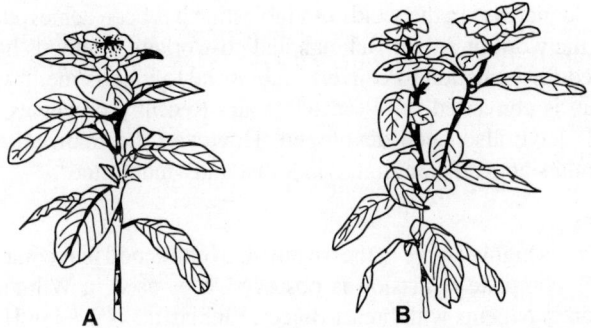

Fig. 3.6. Flowering branches of *Vinca rosea*. A, rose or pink variety; B, white variety.

Catharanthine

Vindoline

	R
Vinblastine	CH₃
Vincristine	CHO

alstonine are already known as they are present in other plants of Apocynaceae, e.g. Rauwolfia, Lochneria and Alstonia, etc. The important alkaloids in Catharanthus are the dimer indole-indoline alkaloids vinblastine and vincristine and they possess definite anti-cancer activity. Other dimer indole-indoline alkaloids also possess anti-cancer activity.

Both vincristine and vinblastine have the same structures with the difference that in vinblastine there is N-methyl group, while in vincristine there is N-formyl group, and both possess different activities. Vincristine is clinically more important and is present in much lower concentration in the plant at a level of about 25 ppm. Out of a ton of dried leaves only 50 mg of vincristine and 2 gm of vinblastine were previously obtainable. A

30–50 fold increase in the yields of vinblastine has been achieved recently through the work of Attaur Rehman and co-workers. Methods have been developed for oxidation to convert vinblastine to vincristine in which N-CR group is converted to N-formyl group. Recently processes for their synthesis have also been developed. However, the main alkaloids in Catharanthus are catharanthine, vindoline and vindolinine.

Uses

Vincristine is highly active in the treatment of childhood leukemia in which case 41% complete remission is observed. It is used in Wilm's tumour regression in patients with breast cancer. Vinblastine is used in Hodgkin's disease and choriocarcinoma. Recently a combination VAMP consisting of vincristine, amephopterine (methotraxate), 6-mercaptopurine and prednisone is being used.

Both vincristine and vinblastine are antimitotic resulting in tumour cell death during replication and they are used intravenously.

Additional note: As stated above **Vinca** is the only drug included as an antitumour drug in the syllabus, even though a large number of natural drugs of plant origin have shown promising rather well-recorded anticancer/ antitumour action. Although a list and/or a brief account of all such drugs does not merit cosideration here, yet it will be pertinent to at least mention **Indian Podophyllum**, which besides being a good antitumour drug, also possesses a number of other important uses and special phytochemical lignan structure. Even otherwise it seems quite strange that Indian Podophyllum does not find a place in the syllabus at all. Hence it is considered appropriate to describe the drug briefly here*.

INDIAN PODOPHYLLUM

Indian Podophyllum Rhizome,
Rhizome Podophylli indicii, Podophyllum indicum

Botanical Source

Indian podophyllum consists of the dried rhizome and root of *Podophyllum hexandrum* Royle. This species was formerly known as *Podophyllum emodi*.

Family

Berberidaceae.

Geographical Source

High slopes of Himalaya, Kashmir, Tibet and Afghanistan.

---

* Footnote under Catharanthus applies here also.

Chemical Constituents

Indian podophyllum contains 10–18% resin. In resin active constituent is 30–40% podophyllotoxin. Podophyllotoxin is a lignan and tetrahydro-naphthalin derivative with OH and lactone groups in *trans* positions which are essential for antimitotic or anticancer property of the drug. In *cis* positions it has only purgative property. It also contains dioxymethylene and lactone groups responsible for the activity. Podophyllotoxin is crystalline, bitter and laevorotatory, and occurs free and combined with sugar as glycoside. Indian podophyllum also contains 4-demethyl podophyllotoxin. It resembles podophyllotoxin except that at 4 position it contains OH instead of OCH_3 group. The drug contains inactive picro-podophyllin, flavone, calcium oxalate and starch. Resin of podophyllum is prepared by extraction with alcohol, precipitating with acidified water, filtering, washing and drying the precipitate. It was official in I.P.

Podophyllotoxin

American podophyllum is obtained from *Podophyllum peltatum*. It contains 3–8% resin and in resin podophyllotoxin is upto 20% and α-peltatin 10% and β-peltatin 5%. Peltatins are lignans similar to podophyllotoxin, but are *cis* isomers and so have no antimitotic property, but have strong purgative property. Peltatins are absent in Indian drug. So Indian drug has no purgative property. American drug is inferior as regards percentage of resin and also as regards percentage of podophyllotoxin.

Uses

It is drastic but slow-acting purgative and has cholagogue action. Podophyllotoxin has antimitotic action and is used in cancer. Sandoz has marketed oral preparations known as S.P.G. Podophyllotoxin benzglycodin glucoside and SP-1 parestial preparation Podophyllic acid ethyl hydrazid. They are used with success. The antimitotic action is due to inhibition of DNA and RNA synthesis. It is used externally in venereal warts.

ANTILEPROTICS
ANTILEPROTIC AGENTS

Leprosy, amongst the infectious diseases, is one of the most serious diseases, a kind of curse. Leprosy (also known as Hansen's disease) is a chronic infectious granulomatous disease caused by bacteria or germs called *Mycobacterium leprae*. It is an infection that affects the skin and the nerves of the hands and feet and can also cause problems in the eyes and nose. The disease develops in two forms: (1) non-lepromatous, and (2) lepromatous. Non-lepromatous is an anaesthetic type, while lepromatous type is a nodular type and is infective. The causative bacteria enter through the skin. In the first stage the sensation of the patient's skin gets dulled and the skin develops small patches of anaesthesia or numbness. The bacteria multiply in the axoplasm of nerve fibres and cause a tingling sensation. In the second stage, skin becomes thick and wrinkled. Ears become swollen and nodules are formed in the skin of nose and throat. These nodules discharge fluid, which is highly infectious. In the third stage the bacteria burst out of the nerve cells and spread to the peripheral tissues and start to proliferate there. This is followed by the formation of deformities in hands, feet, toes, etc. Leprosy is an unfortunate disease, a kind of curse, which develops and progresses very slowly. If uncared from the beginning and untreated in time, it leaves a person crippled. The patients suffering from leprosy are normally isolated and have to undergo long-term treatment.

Leprosy is not an inherited disease. Also, it is rare for more than one person in the same family to have this disease. In most cases, it is spread through long-term contact with a person who has the disease but has not been treated. Also, it is not transmitted through sexual contact or pregnancy. Most people will never develop the disease even if they are exposed to the bactaria. Of the world's population, 95% have a natural immunity to leprosy.

The drugs used to treat the Hansen's disease are called antileprotics and there is only one natural drug, namely Chaulmoogra oil, included in the syllabus.

CHAULMOOGRA OIL

Hydnocarpus oil, Gynocardia oil

Botanical Source

Chaulmoogra oil is the fixed oil obtained by cold expression process from fresh ripe seeds of *Hydnocarpus wightiana*, *H. anthelmintica*, *H. heterophylla* and other species of *Hydnocarpus*. Family is Flacourtiaceae. *Taraktogenos kurzii* (Family: Bixaceae) is another source for the oil.

Geographical Source

The tree is tall and is found in East India, Burma, Thailand and Indochina.

Description

Seeds are ovoid, irregular and angular, 1–1.25 inches long, 0.5 inches wide with smooth skin, grayish colour and are brittle. Kernel is oily and dark brown.

Preparation

Seeds are cleaned, washed and dried. They are cracked to remove testa. The kenels are reduced to a paste and the oil is expressed, filtered and stored in air-tight containers.

Characters

Chaulmoogra oil is a yellow-coloured liquid and at 10°C temperature it becomes whitish solid. It has a characteristic smell and is sharp in taste.

Physical and Chemical Characteristics

Specific gravity at 25°C is 0.937–0.970; Specific rotation of 10% w/w in chloroform +48–60°; Acid value 20–30; Iodine value 96–104; Saponification value 196–213.

Solubility

Sparingly soluble in alcohol but soluble in other fat miscible solvents.

Chemical Constituents

Oil is a mixture of glycerides of fatty acids. The fatty acids are hydnocarpic acid (45%), chaulmoogric acid (20%), gorlic acid (15%), oleic acid and palmitic acid. Hydnocarpic, chaulmoogric and gorlic acids have cyclopentane rings. A double bond is present in gorlic acid. Recently some new cyclopentenyl fatty acids have been worked out for their structures.

These acids seem to be accumulated during the last three to four months of maturation of fruits of these plants. The esterified oil of *H. wightiana*, yielding the pure ethyl hydnocarpate, is now preferably used.

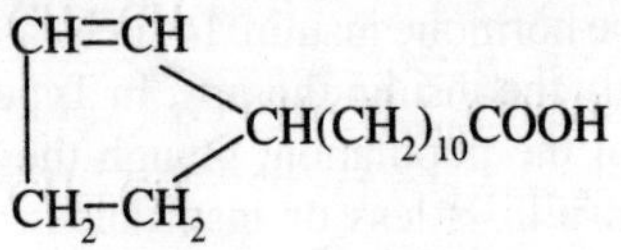

$$\begin{array}{c} CH=CH \\ | \qquad \searrow \\ CH_2-CH_2 \end{array} CH(CH_2)_{10}COOH$$

Hydnocarpic acid

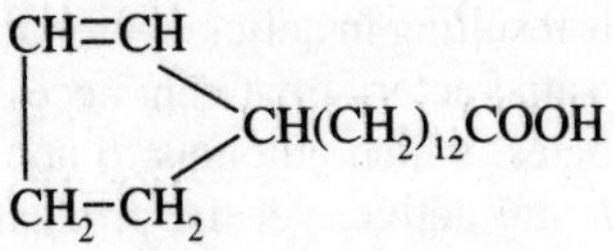

$$\begin{array}{c} CH=CH \\ | \qquad \searrow \\ CH_2-CH_2 \end{array} CH(CH_2)_{12}COOH$$

Chaulmoogric acid

$$\begin{array}{c} CH=CH \\ | \qquad \searrow \\ CH_2-CH_2 \end{array} CH(C_{12}H_{22})COOH$$

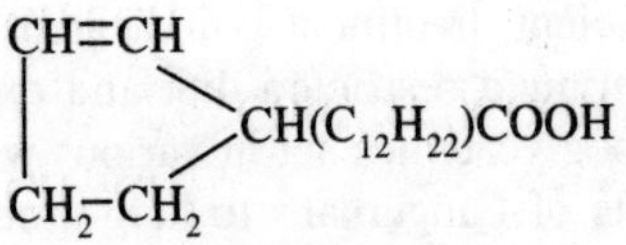

Gorlic acid

Uses

The three fatty acids with cyclopentane ring possess specific toxicity for *Mycobacterium leprae* and *M. tuberculosis* in vitro ten times as powerful as phenol. They are used since a long period in leprosy and tuberculosis. Because of unstable nature of oils, their sodium salts and ethyl esters are used. At present in the treatment of leprosy synthetic sulphones are used.

Chaulmoogra oil is used in endemic area. In lepromatous leprae, it is often effective in early cases in decreasing the size of the nodules, anaesthetic patches and skin lesions. It is administered by direct infiltration injection of the lesions, but for this purpose ethyl ester of hynocarpus oil are generally used.

ANTIDIABETICS
ANTIDIABETIC AGENTS

Antidiabetics or antidiabetic agents are drugs which are used to control **diabetes**. Diabetes, as a disease, has nowadays acquired notoriety; as a fairly large proportion of population throughout the world is suffering from this dangerous incurable disease. The disease is caused by a deficient formation of the hormone **insulin** by the β-cells of the islets of Langerhans in the pancreas, one of the endocrine glands (organs) of the body. Insulin is responsible for the regulation of carbohydrates, triglycerides and protein metabolism at different sites of the body. It finally controls the entry and presence of glucose in the blood. A deficient production of insulin will thus result in hyperglycaemia, a distinct symptom of diabetes. A diabetic person, therefore, shows excess of sugar in the blood and urine, feels hungry and thirsty and loses body weight.

Two types of diabetes occur. Type 1 is the insulin-dependent diabetes and Type 2 is the non-insulin-dependent diabetes. Type 1 includes diabetic children and all others less than 40 years of age, with the exception of some over 40 years of age. In Type 1 diabetes, patient lacks the active β-cells resulting in deficient production of the hormone insulin. In such cases the satisfactory treatment necessitates only the insulin therapy. In Type 2 diabetes, which amounts to about 75% of the population, though the β-cells are active, yet the production of insulin is less or insufficient. In order to cope with the deficiency of insulin the patients are required to control through a suitable diet and exercise. In case the diet regimen and exercise prove insufficient, treatment is indicated by use of oral hypo-glycaemics (with continued restricted diet and exercise). The glucose lowering drugs or hypoglycaemics act in various ways: (i) By activating the β-cells in the islets of Langerhans to help produce more of insulin;

(ii) by reducing or dampening the process of glucogenesis and activating the peripheral utilization of glucose; and (iii) by decreasing the carbohydrate absorption from the alimentary canal leading to the reduction of plasma glucose concentration. In all the above three cases the success still depends upon the production of some insulin by the pancreas. The success of all forms of allopathic drugs used to control diabetes depends upon this condition i.e. production of insulin in whatever amount. In other words the treatment, or to be more correct, control of diabetes by use of medicines, is not possible, if the pancreas has failed to produce insulin.

According to a report from the International Diabetes Federation (IDF), it is now estimated that 20–25% of the world's population suffers from Metabolic Syndrome. People with Metabolic Syndrome have a 500% greater risk of developing Type 2 diabetes, meaning this is fast becoming a substantial burden on global healthcare.

The syllabus includes only two natural drugs – namely Pterocarpus and Gymnema. The former is known as Asana in Ayurvedic medicine, while the latter is known as Gurmar in common Indian languages. They are described below.

PTEROCARPUS

Indian Kino Tree, Malabar Kino (Eng.), Vijasara, Bija (Hindi), Biyo (Guj.), Bijasara (Sanskrit and Urdu).

Botanical Source

Pterocarpus consists of the heartwood of *Pterocarpus marsupium* (other parts of the plant, viz. kino gum, bark and leaves are also used).

Family

Leguminosae (Papilionaceae).

Geographical Source

The plant is found mainly throughout Gujarat, Madhya Pradesh, Bihar and Orissa.

Chemical Constituents

As per the Ayurvedic Pharmacopoeia of India the drug used is only the wood of the plant and it contains alkaloids and resins. However, the bark

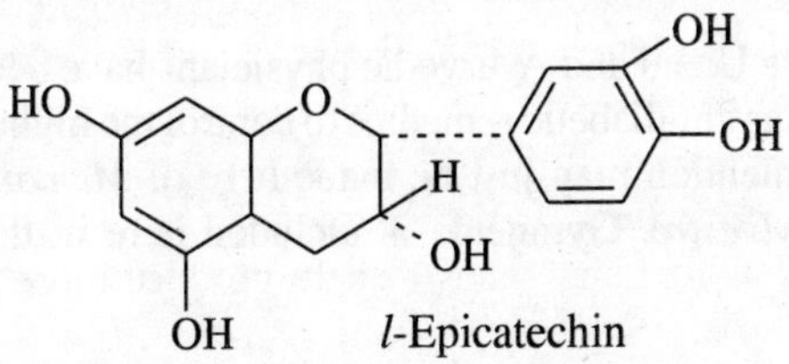

l-Epicatechin

of the same plant is said to contain a reddish-brown colouring matter and *l*-epicatechin. The wood further contains colouring matter, essential oil and also fixed oil.

The heartwood, dissolved in alkali, gives isoliquiritigenin, liquiritigenin and pterostilbine. The sapwood shows the presence of only pterostilbene. The bark contains *l*-epicatechin and pterostilbene. Some workers also obtained a novel isoflavonoid glycol marsupol, carpusin, propterol and propterol B from the heartwood of the tree.

The roots of the plant have also shown a large number of glucosidal and related compounds, including a few mentioned above, but these do not merit their consideration and mention in this book for obvious reasons.

Uses

The wood is considered an antidiabetic and many studies have been undertaken to prove the drug's hypoglycaemic action. An aqueous extract of the plant has shown hypoglycaemic effect in acute as well as chronic experiments on normal rabbits.

Hence, an aqueous infusion or a glass of water with the drug, *P. marsupium*, kept overnight is given for its antidiabetic effect.

(Kino is an astringent and is given in diarrhoea. It is also used for toothache. Powdered leaves are applied as paste to boils, sores and in skin diseases. Even the decoction of the bark is said to be very useful for the diabetic patients.)

GYMNEMA SYLVESTRE

Meshasringi (Sanskrit, Bengali), Gurmar (Hindi),
Kharak (Arabic), Khar-e-khasak (Persian)

Botanical Source

Gymnema consists of the leaves of *Gymnema sylvestre* (Syn. *Asclepias geminata*).

Family

Asclepiadaceae.

Geographical Source

A climbing plant common in central and southern India, Western Ghats and in Goa.

For a long time Unani and Ayurvedic physicians have been using quite a few plant drugs as antidiabetic remedies to control the higher blood sugar levels. Of them mention may just be made here of *Memordia charentia* and *Gymnema sylvestre*. Gymnema is included here in the syllabus of Diploma Course.

Chemical Constituents*

The leaves contain two resins. The larger portion of resin is insoluble in alcohol, while the smaller portion is soluble in alcohol. There are also present a number of other constituents, like a bitter neutral principle, colouring matter, pararobin, glucose, tartaric acid and an organic acid, said to be a glucoside and possessing anti-saccharine property. Also present is gymnemic acid (6%) and quercitol. The presence of lupeol, β-amyrin, stigmasterol and also the gymnemic acid (+)-quercitol has been reported in the drug. The alcoholic extract of the plant has shown the presence of saponins. There are also reports indicating the presence of alkaloid betaine, choline and trimethylamine in the leaves.

Gymnemic acid resembles chrysophanic acid and forms salts with alkaloids.

Uses

The drug is blessed with a number of uses, like astringent, stomachic, tonic, refrigerant and diuretic. *Gymnemic sylvestre* has been shown to cause insignificant reduction in blood sugar in normal rats, but produced marked and significant reduction in anterior pituitary-treated hyperglycemic animals. The leaf is said to stimulate insulin secretion and studies have shown that the active principles of the leaves have blood sugar reducing properties.

The leaves have the property of destroying the taste of sugar, and hence the drug is called Gurmar (meaning sugar destroying). It is, therefore, considered that the drug neutralizes or reduces the excess sugar in the body of a diabetic patient.

Besides, a decoction of the leaves is given in fever and cough. Powdered leaves mixed or triturated with castor oil are also applied to swollen glands. The root of the plant is also used as a remedy for snake bite; either the powder is dusted as such on wound or its paste with water is applied and a decoction can be given internally.

DIURETICS

Diuretics are drugs which increase the output of urine. They may act on the different segments of the nephron, which is the functional unit of the kidney. Diuretics are clinically useful in the following pathological states:

1. Hypertension
2. Congestive heart failure
3. Oedema (due to heart failure or cirrhosis of liver).

---

* For chemical structures the teachers may consult *Pharmacognosy*, 16th ed. by the same author or literature.

Chemically, diuretics are a diverse group of compounds which either stimulate or inhibit various hormones that are naturally occurring in the body to regulate urine production by the kidneys. Herbal medications are not inherently diuretics. They are more correctly called aquadratics.

GOKHRU

Caltrop, Puncture vine, Cathead.

Botanical Source

There are two plants of gokhru:
1. The fruits of *Tribulus terrestris* supplying small or chhota gokhru.
2. The fruits of *Pedalium murex* supplying large or bara gokhru.

TRIBULUS TERRESTRIS (Chhota Gokhru)

Botanical Source

Chhota gokhru consists of dried ripe fruits of *Tribulus terrestris*.

Family

Zygophyllaceae.

Geographical Source

Tribulus terrestris is a plant that grows in many tropical and temperate areas of the world. Weed of pastures is found throughout the farming regions of Australia. The species is also found in Asia, Africa and the Americas. It is also common throughout India and is found especially during the monsoons. It is found upto an altitude of 11000 ft in warm regions of the globe.

Chemical Constituents

The fruits contain furastanol *bis*-glycoside which is identical with protodioscin and on acid hydrolysis it yields spirostanol diosgenin.

Further, fruits contain sapogenins, diosgenin, ruscogenin and gitogenin of the steroid saponins. Fruits contain three flavone glycosides. Two glycosides are kampferol 3-rhamnosides and third tribuloside is kampferol 6-*p*-coumaroyal 3-D-glucoside. It contains traces of an alkaloid, fixed oil and potassium nitrate.

Uses

The drug has diuretic, cooling, demulcent, aphrodisiac and tonic action and is popularly used in Ayurveda. It is used in primary nephritis and also in kidney stone. In Ayurveda entire plant with root is used and is said to be more effective in kidney stone than fruits alone.

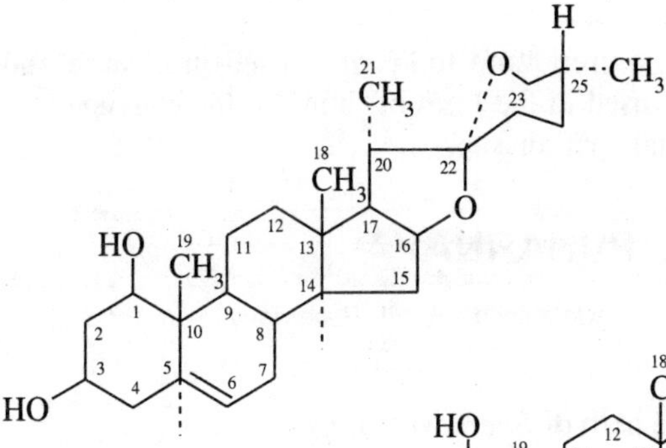

Ruscogenin

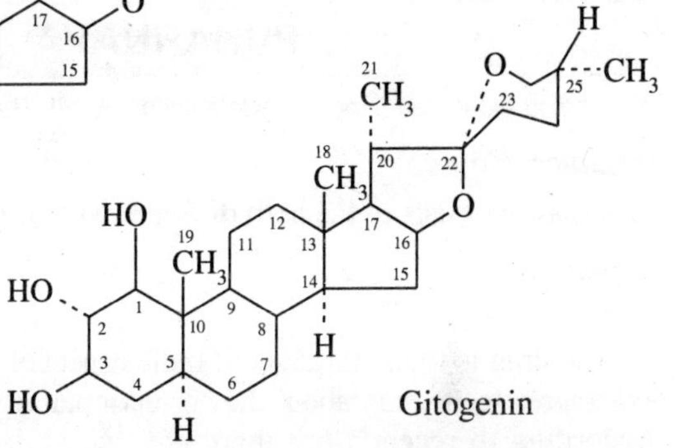

Gitogenin

It improves and restores libido in men as it improves and prolongs the duration of erection. It raises the level of testosterone in men while aiding fertility by enhancing the production of sperms while not causing side effects of other testosterone precursors. It does not limit a decrease in natural testosterone production or testicles shrinkage.

In women it boosts the production of estradiol, a precursor to estrogen and also to testosterone, which has been shown to help with vasomotor manifestation during natural and post-surgical menopause, as well as compliant of insomnia, irritability or apathy. The extract of the *Tribulus terrestris* has been used for centuries as a remedy for impotence and an aphrodisiac for both men and women.

PEDALIUM MUREX (Bara gokhru)

Botanical Source

Bara gokhru consists of dried ripe fruits of *Pedalium murex*.

Family

Pedaliaceae.

Geographical Source

The plant is found near the sea coasts of Saurashtra, Konkan, Deccan peninsula, Sri Lanka and tropical Africa. It occurs widely especially after the monsoons in Delhi, Punjab and Rajasthan.

Chemical Constituents

Fruits contain mucilage, an alkaloid, greenish fatty oil and little resin.

Uses

The drug is demulcent, diuretic and tonic. It is used in dysuria and gonorrhoea. It is usually used in the form of infusion. In Ayurveda it is recommended as tonic and aphrodisiac.

PUNARNAVA

Spreading Hogweed (Eng.), Gadahpurna (Hindi), Punarnava (Sanskrit & Ger.)

Botanical Source

Punarnava consists of the herb of *Boerhavia diffusa*.

Family

Nyctaginaceae.

The drug is found throughout India especially during the rains. There exists great confusion about the correct botanical identity of punarnava. According to recent work there are two varieties, red and white, of punarnava. Red variety is more common and is widely distributed, while the white variety is scarce. The confusion is due to the fact that *Trianthema monogyna* (Ficoideae) also occurring in red and white varieties is often substituted for punarnava and is sold as punarnava, but now *B. diffusa* is more or less established as punarnava.

Some authors earlier reported a new species *Boerhaavia punarnava* with white flowers. It was later found that it was not a new species but was *Boerhaavia erecta* reported earlier.

B. diffusa white differs from *B. erecta* and resembles more red variety of *B. diffusa* and so it is called white variety of *B. diffusa* (see Part III).

Geographical Source

The plant grows throughout India. It is found in abundance in rainy season.

Chemical Constituents

Formerly an alkaloid 'punarnavine' was reported which is probably allantoin, isolated later. Drug contains large amount of potassium nitrate and other potassium salts. It also contains heteroctane, ursolic acid and β-sitosterol which may be partly free and partly as palmitate.

Uses

Punarnava is used as diuretic. Aqueous decoction was found useful in nephrotic syndrome. It gives relief in chronic oedema. It gives overall relief by causing decrease in albuminuria, rise in serum protein and fall in serum cholesterol level. It is found useful also in liver diseases. Action may be attributed partly to potassium nitrate and other potassium salts. Ethyl acetate and methanol extracts were found to possess anti-inflammatory activity.

ANTIDYSENTERIC DRUGS
ANTIDYSENTERICS

Diarrhoea is an acute inflammation of the large intestine characterized by diarrhoea with blood and mucus in the stools. Dysentery may be caused by either bacterial or protozoal organisms. The common bacterial organism responsible for dysentery is *Shigella dysenteriae*. *Entamoeba histolytica* is the causative protozoal organism for amoebic dysentery. Alkaloids of emetine and its derivatives isolated from ipecacuanha are clinically used in hepatic amoebiasis. However, the toxic effects are very high.

IPECACUANHA

*Radix ipecacuanhue, Ipecacuanhae Root,
Ipecac Rio, Brazilian or Johore Ipecac.*

Botanical Source

Ipecacuanha consists of the dried root or rhizome and roots of *Caphaelis ipecacuanha* (Rio or Brazilian ipecac) or of *Cephaelis acuminata* (Cartagena, Nicaragua or Panama ipecac).

Family

Rubiaceae.

Geographical Source

Brazil, Forests of Mattogrosso and Minas, Malaya States (Johore), Burma and Bengal in India.

History

The name of the plant is of Portuguese origin, from the native word, I-pe-kaa-gue'ne, which is said to meam 'road-side sick-making plant'.

The botanical source of Ipecacuanha was the subject of much dispute. It was finally settled by Gomez, a physician of the Portuguese Navy, who brought authentic specimens from Brazil to Lisbon in 1800.

Chemical Constituents

Ipecac root contains 2–2.5% alkaloids emetine, cephaeline, psychotrine and psychotrine methyl ether.

All the alkaloids have isoquinoline ring system and are present in the bark. Emetine, $C_{28}H_{37}O_3N_2OCH_3$ is the active alkaloid and as it does not contain a free phenolic group, it is called non-phenolic alkaloid. Emetine base is non-crystalline, but its salts are crystalline. Rio ipecac contains slightly more than 2% alkaloids from which emetine is two-thirds and

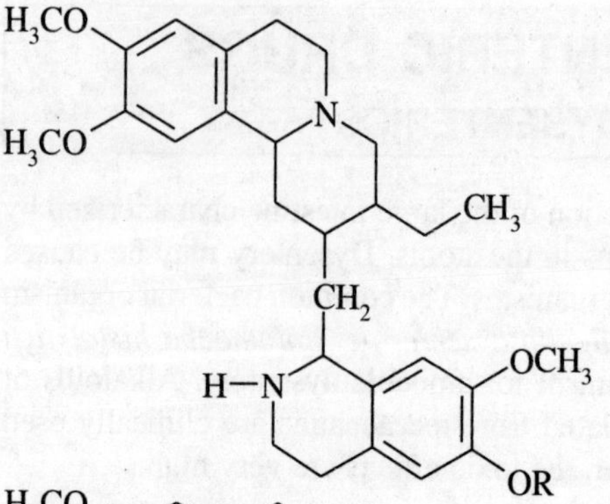

	R
Emetine	CH_3
Cephaeline	H

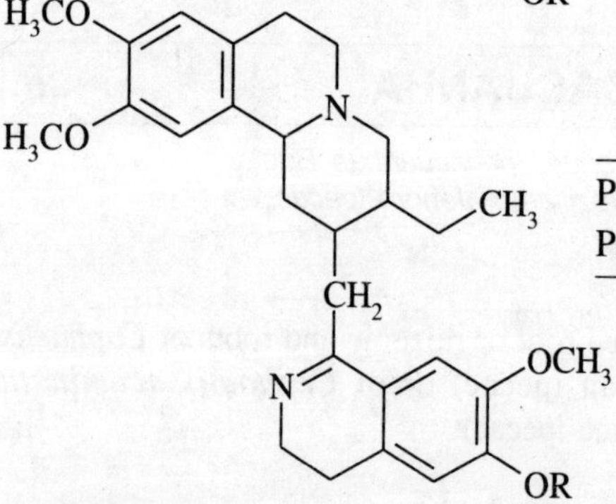

	R
Psychotrine	H
Psychotrine methyl ether	CH_3

cephaeline is one-third. In Cartagena ipecac, alkaloids are up to 2.2% and emetine is about one-third and cephaeline is two-thirds. The other alkaloids are in traces. Because of higher percentage of emetine, at one time, only the Rio ipecac was official, but now in many pharmacopoeias, including I.P., both species are official. Cephaeline is $C_{28}H_{37}O_3N_2OH$ and contains one free phenolic OH group and is called phenolic alkaloid.

Emetine can be obtained from cephaeline by methylation. Psychotrine is $C_{28}H_{35}O_3N_2OH$ and psychotrine methyl ether is $C_{28}H_{35}O_3N_2OCH_3$. The latter two alkaloids contain 2H atoms less than the first two. All the four alkaloids are thus interrelated and can be converted into one another. Ipecac contains a crystalline glycoside ipecacuanhin, as acid sapoain ipecacuanhin acid, starch and calcium oxalate.

Test for emetine

Add 5 ml hydrochloric acid to 0.1 gm of powdered drug, heat and filter. To the filtrate add small crystals of potassium chlorate or chloramine T. The colour of the filtrate becomes yellow-orange and then red.

Uses

The alkaloids have local irritant action and ipecac is used as an expectorant. Emetine like quinine is protoplasmic poison and is used in amoebic dysentery and liver troubles like hepatitis. 2-Dehydroemetine has better amoebicidal action than emetine. Formerly cephaeline was considered more irritant but now both emetine and cephaeline are considered irritant, emetic and toxic. Emetine is administered as injection or orally in the preparation like emetine bismuth iodide. Emetine is excreted slowly from the system and so there is danger of accumulation.

Indian Ipecac

Ipecac is cultivated in Darjeeling district in Bengal. Collection is done from 3-year-old plants. Annual production is more than 45 tons. It contains about 2.1% alkaloids.

ANTISEPTICS AND DISINFECTANTS

Antiseptics

Antiseptics may be defined as substances which inhibit the growth of microorganisms. They are also called bacteriostatic agents since they are not able to kill the microorganisms e.g. alcohol.

Disinfectants

Disinfectants are agents which kill the pathogenic microorganisms. They are used in surgical practice for disinfecting infected wounds, skin or to sterilize surgeons and instruments, e.g. phenol, potassium permanganate and hydrogen peroxide.

BENZOIN

Benzoinum, Sumatra benzoin, Laban (Guj.)

Botanical Source

Benzoin is the balsamic resin obtained from the incised stem of *Styrax benzoin* and *Styrax paralleloneurus*.

Family

Styraceae.

Geographical Source

Sumatra.

Collection

Benzoin is a pathological resin, secreted in secretory ducts and secretory cells of the tree after injury. Fungus also takes part in the production of benzoin. In Sumatra, benzoin is obtained from cultivated trees. Collection of the resin is carried out from trees of 7–20 years. All kinds of the exudations are sent to Palembang after collection, mixed there in definite proportions, softened by keeping in the sun and allowed to solidify. From each tree about 10 kg of benzoin is produced every year.

Characters

Benzoin consists of mass of brittle, opaque, hard, white or red tears. This mass is embedded in translucent, reddish-brown resinous matrix. Fractured surface is uneven. Odour is balsamic, aromatic, and agreeable and taste is slightly acrid. When heated irritating fumes of benzoic and cinnamic acids are produced.

Chemical Constituents

Sumatra benzoin contains 23% free balsamic acids containing mainly cinnamic acid. It contains 70–80% resin consisting of triterpenoid acids, siaresinolic acid (19-hydroxy oleanolic acid) and sumaresinolic acid (6-hydroxy oleanolic acid) and their esters with balsamic acids at hydroxy group.

It also contains vanillin. styrol (phenyl ethylene) and phyenyl propyl cinnamate responsible for the aromatic smell.

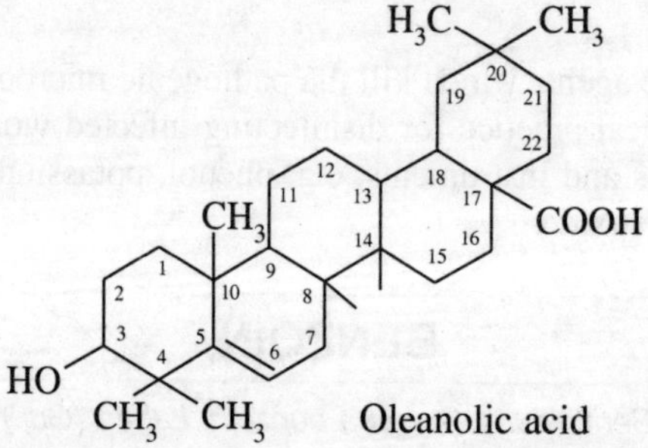

Oleanolic acid

Uses

It is used as antiseptic, exectorant, stimulant and healing agent. It is used in the preparation of compound benzoin tincture. This tincture contains benzoin, aloe, storax and tolu balsam and is used as topical protectant, antiseptic and expectorant. It is used as inhalation in respiratory diseases. In pharmacy only the Sumatra benzoin is used.

SIAM BENZOIN

Botanical Source

Siam benzoin is the balsamic resin of *Styrax tonkinensis*. It is official in French and many European Pharmacopoeias.

Family

Styraceae.

Geographical Source

North Laos and North Vietnam at an altitude from 600–1200 metres. It is exported from Bangkok of Siam hence the name Siam benzoin.

Collection

It is a pathological resin. Fungus also plays a part in its forrnation. Incisions reaching upto xylem are made in 6–10 years old trees. Because of the injury cambium produces secondary tissues, rich in secretory ducts which may become lysigenous and extend upto medullary rays. Balsam exude, which is first liquid and then solidifies, is similar to Sumatra benzoin. First exudation is not used but second and subsequent exudations are used as a drug.

Chemical Constituents

Siam benzoin contains about 70% crystalline and 10% amorphous coniferyl benzoate. It contains 10% free benzoic acid, 6% D-siaresinolic acid, vanillin and cinnamyl benzoate.

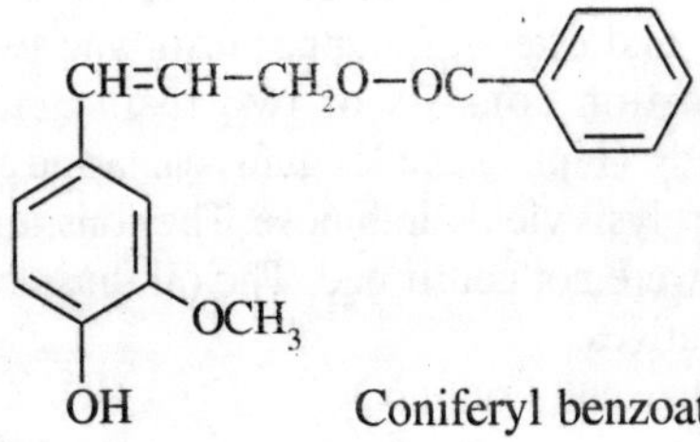

Coniferyl benzoate

Uses

Benzoin is used as antiseptic and expectorant. It is used externally as mild disinfectant. Siam benzoin is used in the preparation of benzoinated lard. In perfumery and in cosmetics as a fixative.

MYRRH

Myrrh, Myrrha, Arabian Myrrh, Somali Myrrh, Hirabol (Guj.), Bol (Hindi)

Botanical Source

Myrrh is the oleo-gum-resin obtained by incision from the stem of *Commiphora molmol*, *C. abyssinica* and other species of *Commiphora*.

Family

Burseraceae.

Geographical Source

Somalia (Northeast Africa).

Collection

The tree is small about 3 metres in height. The phloem contains schizogenous ducts and lysigenous cavities which are filled with yellowish granular resinous liquid. Incision is made in the bark, the oleo-gum-resin which is liquid exudes and hardens to a reddish-brown mass which is collected by the natives in the goat skin. Some of the resin is collected from spontaneous exudation from the cracks or fissures which are formed in the bark. The natives simultaneously collect **bdellium**, another drug, which they separate later. However, sometimes bdellium gets admixed in the drug.

Chemical Constituents

Myrrh contains volatile oil 7–17%, resin 25–40% and gums 57–61% and 3–4% impurities. Volatile oil contains cuminic aldehyde, eugenol, meta-cresol, pinene, limonene, dipentene and two sesquiterpenes. Volatile oil resinifies on exposure to air. Because of volatile oil, myrrh should be stored in lumps in airtight containers. Resin is complex and a greater part of it is soluble in ether and consists of three free resin acids, α-, β- and γ-commiphoric acids, and esters of another resin and two phenolic resins. Ether insoluble portion consists of two resin acids, α-, β- and γ-herabomyrrholic acids. Gum resembles gum acacia and contains an enzyme oxydase and on hydrolysis yields arabinose. The constituents of the volatile oil reported earlier were not confirmed. The oil thus contains exclusively sesquiterpene derivatives.

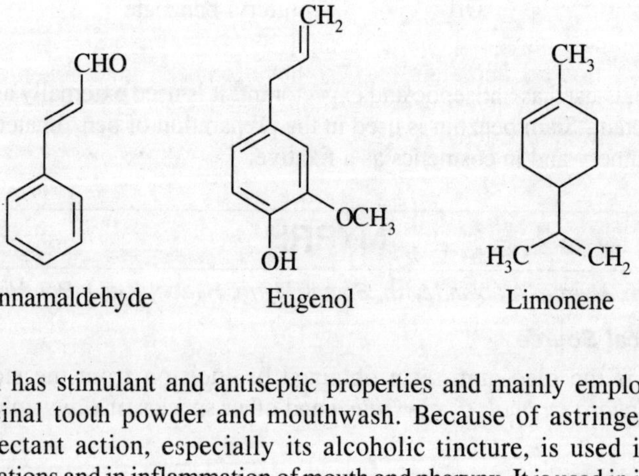

Cinnamaldehyde   Eugenol   Limonene

Uses

Myrrh has stimulant and antiseptic properties and mainly employed in medicinal tooth powder and mouthwash. Because of astringent and disinfectant action, especially its alcoholic tincture, is used in skin applications and in inflammation of mouth and pharynx. It is used in incense and perfumes.

NIM LEAF

Nim, Nimba (Hindi and Punjabi), Margosa tree (Eng.),
Kohumba (Guj.), Neem (Unani)

Botanical Source

Nim consists of the dried leaves of *Azadirachta indica* (Syn. *Melia azadirachta*).

Family

Meliaceae.

Geographical Source

A fairly large evergreen tree, about 15 metres in height, occurs throughout India and other countries of South-East Asia.

Chemical Constituents

Neem is one of such important trees whose all parts are esteemed, as they i.e. the parts or organs – leaves, flowers, young fruits, nuts or seeds, including the barks of the stems and roots and gum and toddy – have been chemically investigated and they have shown the presence of varied phyto-chemicals. Surely their (azadirachtin, nimbin, nimbidin, etc.) mention here, especially with chemical structures, is beyond the scope of the book, which is considered here under the class of antiseptics and disinfectants in the prescribed syllabus.

The leaves have been shown to contain quercetin and β-sitosterol, besides ascorbic acid, carotinoides and amino acids.

The neem oil contains sulphur-containing constituents and some very bitter principles. The bitter principles, also said to be present in the trunk bark, are called nimbin and nimbinin, nimbidin and nimbidol.

Work on flowers and stem exudate has also been undertaken and reported. Of the other constituents nimatone, margosine, essential oil and tannins have been reported.

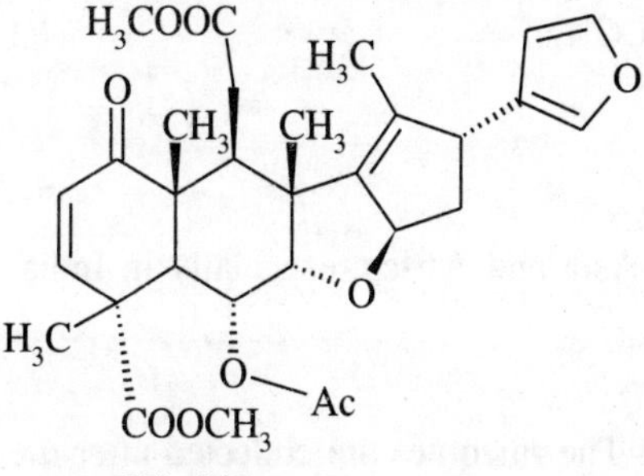

Nimbin 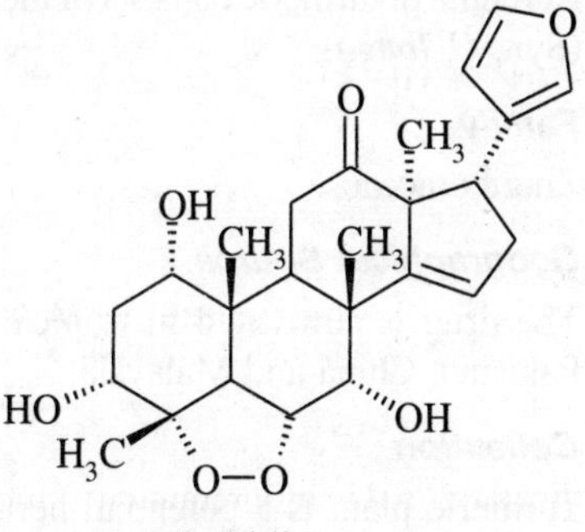   Nimbidin

Uses

Nim tree and its different organs are known for their antiseptic, insecticidal, anthelmintic, deodorant, diuretic, emmenogogue and febrifuge properties. Nim leaves have exhibited antibacterial activity. Nim oil and its bitter constituents, namely nimbidin and nimbidol, have shown antifungal and spermicidal activity and is found effective in skin diseases. The leaf extract fractions delay blood clotting time. Besides:

- Neem twigs are used for brushing teeth in India and Pakistan. This practice is perhaps one of the earliest and most effective forms of dental care.
- All parts of the tree (seeds, leaves, flowers and bark) are used for preparing many different medical preparations.
- Neem oil is used for preparing cosmetics (soap, shampoo, balms and creams).
- Besides its use in traditional Indian medicine, the neem tree is of great importance for its anti-desertification properties and possibly as a good carbon dioxide sink.
- Neem oil is useful for skin care such as acne, and keeping skin elasticity.
- Traditionally patients suffering from chickenpox sleep on the leaves in India owing to its medicinal value.

From time immemorial the insecticidal and insect-repellant properties of nim leaves have been known to forefathers who have been using the dry leaves and young branches to preserve the woollen clothes in place of now commonly used phenyl balls.

CURCUMA

Turmeric (Eng.), Haldi (Hindi and Unani),
Zardchob (Pers.), Arqussofar (Arab.)

Botanical Source

Curcuma or turmeric consists of the dried rhizomes of *Curcuma domestiaca* (Syn. *C. longa*).

Family

Zingiberaceae.

Geographical Source

The drug is cultivated in tropical Asia and Africa, especially in India, Pakistan, China and Malaysia.

Collection

Turmeric plant is a perennial herb. The rhizomes are collected after the aerial plant dies. Roots and aerial plants are removed and rhizomes are boiled for 12–14 hours in their own juice or with (addition of) water. They are then dried in the sun or in ovens. The process results in the starch getting gelatinized and also bringing out the yellow colour from the secretory cells, which spreads in the entire lot of rhizomes.

Chemical Constituents

Turmeric contains volatile oil, colouring matter curcurrun and resin. Volatile oil contains phellandrene d-sabinene, borneol and cineole. However, it contains mainly sesquiterpene hydrocarbon zingiberene and 65% two ketones, turmerone and ar-tumerone. All the three substances are related to each other.

Curcumin is responsible for the colour of the drug and consists of curcumin I, II and III. Curcumin I is 60% and is deferuloylmethane, curcumin II is 24% and is hydroxycinnamoyal feruloylmethane and curcumin III is 14% and is dihydroxy dicinnamoylmethane.

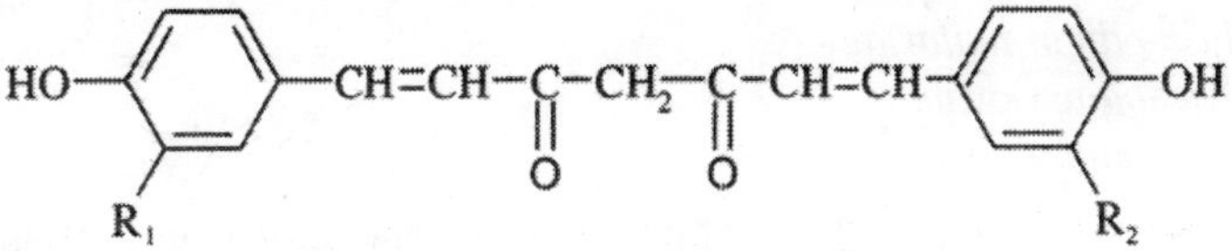

	R_1	R_2
Curcumin I	OCH_3	OCH_3
Curcumin II	OCH_3	H
Curcumin III	H	H

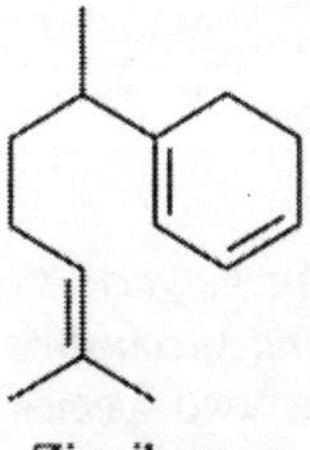

Zingiberene 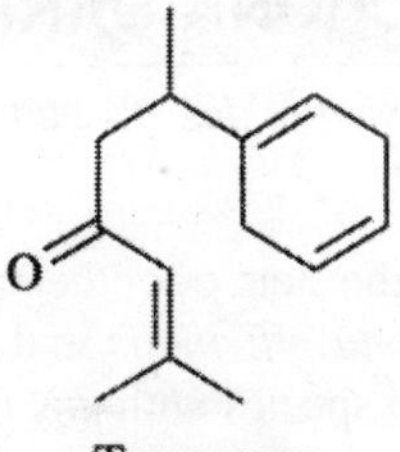   Turmerone 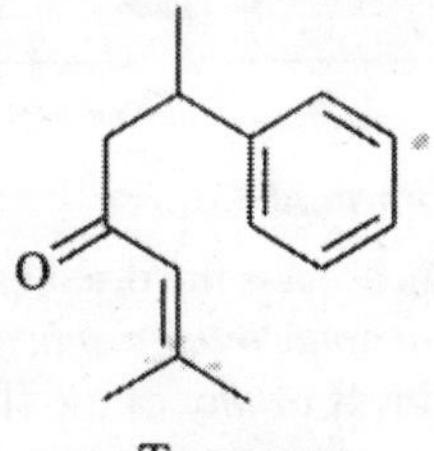   ar-Tumerone

Uses

Volatile oil is responsible for the aromatic and pungent properties of the drug. Curcumin I and II have choleretic and cholagogue action while curcumin III has anticholeretic action and so in some pharmacopoeias *C. domestica* is not official but only Java curcuma is official.

It is, however, used as choleretic and cholagogue and is used in liver diseases. Turmeric has anti-inflammatory action and compares favourably with phenylbutazone. It is useful in cough and bronchitis. It has great reputation in Ayurveda and is used in diabetes and liver diseases. Turmeric is one of the ingredients of a spice known as Curry powder used in India and abroad and consists of equal parts of coriander, cinnamon pimento, clove, nutmeg, ginger and turmeric. Curcuma is said to be an antiseptic and disinfectant.

Turmeric is used for identification of boric acid and ammonia. Turmeric paper gives red colour with boric acid and with fumes of ammonia becomes blue. Further turmeric is used as a dye for food materials such as cheese and sweets and for fabrics of wool and silk.

ANTIMALARIALS

Malaria is a protozoal disease caused by *Plasmodium* species namely:

1. *Plasmodium falciparum*
2. *Plasmodium malariae*
3. *Plasmodium ovale*
4. *Plasmodium vivax*

The disease is transmitted by the bites of female *Anopheles* mosquito. The protozoa mainly affects the liver and red blood cells of the infected person. The clinical symptoms of malaria include fever, chills, headache, nausea, vomiting, anaemia and enlarged spleen and liver. Alkaloids of cinchona are very useful in malaria.

CINCHONA BARK

Countess, Peruvian or Jesuit's bark, Cinchona

Botanical Source

Cinchona is the dried bark of the stem or of the root of *Cinchona calisaya*, *Cinchona ledgeriana*, *Cinchona officinalis* and *Cinchona succirubra* or hybrids of any of the first two species with any of the last two species.

Family

Rubiaceae.

Plants are tropical shrubs or trees. Members of the family contain alkaloids of quinoline ring as quinine, isoquinoline ring as emetine and indole ring as yohimbine.

Geographical Source

Cinchona is a native of South America occurring wild there. At present, it is mainly cultivated in Indonesia (Java), Zaire, India, Guatemala and Bolivia.

Cultivation

Cinchona is cultivated by planting the seeds. Seeds which produce bark rich in alkaloids are selected. Better quality of the drug is obtained by hybridization. Cinchona plants require hot humid and tropical climate. The average temperature should be 15–20°C, which by day should be 20–30°C and 10–15°C by night. Rainfall should be heavy, i.e., from 75″ to 180″ per year. Plants do not tolerate frost. Selected strains of seeds are sown in seed beds, protected from rains by roof. Seedlings are transplanted twice till they are about 1½ years old. Then they are transplanted at a distance of 1 metre in rich, porous and well-drainted soils in slopes or terraces at altitude of 1,000 to 2,000 metres. In the first few years, protection especially from wind is given to the plants by planting banana trees in between them.

Collection

Cinchona bark is collected in rainy season from 6–9 years old plants by uprooting or coppicing methods and plants are gradually thinned. Bark from branches, stem and root is collected by making suitable incisions and dried. During drying, pale colour of inner surface of fresh bark is changed to red because of the formation of cinchona red from cinchotannic acid.

Chemical Constituents

Cinchona bark contains about 25 alkaloids of which main crystalline alkaloids are quinine, quinidine, cinchonine and cinchonidine. These alkaloids contain quinoline ring and a quinuclidine ring with vinyl group attached to it.

The alkaloids are formed in the middle layer of the parenchyma tissue of the bark.

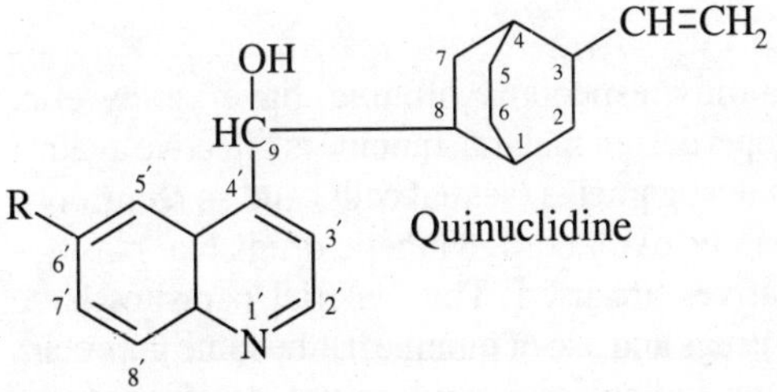

Quinoline   Quinuclidine   Quinic acid

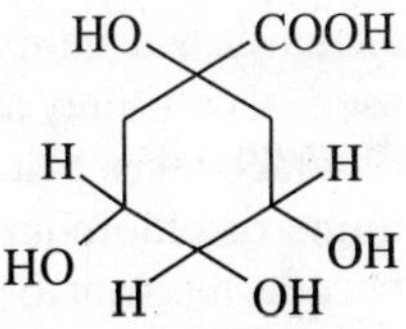

Quinine

Quinine and quinidine contain methoxy groups and are stereoisomers. Quinine and quinidine show blue fluorescence with oxygenated acids like sulphuric acid in filtered ultraviolet light. Cinchonine and cinchonidine do

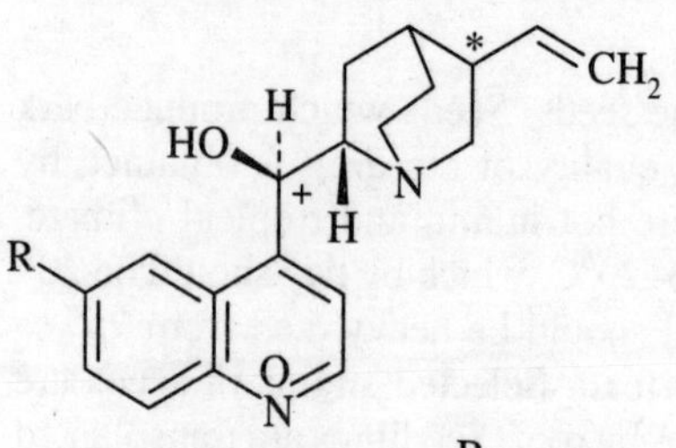

Quinine	OCH$_3$		Quinidine	OCH$_3$
Cinchonidine	H		Cinchonine	H

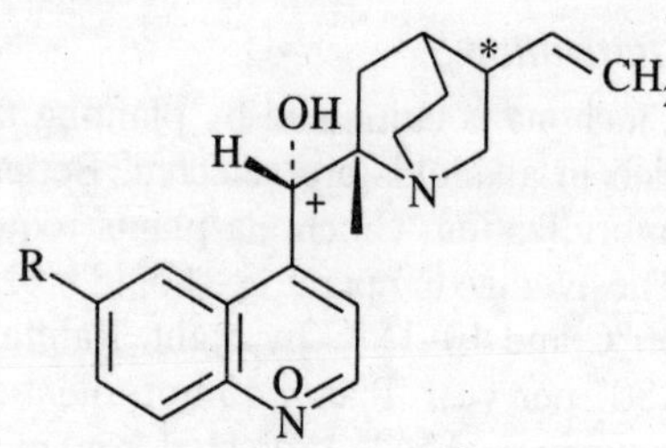

not contain methoxy groups and are stereoisomers and do not show fluorescence.

Quinine and cinchonidine with tartaric acid form insoluble salts, and are levorotatory, while quinidine and cinchonine with tartaric acid form soluble salts and are dextrorotatory.

Alkaloids are in combination with quinic acid and cinchotannic acid. Cinchotannic acid decomposes into insoluble phlobaphene cinchona red and is responsible for the red colour of the bark, and may be present upto 10% in *C. succirubra*. Quinovin, a bitter glycoside, calcium oxalate and starch are also present.

Tests

1. Cinchona bark powder when heated in a dry test tube, preferably with little glacial acetic acid, forms reddish fumes which are condensed on the upper side of the test tube.
2. Cinchona bark, on being moistened with sulphuric acid, shows a blue fluorescence in ultraviolet light.

Uses

Cinchona bark and its alkaloids, especially quinine, have antipyretic, analgesic and antimalarial properties. In malaria, quinine is effective against asexual cells only and not against gametes (sexual cells) and so recurrence of attack takes place. This can be avoided if synthetic drugs like plasmo-quine or chloroquine derivatives are used. The malarial parasites have become resistant to synthetic drugs and use of quinine has become important again. Quinine is anti-infective and analgesic and is used in cold sickness and flu. Quinine is also protoplasmic poison and oxytocic. Cinchonidine has weaker action than quinine, but is used in rheumatism, neuralgia and sciatica. It is used as antispasmodic in whooping cough. Quinidine is cardiac depressant and is used to inhibit auricular fibrillation. Cinchona alkaloids are used as stomachic and bitter tonic. Quinine is used in USA in the preparation of effervescent appetite stimulant tonic drinks.

Allied Drugs

Cuprea bark.

Cuprea Bark

It is obtained from *Remijia pedunculata.*

Family

Rubiaceae.

Geographical Source

Columbia.

Characters

The colour of the bark is copper-red. It is very hard and breaks with granular and splintery fracture.

It contains numerous transversely elongated stone cells which are absent in cinchona. It contains quinine and quinidine and is used as a source of quinidine. Bark of *R. purdieana* known as false Cuprea bark contains no quinine.

OXYTOCICS

Oxytocics are drugs which cause contraction of uterus muscle. These agents are used to induce labour. They are also used to treat post-partum haemorrhage.

Methyl ergometrine tablet and Methyl ergometrine maleate injection are clinically used in the active management or 3rd stage of labour.

ERGOT

Ergot of Rye, Ergot

Botanical Source

Ergot is the dried sclerotium of the fungus *Claviceps purpurea* Tulsanse, arising in the ovary of rye plant *Secale cereale* (Family Gramineae).

Family

Clavipitaceae (Ascomycetes).

Geographical Source

North-West Spain (exported from Portugal) and Russia. Now large quantities are cultivated in Czechoslovakia, Germany, Hungary, Switzerland and India.

Collection

The life cycle of *Claviceps purpurea* shows the following three distinct stages:

1. Sphacelia or Honeydew stage
2. Sclerotium (Ergot) stage
3. Ascospore stage

1. **Sphacelia or Honeydew Stage:** The rye plant bears flowers at the end of spring or in early summer. During this period spores of the fungus from ascospore stage are carried by insects or wind currents, reach the flowers of the rye plant and deposit at the base of the ovary of the flowers. Spores germinate, forming hyphal strands which penetrate the walls of the ovary by enzymatic action and form a soft white mass on the surface of ovary known as sphacelia. This sphacelia secretes a sweet saccharine yellow-coloured liquid called honeydew. Hence this stage is called sphacelia or Honeydew stage. Insects are attracted by the honeydew because of its sweet taste. Insects suck the sweet liquid containing the abstracted conidia, the asexual spores, and carry them to other plants and spread the disease.

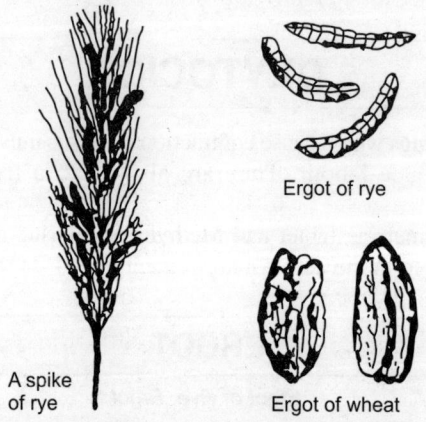

Ergot of rye

A spike
of rye

Ergot of wheat

Fig. 3.7. Ergot, *Claviceps purpurea.*

2. **Sclerotium Stage:** In the first stage hypha penetrates only the walls of the ovary. Gradually it penetrates deeper and deeper into the ovary and develops further feeding itself on the mass of the ovary and in the end replaces the entire mass of the ovary by a new hard compact dark purple parenchymatous mass. Thus elongated sclerotium, known as ergot, is produced. This stage is called Sclerotium stage or Resting stage. In the beginning sclerotium is small in size and projects on the rye plant, showing remains of sphacelia on its apex. It is collected. For medicinal purposes this sclerotium is used.

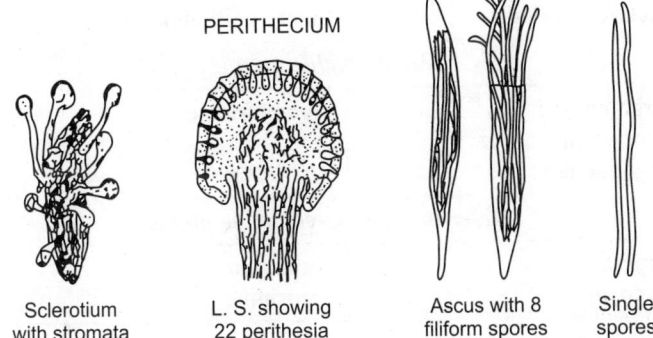

Fig. 3.8. Ergot, *Claviceps purpurea*. Germination of sclerotium, showing different stages – stroma, fruitification with perithesia and ascus with eight spores and single spore.

3. **Ascospore Stage:** Some sclerotia are not collected and fall on the ground and these sclerotia produce next year stromata. These stromata have a stalk and a round head. The head contains flask-shaped pockets known as perithecia. A number of asci are found in perithecia and each ascus (sporangium) contains eight filamentous ascospores. As mentioned in the first stage these ascospores are carried by insects or wind currents to the flowers of the rye plants and life cycle of the fungus is completed in this way.

Collection

Ergot, which is projecting and fully developed, is collected either by hand or by machine in summer in the month of July or August. Ergot is sometimes collected along with rye cereal and subseguently separated by sieving. Ergot is then dried well to remove moisture.

Chemical Constituents

The ergot alkaloids hold a vital position as medicinals which are being used in internal medicine, neurology and psychiatry. More than a score of alkaloids have been obtained from the fungus *Claviceps purpurea*.

Ergot contains six pairs of indole alkaloids out of which alkaloids of only one pair i.e. ergometrine and ergometrinine is water-soluble, while alkaloids of the remaining five pairs are water-insoluble. Each pair has an active alkaloid and a corresponding inactive alkaloid. Active alkaloids are derivatives of lysergic acid, while inactive alkaloids are derivatives of iso-lysergic acid. Ergotoxine, which was formerly considered to be a single alkaloid, has now been shown to be a mixture of three alkaloids, namely ergocristine, ergocornine and ergocryptine. The structure of active and inactive alkaloids of ergot given here should be clearly understood. Ergo-metrine and ergometrinine are lysergic and isolysergic acid derivatives in

	Active alkaloids	Inactive alkaloids
	Water-soluble group	
1.	Ergometrine (known in USA as ergonovine)	Ergometrinine
	Water-insoluble ergotamine group	
2.	Ergotamine	Ergotaminine
3.	Ergosine	Ergosinine
	Water-insoluble erogotoxine group	
4.	Ergocristine	Ergocristinine
5.	Ergocryptine	Ergocryptinine
6.	Ergocornine	Ergocorninine

which carboxyl group is combined with amino alcohol. They are acid amide alkaloids, combined with 2-aminoporpanol. Alkaloids of ergotamine and ergotoxine groups are polypeptides of lysergic acid and isolysergic acid with amino acids (see chemical structures).

Ergometrine (ergonovine), the specific uterotonic alkaloid, is found in ergot along with a small quantity of ergometrinine (ergonovinine). The alkaline hydrolysis of ergometrine gives lysergic acid and L(+)-2-amino-propanol.

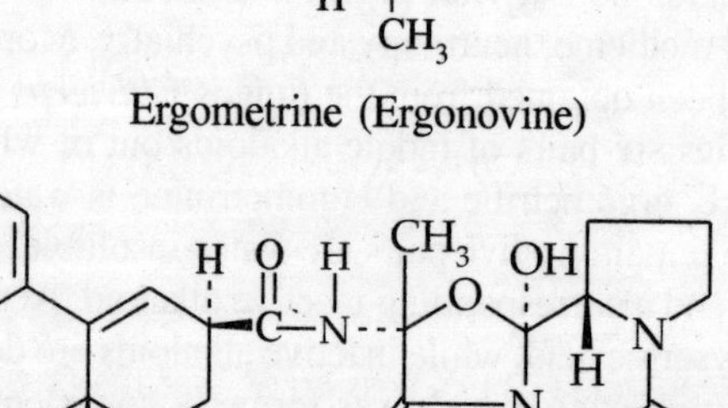

Ergometrine (Ergonovine)

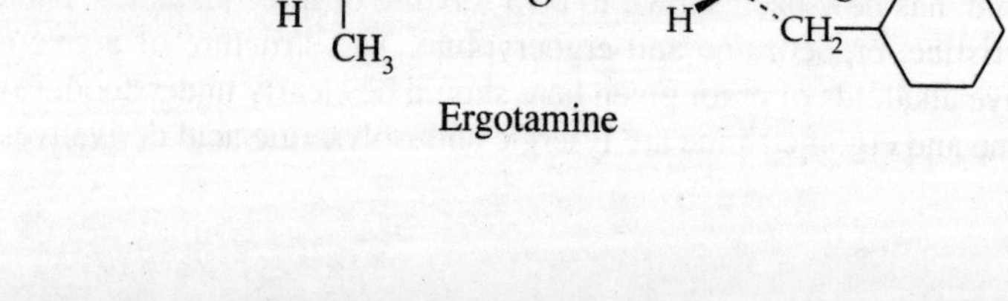

Ergotamine

R	COR structure (9,10 positions)	COR structure (9,10 positions)
	(numbered positions 9, 10; N–H indole)	(numbered positions 9, 10; N–H indole)
—OH	(+)-Lysergic acid	(+)-Isolysergic acid
—NH$_2$	Lysergic acid amide (Ergine)	Isolysergic acid amide (Erginine)
—N(C$_2$H$_5$)$_2$	Lysergic acid diethyl-amide (LSD)	
—NH—CH(CH$_3$)(OH)	Lysergic acid methyl-carbinolamide	
—NH—C(H)(CH$_3$)(CH$_2$OH)	Ergonovine (Ergometrine)	Ergometrinine
—NH—C(H)(CH$_2$CH$_3$)(CH$_2$OH)	Methylergonovine	
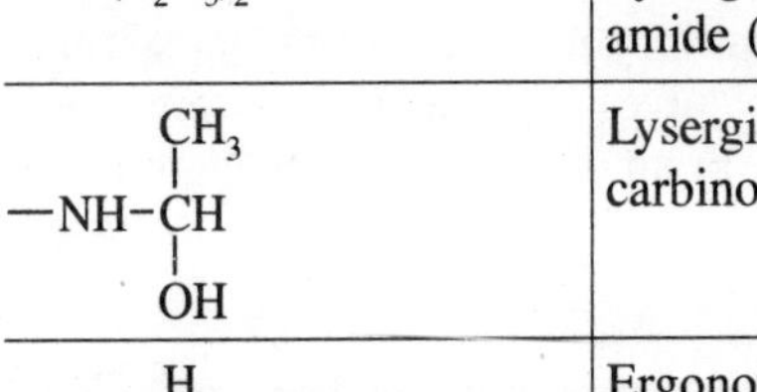 (complex structure)	Ergotamine	Ergotaminine

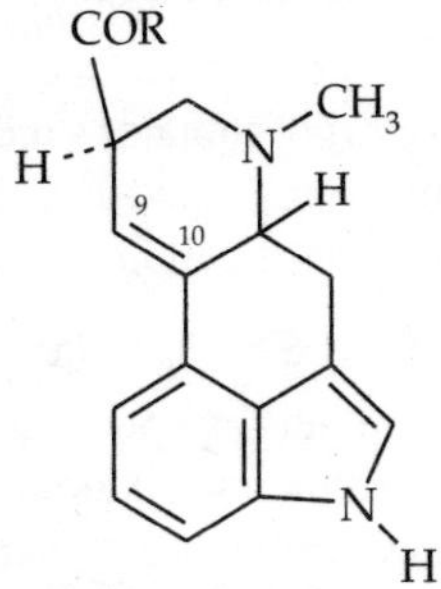

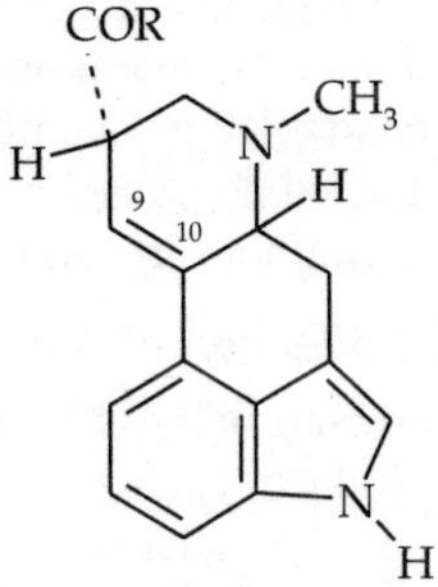

Ergotamine, obtained from Swiss ergot, was the first ergot alkaloid to find widespread medical application. Cleavage products resulting from hydrolytic degradation of ergotamine are lysergic acid, proline, ammonia, pyruvic acid and phenylalanine.

Ergot also contains 30–40% of fixed oil. The unsaponifiable part of the fixed oil contains about 1% ergosterol and other sterols. Ergosterol yields on irradiation vitamin D_2. Ergot contains a red colouring matter, sclereythrin and amino acids, histamin, tyrosin and acetylcholine. The cell wall of ergot is chitinous in nature instead of cellulosic, usually found in plants.

Production of Alkaloids in Saprophytic Culture

By saprophytic culture of ergot spore, mycelium is produced which produces conidiospores. Medicinal alkaloids are produced only in the next parasitic sclerotium stage. Ergot is produced by inoculation of cultured conidiospores on rye plant and ergot sclerotia are produced in about 6 weeks which are collected. Large scale production of ergot is carried out in many European countries by this method.

By saprophytic culture of *Claviceps purpurea* lysergic acid alkaloids are not produced but instead related clavine alkaloids are produced which have no medicinal importance.

In 1960, it was shown that by saprophytic culture of potent strain of *Claviceps paspali* lysergic acid derivatives especially (+)-lysergic acid methyl carbinol amide are produced. From these derivatives ergometrine and ergotamine are synthesized.

Storage

Ergot deteriorates in the presence of moisture, light, higher temperature, air, bacteria, mould and insects. Ergot if stored in entire condition should not have more than 8% of moisture content. If stored in powdered condition it should be defatted and moisture should not exceed 6%. Fixed oil in the presence of moisture, light, air, etc. becomes rancid and free fatty acids are liberated. The fatty acids cause further deterioration. The alkaloids of ergot and chitin, if not property stored, also undergo decomposition and liberate ammonia. Since ergot is often attacked by insects, carbon disulphide, camphor, chloroform or mercury in definite proportion is added to prevent the same. Ergot should be stored as far as possible in fully well-closed containers at low temperature protected from moisture, air and light.

Chemical Tests

1. Ergot when seen in filtered ultraviolet light shows a red-coloured flourescence. Rye flour is used as food in many European countries and contamination with ergot can be easily detected by this test.
2. **Ergotoxine test:** Extract ergot powder with chloroform and sodium carbonate. Separate the chloroform layer and add to it the reagent consisting of 0.1 gm of *p*-dimethyl aminobenzaldehyde, 100 ml 35% v/v sulphuric acid and 1.5 ml of 5% ferric chloride. A deep blue colour is produced. This reaction is also used for the quantitative estimation of alkaloids by colorimetric method using ergotoxine ethanesulphonate as the standard.

Uses

Ergometrine has oxytocic action and produces much faster uterine stimulation than other alkaloids. It is used for hastening the delivery. By increasing the tone of uterine muscles it prevents postpartum bleeding. The activity of ergometrine increases with methyl group and activity of methyl ergometrine is more and lasts for a longer period. Only peptide alkaloids including 9,10-dihydroergotamine possess sympatholytic action. Action is due to competitive blocking of α-adrenergic and serotonergic receptors i.e. inhibition of adrenaline, noradrenaline and serotonin. This causes lowering of blood pressure.

Polypeptide alkaloids have uterine contracting and sympatholyic properties. By hydrogenation of 9-10 bond oxytocic property decreases and sympatholytic properties increase and 9,10-dihydroergotamine is used in migraine. Similar to Belladonna, dihydroergotamine is used as sedative and is used in Basedow's sickness, tachycardia, menopause and other disturbances of nervous system.

Mixture of equal parts of dithyroergocristine, dihydroergocryptine and dihydroergocornine produces vasodilatation, increase of cerebral blood flow, lowering of systemic blood pressure and bradycardia and is used in elderly patients. Recently ergocristine and ergocryptine by reduction of prolactin formation have shown to inhibit the growth of mammal tumours. Bromocryptine is also used for the above purpose. Bromocryptine is also used in Parkinson's disease.

As the alkaloids of ergot possess different pharmacological actions instead of the drug, in therapy definite alkaloids are used.

Polymorphism: The different stages of life cycle of ergot show distinct and different forms. It thus shows phenomenon of polymorphism.

Ergotism: Formerly sometimes ergot got mixed with rye flour and caused poisoning. This poisoning was known as ergotism and was either gangraneous (holy fire) or convulsive. In the gangraneous type because of the incomplete circulation of blood, the extremities of the limbs got paralysed, there was intense burning pain, they lost their feeling and ultimately they got detached. The cause at that time was not known and this was also known as **holy fire**. Convulsive type of ergotism was caused by the simultaneous deficiency of vitamin A.

LSD (Lysergic acid diethylamide): In the synthesis of ergometrine LSD was prepared which in small doses showed hallucinogenic property. Lysergic acid amide is found in a hallucinogenic drug used in Mexico called **ololiuqui**, consisting of seeds of *Rivea corymbosa* (Convolvulaceae) and used in Mexico for religious and magic purposes.

VITAMINS

The word **vitamins** refers to a group of essential substances which are vital for maintaninig normal cell functions, growth and development of the body. Vitamins are organic compounds required as nutrients in minute amounts by living organisms. They are called vitamins when they cannot be synthesized in sufficient quantities by an organism, and must be obtained from the diet and/or supplied from outside. They are needed in small amounts. They do not supply energy and are not much concerned with building of cellular structures. Each vitamin has specific functions to perform. Thus, the absence of vitamins or deficiency of any one of the vitamins in diet results in vitamin deficiency diseases such as scurvy, beriberi, rickets, exophthalmia, pellagra, etc. There are 13 essential vitamins which are needed for the proper body function. They are grouped into two categories:

1. **Fat-soluble vitamins**, which are stored in the body's fatty tissues.
2. **Water-soluble vitamins**, which are used by the body as such straightaway.

Any leftover water-soluble vitamins leave the body through the urine. Vitamin B_{12} is the only water-soluble vitamin that can be stored in the liver for many years.

Vitamins are classified by their biological and chemical activity and not by their structure. Thus, each 'vitamin' actually refers to a set of distinct chemical compounds which show the biological activity of a particular vitamin. Such a set of chemicals are grouped under an alphabetized vitamin generic title, such as "Vitamin A", which, for example, includes retinal, retinol and other carotinoides. 'Vitamin C' is ascorbic acid which occurs in nature and besides being an antioxidant it prevents scurvy. The term vitamin does not include other essential nutrients such as dietary minerals, essential fatty acids or essential amino acids, nor does it encompass the large number of other nutrients that promote health but are otherwise required less often.

SHARK LIVER OIL
OLEUM SELACHOIDI

Zoological Source
Shark liver oil is the fixed oil obtained from the fresh or carefully preserved livers of shark, *Hypoprion brevirostris* and other allied species.

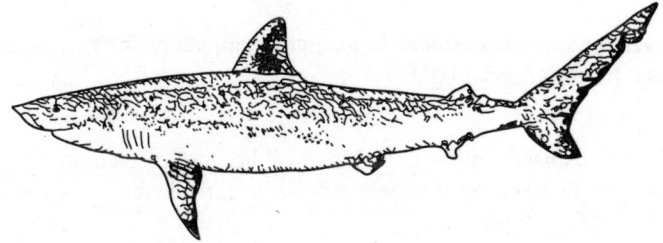

Fig. 3.9. The Shark, *Hypoprion brevirostris.*

Family

Carcharhinidae.

Geographical Source

Sea coasts of India and other European countries.

Preparation

Shark liver oil is prepared after removing the livers from the fish. The healthy liver (without gall bladder) is heated with steam. Oil exudes. It is filtered, washed and freed from water. Heating destroys the enzyme lipase. Water is removed using a dehydrating agent and the oil is chilled to separate stearin and centrifuged to remove impurities.

Chemical Constituents

Shark liver oil is rich in vitamin A. According to pharmacopoeia 1 gm contains 6,000 I.U. of vitamin A. In a good sample vitamin A may be present upto 20,000 I.U. per gram. It does not contain vitamin D and thus it is not a true substitute of cod liver oil. It contains glycerides of both saturated and unsaturated acids.

Vitamin A alcohol (Retinol)

Vitamin D_3 (Cholecalciferol)

Storage

Shark liver oil should be stored in air-tight completely filled, coloured containers, protected from light.

Uses

Shark liver oil is used similar to cod liver oil because of vitamin A after adding vitamin D. It is used as a tonic and nutritive in tuberculosis, wasting disease and malnutrition.

AMLA

Embelic myrobalan (Eng.), Amala (Hindi and German); Amlaki (Beng.); Aamlah (Urdu and Pers.); Amlaj (Arab.); Nelli (Tamil)

Botanical Source

Amla consists of fresh or dried fruits of *Emblica officinalis* (*Phyllanthus emblica*).

Family

Euphorbiaceae.

Geographical Source

The plant is widely distributed throughout the tropical and subtropical countries such as India, Sri Lanka, China and Malaysia.

The plant, which is a small to middle-sized tree plant, is found both in wild and cultivated state, common in the mixed deciduous forests in India.

Chemical Constituents

Fruit is a rich source of vitamin C. 10 gm of fresh fruits contain 600–900 mg of vitamin C. Small fruits contain more vitamin C than large fruits. Fruits contain pectin in good quantity, **glucose** and tannins **gallic acid**, **phyllemblin** and other tannins. Phyllemblin has adrenergic potentiating action as reported earlier. According to recent work fruits lose vitamin C more when dried in the sun than in the shade.

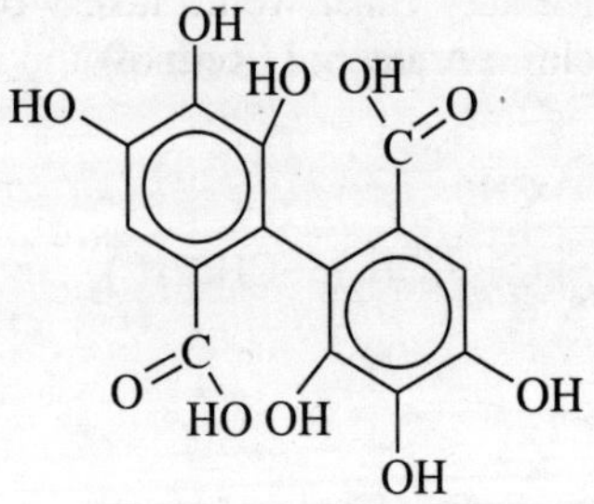

Hexahydrodiphenic acid

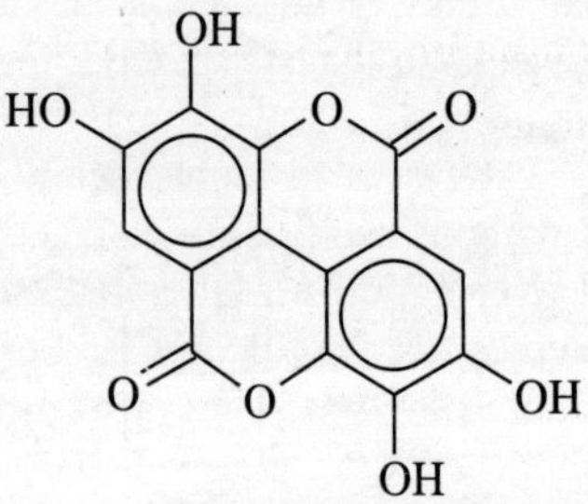

Ellagic acid

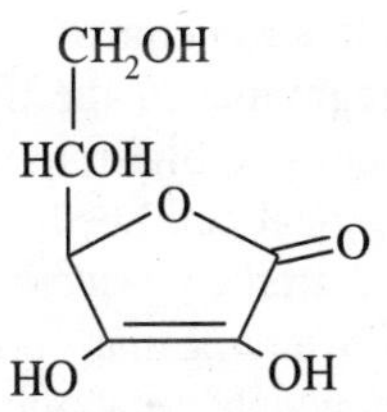

Vitamin C 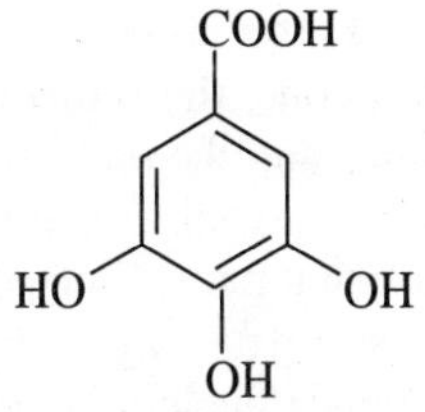   Gallic acid

Ellagic acid

Ellagic acid is present in **ellagitannins** and is obtained by hydrolysis from ellagitannins. Ellagic acid is not originally present in tannins but is formed as secondary substance from **hexahydrodiphenic acid** by loss of two molecules of water. Ellagic acid is also found in the bark of pomegranate tree, galls, chestnut, myrobalans and other fruits of Combretaceae.

Uses

Amla is a popular medicine in Ayurveda and Chyavanprashavaleh is a known preparation and is used in cough, bronchitis, haemoptysis, tuberculosis and as a rejuvenating tonic. Its action is attributed to vitamin C. It is used in scurvy. Amla is used in liver diseases including diabetes often combined with turmeric. Amla potentiates the action of adrenaline in vitro and in vivo. Amla is one of the most celebrated herbs in the Indian traditional medicine systems. Amla's traditional uses include as a laxative, eye wash, appetite stimulant, restorative tonic and to treat anorexia, indigestion, diarrhoea, anaemia and jaundice. Amla is becoming increasingly well-known for its unusually high level of vitamin C, which is resistant to storage and heat damage due to cooking.

ENZYMES

Enzymes are biological catalysts. They speed up the chemical reactions in living things. Without enzymes our alimentary canal would take weeks and weeks to digest our food. Our muscles, nerves and bones would not work properly and we would not be living properly or at all.

A catalyst is any substance which makes a chemical reaction go faster and without itself being changed. A chemical catalyst can be used over and over again in a chemical reaction without being getting used up. Enzymes act very much in the same way except that they are easily denatured by heat. They work best at body temperature and also have to have the correct pH.

Enzymes are proteins that catalyze or accelerate chemical reactions. In enzymatic reactions, the molecules at the beginning of the process are called substrates and the enzyme converts them into different molecules, the products. Almost all processes in a biological cell need enzymes to occur at significant rates. Since enzymes are extremely selective for their substrates and speed up only a few reactions from among many possibilities, the set of enzymes made in a cell determines which metabolic pathways occur in that cell.

Human saliva contains an enzyme called amylase. This enzyme helps to change (digest) starch into a sugar called maltose. Amylase works best in neutral or slightly alkaline conditions, i.e. at about pH 7. When the food reaches the small interstine, more amylase is made available by the pancreas and this changes the remaining starch into maltose. Another enzyme, maltase, changes all this maltose into glucose. Glucose is then absorbed into the blood. The human alimentary canal contains amylase, maltase, sucrase, lipase and pepsin and these are responsible for the digestion of starch, maltose, sucrose, fats and proteins, respectively.

All animals, green plants, fungi and bacteria produce enzymes. Enzymes, therefore, are not just there for the digestion of food. The enzymes which digest our food are extracellular, which means that they are found outside the cells. There are enzymes inside the cells and these are called intracellular enzymes. Enzymes are used in all chemical reactions in living processes, including respiration, photosynthesis, movement, growth, getting rid of toxic chemicals in the liver, etc.

They are made of proteins with molecular weights ranging from 13,000 to 8,40,000. Proteins are very easily affected by heat, pH and heavy metal ions. Enzymes must have the correct shape to do their job. Enzymes change their shape if the temperature or pH changes, and hence they have to have the right conditions for performing their functions. Many enzymes consist of a protein and a non-protein (called the cofactor). The proteins in enzymes are usually globular. The intra- and intermolecular bonds that hold proteins in their secondary and tertiary structures are disrupted by changes in temperature and pH. This affects shapes and so the catalytic activity of an enzyme is pH and temperature sensitive.

Enzymes are present in all biological systems and are found in all tissues and fluids of the body. They come from natural systems and when they are degraded, the amino acids, of which they are made of, can be readily absorbed back into nature. Intracellular enzymes catalyze the reactions of metabolic pathways. Plasma membrane enzymes regulate catalysis within cells in response to extracellular signals, and enzymes of the circulatory system are responsible for regulating the clotting of blood. Almost every significant life process is dependent on enzyme activity.

Enzymes work only on renewable raw materials. Fruits, cereals. milk, fats. meat, cotton, leather and wood are some typical candidates for enzymatic conversion in industry. Both the usable products and the waste of most enzymatic reactions are non-toxic and readily broken down.

The enzymes are classified, based on their action by a complex system determined by a commission on enzymes, into six major classes. The enzymes are named usually by using the ending -ase or -in.

There are three drugs (enzymes) that are included in the syllabus under the category of enzymes. They are discussed in the following pages.

PAPAYA / PAPAIN

Papaw (Eng.); Papaya (Beng., Guj., Hindi); Amba Hindi (Arab., Pers.); Arandkharbuza (Unani); Melonenbaum (Germ.); Pappali (Tamil).

Botanical Source

Papaya fruit and the enzyme papain are obtained from *Carica payapa*.

Family

Caricaceae.

Geographical Source

The plant is said to be originally from southern Mexico and America. The papaya plant is now cultivated in most countries with a tropical climate, including India, Pakistan, Bangladesh and Sri Lanka.

Chemical Constituents

Fruit's pulp contains a caoutchouc-like substance, a soft yellow resin, fat, albuminoids, sugar, pectin, citric, tartaric and malic acids and dextrin. Seeds contain an oil. Leaves contain an alkaloid known as carpaine and a glucoside carposide.

Papain (papayotin) is usually produced as a crude, dried material by collecting the latex from the fruit of the papaya tree. The latex is collected after scoring the neck of the fruit (shallow incision on four sides) where it may either dry on the fruit or drip into a container. This latex is then further dried in the sun or by artificial heat to get it as a dried, crude material. A purification step is necessary to remove contaminating substances. This purification consists of solubilization and extraction of the active papain enzyme system through a special process. This purified papain may be supplied as powder or as liquid. The powder is white or greyish white and is somewhat hygroscopic. It is not completely soluble in water and glycerin. Papain is capable of digestion of 35–40 times of its weight of lean meat. Papayotin is rich in several enzymes.

Papain is a cysteine protease. It consists of 212 of amino acids stabilized by 3 disulfide bridge. Its 3D structure consists of 2 distinct structural domains with a cleft between them. This cleft contains the active site, which contains a catalytic triad that has been likened to that of chymotrypsin. Its catalytic triad is made up of 3 amino acids: cysterine-25 (from which it gets its classification), histidine-159 and asparagine-158. Papain is rich in several enzymes, one of which is peptidase I, which is capable of converting proteins into dipeptides and polypeptides; a rennin-like coagulating enzyme that acts on the casein of milk, an amylolytic enzyme; a clotting enzyme similar to pectase and an enzyme that has a feeble activity on fats (also see general description on enzymes above).

Uses

The primary use of papaya is as an edible fruit. The ripe fruit is usually eaten raw, without the skin or seeds. The unripe green fruit of papaya can be eaten cooked, usually in curries, salads and stews.

Papaya is rich in papain, a protease, which is useful in tenderizing meat and other proteins. Its ability to break down tough meat fibres was utilized for thousands of years by indigenous Americans. It is included as a component in powdered meat tenderizers, and is also marketed in tablet form to remedy digestive problems. Papain is also popular (in countries where it grows) as a topical application in the treatment of cuts, rashes, stings and burns. Papain ointment is commonly made from fermented papaya flesh, and is applied as a gel-like paste.

Women in India, Pakistan, Sri Lanka and other parts of the world have long used papaya as a folk remedy for contraception and abortion. Medical research in animals has confirmed the contraceptive and abortifacient capability of papaya, and also found that papaya seeds have contraceptive effects in adult male langur monkeys, possibly in adult male humans as well. Papain has been employed to relieve the symptoms of episiotomy (surgical incision of the vulva for obstetric purpose). The black seeds are edible and have a sharp, spicy taste. They are sometimes ground up and used as a substitute for black pepper.

Papain (and fruit) is also used in attacks of insects, ascarides, oxyurens, trichocephalens and nematodes. Preparations are used in attacks of stomach and intestine by round worms and a number of other worms.

In short it can be said that papain is used in biochemical research involving the analysis of proteins in the preparation of various remedies for indigestion, in tenderizing meat and in enzyme-action cleansing agents for soft contact lenses.

DIASTASE

Amylase, Malt Diastase, Maltin, Ptyalin

A diastase (from Greek meaning "separation") is any one of a group of enzymes which catalyses the break down of starch into maltose. It was the first type of enzyme discovered in 1833 in malt solution. Today diastase means any α-, β-, or γ-amylase (all of them hydrolases) that can break down carbohydrates.

Amylases are enzymes that catalyze or accelerate the hydrolysis of starch. These are a widespread group of enzymes that hydrolyse the glycosidic bond between two or more carbohydrates or between a carbohydrate and a non-carbohydrate moiety.

Malt diastase is a carbohydrolytic enzyme useful for digestive support and general nutrition support. Malt diastase is characterized by the ability to break down amylose and other polysaccharides. The enzyme works with amylase and glucoamylase to digest carbohydrate-rich foods such as grains as well as malt, maltose and sugars. Malt diastase is also known as maltase. It is produced by the cells lining the small intestine.

Botanical Source

Diastase is obtained from barley, which is the dried grain of one or more varieties of *Hordeum vulgare*. Malt or malted barley is artificially germinated barley grain.

Family

Gramineae.

Preparation

Malt is prepared from heaps of barley grains which are kept with water in a warm room, till they protrude caulicles. The grain is quickly dried. The enzyme diastase, which is present in the moist and warm grains, converts the starch into maltose. This stimulates the embryos to grow. The embryos are killed when the grains are dried.

Characters

The malt resembles barley and has an agreeable odour and sweet taste. It contains 50–70% of the sugar, maltose; 15% of dextrins; 8% of proteins and enzymes diastase and peptase.

Malt extract is produced by extracting malt from the varieties of *Hordeum vulgare* by the infusion process. The infusion is made with water at 60°C. The expressed liquid is concentrated at the same temperature, preferably under reduced pressure. The extract is mixed with 10% of glycerin by weight. It contains dextrins, maltose, small amounts of glucose and amylolytic enzymes. It can convert five times its weight of water-soluble sugars.

Diastase: Malt diastase is a light tan or yellowish-white amorphous powder extracted from barley by infusion process. It is soluble in ethanol. Malt diastase is active in the temperature range 20–50°C. Optimum pH range is 4–8. The product is standardized to 4000° Lintner. It can convert 50 times its weight of potato starch into sugars.

Uses

Diastase as such is made use of for manufacturing starch and for conversion of starch into sugar. It is also utilized to remove starch from fabrics.

Malt extract is used as an easily digested nutritive and as an aid in digesting starch.

YEAST

Farex medicinalis, Cerevisiae fermentum

Botanical Source

Yeast consists of unicellular fungi and is obtained from *Saccharomyces cerevisiae* and other species of *Saccharomyces*.

Family

Saccharomycetaceae and the Order is Ascomycetes.

Preparation

Yeast available in the market is brewer's or baker's yeast and is obtained as by-product in the manufacture of alcohol or it can be obtained as the sole product of manufacture. Yeast is grown in a suitable medium containing sucrose, nitrogenous matter and inorganic salts. If yeast is grown at a temperature 20–25°C it multiples rapidly by the process of gemmation. Yeast is separated from the medium, washed, and passed through filter press. Yeast obtained in this way is known as 'compressed yeast' or 'baker's yeast' and contains 70% moisture and is converted into dried yeast by heating at a temperature below 30° C until the moisture content is 9%.

Characters

Dried yeast occurs as buff or brownish powder, consisting of dead cells. Under the microscope, it shows spherical, elliptical or ovate cells up to 8 μm long, some showing budding. Yeast should not contain starchy material.

Chemical Constituents

Dried yeast contains constituents of vitamin B-complex like vitamins B_1, B_2, B_6, B_{12}, nicotinic and folic acids. It contains nucleoprotein, carbohydrates, particularly glycogen, fat sterol and numerous enzymes including zymase, diastase and invertase.

Storage

Yeast should be stored in a cool dry place protected from light and moisture.

Uses

Yeast is important in the manufacture of alcohol and bread. Dried yeast is used as a source of B vitamins. It is rich source of biologically complete protein and is used in the manufacture of nucleic acid. As a nutritional diet supplement, called "nutritional yeast", it is used by strict vegetarians as a rich source of proteins and vitamins. It is considered a substitute for proteins.

PERFUMES AND FLAVOURING AGENTS

Ancient Egypt is said to be the original place where the primary recognized application of women's perfume was made use of. Firstly, they, the Egyptians, used it medically in their application of balms and ointments and for religious rites by burning incense.

They used perfumes as cosmetics, or in the treatment of sickness and injuries as balms and ointments. During various rituals perfumes were used as implements for clearance and purification. During the first one and half millennia before the Common Era, they applied them for increasing sexual thrills and utilized them in festivals and parties.

In succession Greece, Rome and the Islamic empires eventually heard about the ancient Egyptians' use of fragrances and they followed them. Although the Arabs maintained consistent use of women's perfumes, the increasing followers of Christianity considered them wicked and irrelevant. However, the knowledge and renown of perfumery sprung up anew approximately in the twelfth century in a new commercial upswing.

In France scented gloves became popular, and this was followed in the second half of the seventeenth century by the establishment of women's perfume manufacturers. The perfumed odour continued to increase in popularity among the aristocracy and common people at the same rate and developed into an obsession to add fragrance to everything by everybody.

It was in the nineteenth century when the discovery of eau de cologne became a turning point that the fruit and natural herbs were utilized for the enhancement of production of different fragrant and odorous materials. Some people even made injections of these apart from adding them to their bath water, wine, using it for washing out the mouth, enemas and additions to sugar.

The scent was frequently packed into a small bottle or package or applied to a saturated sponge. As more and more people wanted to package their assorted odours, glass suddenly grew in demand. The industry began to rapidly change in the wake of the modern chemistry's developments. The design of special glass containers was taken up by the renowned Baccarat company as the package grew in importance.

Gabriel Chanel's renowned Chanel No. 5 was introduced into the market in 1921. From that moment on perfumes appeared with added fruits, fresh herbs, flowered fragrances and touches of leather. Like wild flowers the fashion took off, and the women's perfume market was jointed by any designer who had become famous. Pierre Bal, Nina Ricci and Christian Dior are just some of the names producing perfumes everywhere. And today these are the brand names we are so aware of.

Aromatherapy

With the application of aromatherapy as one of the newly practised therapeutic sciences of the complementary and alternative medicines (CAM), the use of natural aromatic plants and their essences have acquired all the more importance. This branch of CAM i.e. aromatherapy has resulted in the widespread use of aromatic plants and their volatile oils and essences and has therefore made the perfumes and flavoring agents highly valuable. These volatile oils and essences are made use of through the stimulation of the sense of smell using pungent material. The vital material in this treatment are the essential oils obtained from the plant sources.

The research in perfumery industry is highly industrialized and enormous. It cannot be discussed here in any detail for obvious reasons. Suffice here to mention that fragrant plants and especially those which contain essential/volatile/ethereal oils are the ones which provide the best natural resources for research and industry interested in perfumes and flavourings agents. As regards the description and chemical background of this group of compounds is concerned, the readers are advised to look into the chapter of phytochemicals under the heading of volatile oils.

There are five drugs included under this therapeutic category and these – Peppermint oil, Lemon oil, Orange oil, Lemon grass oil, Sandal oil – are discussed one by one in the following pages.

PEPPERMINT OIL
MENTHA PIPERITA OIL

Pudina (Hindi, Beng., Arabic, Unani), Corn. Mint (Eng.)

Botanical Source

Peppermint oil is obtained by steam distillation from fresh aerial parts of *Mentha piperita*, rectified and not dementholized partially or wholly.

Family

Labiatae.

Geographical Source

The following species contain high percentage of menthol. They are cultivated in different countries.

1. **Mentha piperita:** It is cultivated widely in USA, USSR, Central, Western and Eastern European countries, England, France and Germany.
2. **Mentha arvensis var. piperascens:** It is cultivated in Japan, Brazil, South California, India (Jammu).

Characters

It is pale yellow or greenish yellow oil. It has strong penetrating odour of peppermint and pungent aromatic taste followed by sensation of cold. Its odour is mainly due to menthol.

Menthol is an alcohol obtained from different mint oils or prepared synthetically. Natural menthol is laevorotatory while synthetic menthol is racemic. Menthol is prepared from mint oils by refrigeration (–22°C). Menthol occurs in colourless, hexagonal crystals usually needle-like or as crystalline powder and has pleasant peppermint-like smell. It is antipuritic locally and is used on skin or mucous membrane as counter-irritant, stimulant and antiseptic.

Chemical Constituents

Peppermint oil contains 50–60% free menthol. American oil contains up to 78% and Japanese oil contains 70–90% menthol. Indian Pharmacopoeial limit of menthol is 50%. Esters of menthol with acetic acid and valeric acid are not less than 5% but are usually 5–15%. Menthone is about 10%. Further, the oil contains menthofuran, jasmone, a ketone and phellandrene, pinene, cineole and piperitone. Jasmone and esters of menthol are responsible for aromatic smell. If menthofuran is more, smell is unpleasant and oil gets resinified.

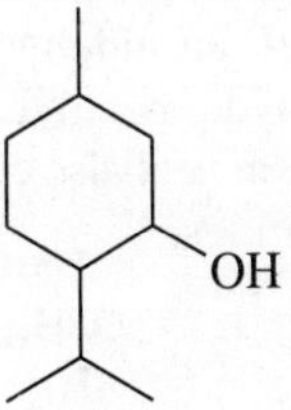

Menthol 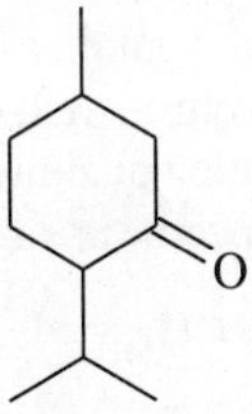   Menthone 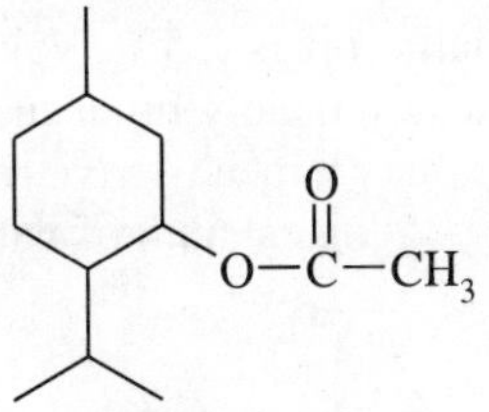   Menthyl acetate

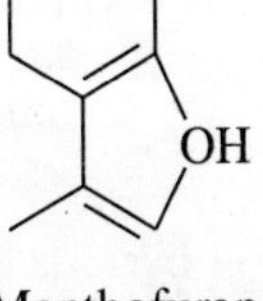

Menthofuran 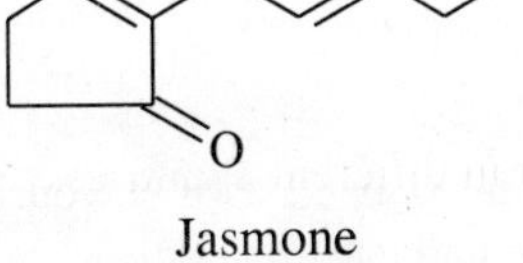   Jasmone

Uses

Peppermint oil is used in perfumery, cosmetics and in pharmaceutical and food industries. It is used as a flavouring agent, aromatic, carminative, stimulant and counter-irritant. It is used in toothpaste, candies, chewing gum and confectionary like jellies.

LEMON OIL

Oleum cortex limonis

Botanical Source

Lemon oil is the oil expressed from the fresh peel/outer part of pericarp (rind) of *Cirrus limonia* (*C. medica* var. *limonum*, *C. limon*).

According to Pharamacopoeias lemon oil (as well as some other oils) is to be obtained by mechanical means and without the aid of heat.

Family

Rutaceae.

Geographical Source

Plant is a native of India. It is now cultivated in subtropical countries, especially Mediterranean such as South Italy, Sicily, Spain, Portugal and also in Florida, California, Jamaica, and Australia. The plant is a small evergreen tree, about 4 metres in height. Fruits are collected before they are completely ripe and when their colour changes from green to yellow from October to January.

Chemical Constituents

Volatile oil is 2.5%. Volatile oil contains 4% citral, an aldehyde, and terpenes, mainly limonene 90%, citronellal, an aldehyde, geranyl acetate and other terpene derivatives in small quantities. Lemon peel also contains hesperidin, calcium oxalate and pectin in small quantities.

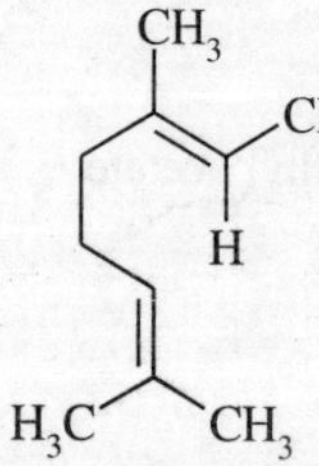

Citral 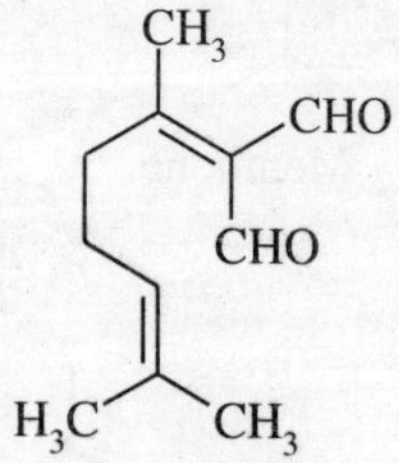   Citronellal 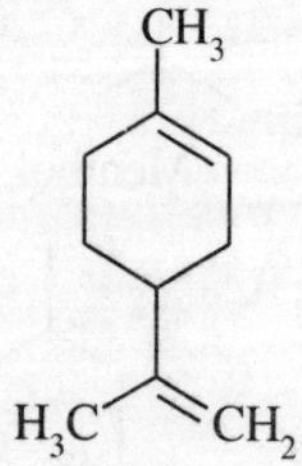   Limonene

Uses

Lemon peel is used as a flavouring agent and in perfumery. It is also stomachic and carminative.

ORANGE OIL

Botanical Source
Orange oil is the oil obtained by expression from the fresh peel of the ripe fruit of the tree, *Citrus aurantium* var. *amara* or *Citrus sinensis*.

Family
Rutaceae.

Geographical Source
The tree is native to North India, but is now cultivated in subtropical countries, especially South Spain (Seville), Sicily, Malta and Morocco. *C. sinensis* is grown in California, Florida, Brazil and West Indies.

Characters
It possesses characteristic pleasant aromatic odour and aromatic somewhat bitter taste.

Chemical Constituents
It contains 1–2% decanal and more than 90% limonene.

Uses
It is used as a flavour in perfumery and allied industries.

LEMON GRASS OIL

East India Lemon Grass oil, Indian Oil of Verbena

Botanical Source
There are two plants from which lemon grass oil is obtained. East Indian lemon grass oil is obtained from *Cymbopogan flexuosus* and West Indian lemon grass oil is obtained from *Cymbopogan citratus*.

Family
Gramineae.

Geographical Source
East Indian oil is mainly obtained from cultivated plants in Kerala in South India. West Indian oil is obtained from cultivated plants in Guatemala, Haiti, West Indies and Kenya and Zaire in Africa.

Recently in Kerala an improved variety OD-19 has been developed by selection. It contains more oil and citral content is 85–90% as against 70–75% citral of other local types.

Characters

The oil is reddish yellow to brown. It possesses an odour similar to the lemon oil. It is soluble in usual solvent and 70% alcohol.

Chemical Constituents

Leaves of both the species contain 1–2% volatile oil and volatile oil contains 70–80% citral. Oil is used as stimulant and carminative.

Uses

It is used in perfumery industry and finds a variety of uses in different fields.

Citral is a suitable substance for the synthesis of β-ionone used in the synthesis of vitamin A. So the importance of lemon grass oil has increased. β-ionone synthesized from citral is also exported from India.

SANDALWOOD OIL

*Safed Chandan (Hindi); White Sandalwood (Eng.),
Sandal Safed (Pers., Unani)*

Botanical Source

Sandalwood oil is obtained by distillation from the small chips and billets cut out of the heart wood of *Santalum album*.

Family

Santalaceae.

Geographical Source

The plant is a small evergreen parasitic tree growing wild and is also systematically cultivated in Karnataka, Coimbatore, Salem and other parts of Tamil Nadu state.

Characters

The volatile oil is present in all the elements of the wood. The sandalwood oil is viscous, with a light yellow colour and possesses a characteristic roseate and penetrating adour. It is slightly acrid and somewhat bitter in taste. It is soluble in 3–6 volumes of 70% alcohol at 20°C. It has sp. gr. 0.9732–0.985; optical rotation 14–21, refractive index 1.5040–1.5100 and acid value 0.5–0.8.

Chemical Constituents

The main chemical constituent of the oil is santalol, a mixture of isomeric sesquiterpene alcohol with different boiling points. The main sesquiterpene alcohol accounts for more than 90% of the oil. It is a mixture of two isomers known as α-santalol and β-santalol. The rest of the oil is composed of

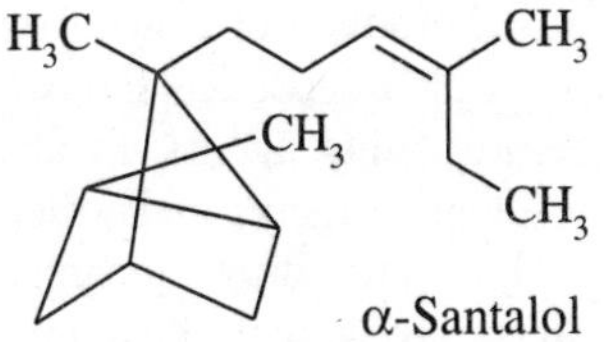

α-Santalol

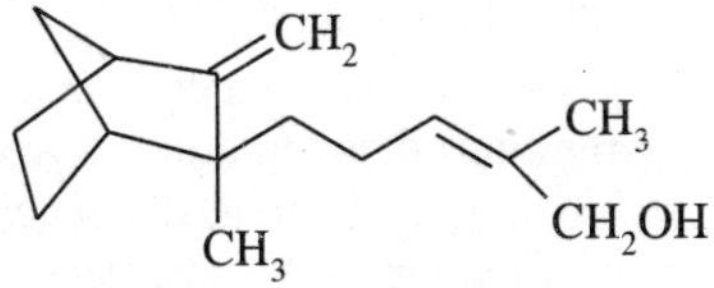

β-Santalol

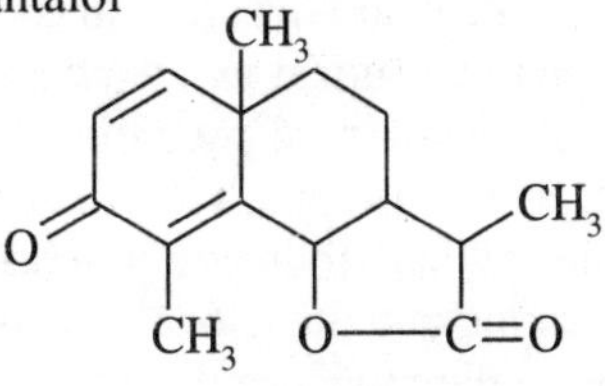

α-Santonin

aldehydes and ketones, isovaleric aldehyde, centonone, esters and free acids.

Uses

The wood is a bitter cooling sedative and astringent. Sandalwood oil is astringent and disinfectant to the mucous membranes of the genitourinary and bronchial tract. It is also diuretic, expectorant and stimulant. The oil is also used as a diaphoretic and as an aphrodisiac. Externally, the oil is used as an excellent remedy in scabies in every stage and form.

PHARMACEUTICAL AIDS

The Category (t) concerning drugs under Pharmaceutical Aids of the Syllabus deals with 14 drugs/technical materials, which are though clubbed together within this Common category, show no logical arrangement. Even if they are all justifiably belonging to more of Pharmaceutical aids' category, yet their arrangement should have some sort of scientific sequence. The best arrangement, as one will see and feel to be logical, followed hereunder is based on the phytochemical ground (which incidentally also conforms to a great extent to morphological, and to be more exact, to the unorganized class of drugs' classification).

Thus these 14 drugs are rearranged in this book as follows and will be described below one by one. As regards their detailed phytochemical nature and description is conerned, the readers' attention is drawn to Chapter 5, entitled phytochemistry.

The arrangement followed is: Honey, Starch, Acacia, Tragacanth, Guar gum, Pectin, Sodium alginate, Agar, Gelatin, Arachis oil, Olive oil, Beeswax, Lanolin and Kaolin.

The above mentioned materials are also natural products obtained from plants and animals, but their predominant use in the pharmaceutical industry as binding, disintegrating, suspending and emulsifying agents, as also stabilizing, thickening, deflocculating and sweetening agents make them more important in the pharmaceutical industry. Quite a few drugs (technical products and/or the so called pharmaceutical aids) have a dual role to play, both as a drug and a pharmaceutical aid, such as honey (as sweetening, laxative and universally acclaimed medicine for many ailments and treatment of wounds); fixed oils e.g. olive oil, almond oil, arachis oil (as emollients, vehicles, nutritional products and lubricants); agar, gelatin (as suspending, capsule making and nutritional agents).

A detailed account on the topic of pharmaceutical aids is given in the Chapter 1, dealing with the General Introduction to the book. Since the drugs included in this Category (t) of the syllabus are to be described in detail, it is considered necessary to again dilate upon the topic "Pharmaceutical aids" here, before individually describing the drugs.

Pharmaceuticals Aids

Some of the natural products obtained from plants and animals are used as pharmaceutical aids. Thus

- Gums like acacia and tragacanth are used as binding, suspending and emulsifying agents. Guar gum is used as a thickening agent and as binder and as disintegrating agent in the manufacture of tablets. Sterculia and tragacanth because of swelling property are used as bulk laxative drugs.
- Starch is used as a disintegrating agent in the manufacture of tablets and because of its demulcent and absorbent properies it is used in dusting powders.
- Sodium alginate is used as a stabilising, thickening, emulsifying, deflocculating, gelling and filming agent.
- Drugs like glucose, sucrose and honey are used as sweetening agents and as laxatives by osmosis.
- Agar is used as a laxative and emulsifying agent and in culture media in microbiology.
- Fixed oils and fats are used as emollients and as ointment bases and vehicles for other drugs. Volatile oils are used as flavouring agents.
- Gelatin is used in coating of pills and tablets and in the preparation of suppositories, as culture media in microbiology and in the preparation of artificial blood plasma.
- Beeswax is used as ointment base and thickening agent in ointments.
- Wool fat and wool alcohols are used as absorbable ointment bases.

Thus many of the natural products have application as pharmaceutical aids.

HONEY

Madhu, Mel, Shehad, Asal (Arabic)

Biological Source

Honey is the saccharine liquid prepared from the nectar of the flowers by the hive bee *Apis mellifica* and bees of other species of *Apis*.

Family

Apidae.

Order

Hymenoptera.

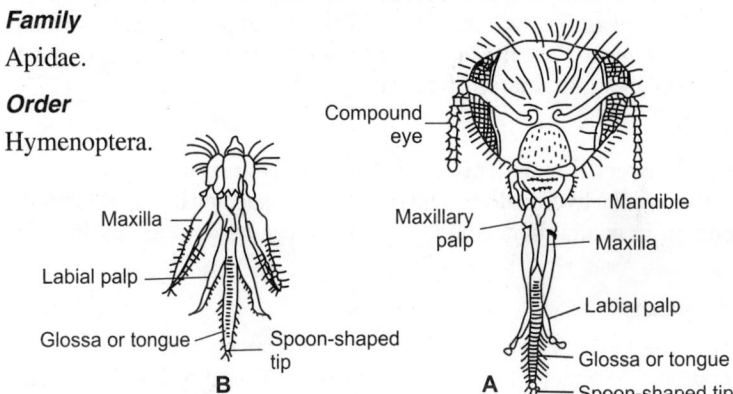

Fig. 3.10. *Apis mellifica* (Honey bee). **A.** Head of a worker bee; **B.** Proboscis.

Geographical Source

Honey is produced in certain parts of West Indies, California, Chile, Africa, Australia, New Zealand and also in India.

Preparation

Nectar of the flowers is mainly watery solution of sucrose and contains about 25% sucrose and 75% water. The worker bee sucks the nectar from the flowers by means of a long hollow tube, formed from the maxilla and labium, passes it through the mouth proboscis and the oesophagus into the honey sac or crop.

The saliva of the bee contains enzyme invertase. Sucrose along with invertase goes to the honey sac which is located in the abdomen of the bee and is hydrolyzed by invertase into invert sugar. Some invert sugar is utilized by the bee for its nutrition. The bee reaches the honeycomb and regurgitates the remaining invert sugar and deposits it into a special cell prepared earlier. In the next three days, at the temperature of honeycomb, invert sugar is converted into honey and the water is lost by evaporation. In this process honey contains about 80% invert sugar and 20% water. When the honey cells are completely filled, the bee closes it by a cap of wax. Collection is made by means of sharp knife previously immersed in hot water.

The wax cap is removed and honey is separated by keeping hive-comb in a centrifuge. Sometimes honey is separated by means of pressure. By this method honeycomb breaks and wax finds its way in honey as an impurity.

Constituents

Honey contains about 80% natural invert sugar which is a mixture of glucose and fructose. Its optical rotation is opposite to sugar and so it is called invert sugar. Sucrose, dextrin, volatile oil and pollen grains are also present in honey. Pollen grains, when seen under microscope, give information about the source of honey.

Adulterant

Artificial Invert Sugar: This is obtained by hydrolysis of sucrose by mineral acids like hydrochloric acid or sulphuric acid and contains furfural not present in natural honey and its presence can be detected by Fiche's test.

Uses

Honey is used as nutritive, demulcent and mild laxative. It is used in the preparation of oxymels. Because of osmosis it is used internally in cold sickness and externally in wound treatment. It acts as a mild antibacterial.

STARCH
Amylum

Botanical Source

Starch consists of polysaccharide granules which on complete hydrolysis yields glucose.

Starch and amylum, both the names, have historical importance. Starch was used for giving stiffness or strength to clothes for laundry purpose. The German name for starch is Starke which means strength. Amylum means without mill. In the early period, starch was prepared by softening wheat grains with water and crushing them without powdering in the mill and hence the name.

Starch is the first or primary product of photosynthesis. According to its origin and size starch is either assimilatory or reserve starch. Assimilatory starch is produced in chlorophyll containing parts of plants like stem or leaves and consists of small granules and is again utilized in the metabolism of plant after formation. Reserve starch is present in non-chlorophyll parts of the plants like root, rhizome, tuber and consists of larger granules and usually not utilized or metabolized by the plant.

Starch is obtained from:
1. Wheat
2. Maize
3. Rice
4. Potato.

The following are the botanical and geographical sources. Wheat, maize and rice belong to the same Family Gramineae.

	Species	Family	Geographical Source
Wheat	*Triticum sativum*	Gramineae	Many temperate countries of the world
Maize	*Zea mays*	Gramineae	USA, Argentina, India and other tropical and subtropical countries
Rice	*Oryza sativum*	Gramineae	India, China, Japan and other tropical and subtropical countries
Potato	Tubers of *Solanum tuberosum*	Solanaceae	Many countries of the world

Preparation of Starch

In wheat, maize and rice starch is present in the endosperm along with the proteins, mainly gliadins and glutelins collectively known as gluten. In the preparation of starch, it is necessary to remove the protein. Gluten forms with water sticky, elastic mass or swells with water and can be removed by filtration. Gluten dissolves in dilute alkali while starch is insoluble. Starch is heavier than gluten. Thus by filtration, solubility or centrifugation protein can be separated.

1. **Maize Starch:** Maize fruits are thoroughly washed to remove dirt and adhering material. Then they are macerated with water containing 1% sulphurous acid at 40–60° for two to four days. Fruits get softened. They are taken out and the liquid containing minerals, sulphur, organic phosphorous proteins and carbohydrates, etc., known as corn-steep liquor, is used as culture medium for the production of penicillin. The softened fruits are crushed in rollers and as a result embroys containing fixed oil, known as germ, is separated. On addition of water the germ floats and is skimmed off. From the germ, maize oil is obtained using oil expellers. This fixed oil contains unsaturated fatty acids, linoleic and linolenic acids and may be used as a cholesterol-transporting or suppressing fat in the blood as well in the manufacture of soap.

After removing the germ, the milky liquid is filtered through sieves of small mesh when cell-tissue and most of the gluten separates. The cell-tissue is mainly cellulosic and is used as an animal food. The milky liquid of impure starch contains proteins which are removed by the so-called tabling operation. The liquid is slowly poured in shallow tables, about 40 metres long, 20–30 cm deep and 30–60 cm broad. Starch being heavier deposits in the tables while protein falls on the sides. Traces of protein are again removed either by repeating the tabling operation as above or by treating with dilute alkali when gluten dissolves or swells and can be separated by filtration. The starch is then washed with water and dried. In modern factories instead of tabling operation protein is separated from starch by successive centrifugation.

2. **Rice Starch:** Rice starch is prepared from broken pieces of rice, which remain behind after polishing rice. Pieces of rice are macerated with 0.5% caustic soda solution. Gluten softens or dissolves. Rice pieces are taken out, crushed and macerated with water. Starch is separated from the milky starchy liquid by keeping it for some time or by centrifugation. It is then washed, dried and powdered.

3. **Wheat Starch:** Wheat is used as a food and so practically no starch is prepared from wheat. In the preparation of starch wheat flour is made into a dough by adding water and kept for about an hour when gluten in the dough swells. Lumps or balls of the dough are put into grooved rollers moving to and fro and simultaneously water is poured over them. Starchy liquid falls below from which it is separated by centrifugation. It is washed and dried.

4. **Potato Starch:** The method of preparation of potato starch is slightly different as gluten is absent in potatoes. Potatoes are washed and made into pulp by crushing in a rasping machine. Water is added to it and the solution filtered through sieve when the cellular tissue separates. The milky starchy liquid is purified by centrifugation. The washed starch it dried and powdered.

Constituents

Starch contains amylose or β-amylose and amylopectin, which are chemically two different substances. Amylose consists of straight-chained glucose units liked by α-1,4-glucosidic bonds. It is present in the inner part of the granules and is of high molecular weight and is responsible for the soluble property of starch. It is soluble in water and gives bright blue colour with iodine. Amylose undergoes hydrolysis with malt extract or β-amylose and forms maltose. Amylopectin consists of both straight as well as branched chains of glucose units, present in the outer part of granules. It consists of α-1,4 linked glucose units in straight chains and α-1,6-glucose units in branched chains. It is insolube in water and swells with water and is responsible for the gelatinizing property of the starch. It gives bluish-black colour or precipitate with iodine. Amylopectin is more and it is responsible for the framework of the starch.

Uses

Starch is nutritive, demulcent, protective and absorbent. Starch is an important food of human beings and animals and during digestion it is

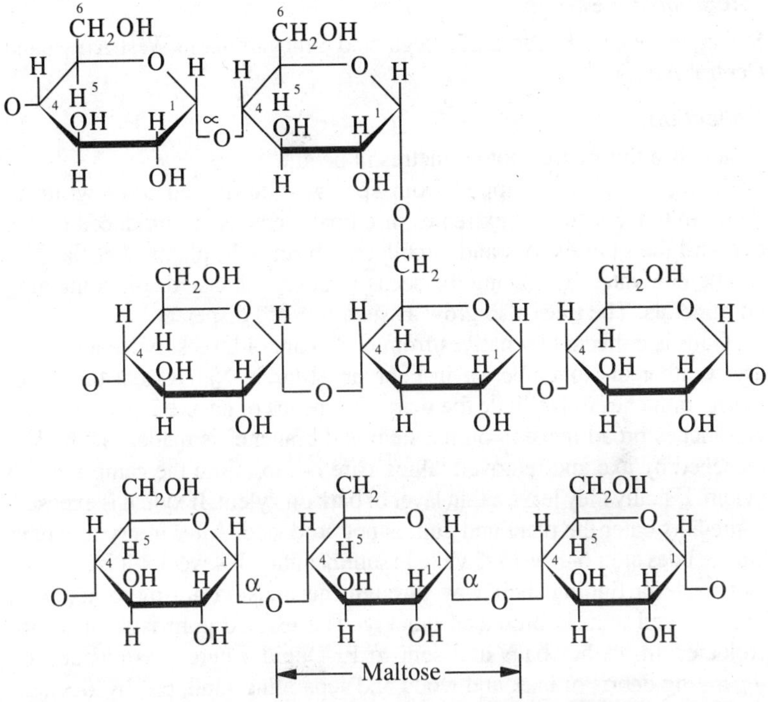

β-amylose and amylopectin

converted into glucose which is absorbed in the small intestine. Starch has demulcent action on skin and mucous membrane. It is used as a dusting powder in skin irriation, in swelling and inflammation. Starch is used as an antidote in iodine poisoning. It is used as a disintegrating agent in pills and tablets and as an indifferent diluent in solid extracts of drugs and medicinal powders. Starch is an important diagnostic agent in identification of crude drugs in pharmacognosy.

GUM ACACIA
Gum Arabic

Botanical Source

Acacia gum is the dried gummy exudation obtained from stem and branches of *Acacia senegal* and other *Acacia* species.

Family

Leguminosae.

Geographical Source

Sudan, especially Kordofan, Senegal and Senegambia in West Africa and Central Africa.

Collection

Acacia is a thorny tree upto 6 metres in height.

In Sudan, gum is tapped from specially cultivated trees while in Senegambia, because of extremes of climate, cracks are produced on the tree and the gum exudes and is collected from wild plants. Acacia trees can be cultivated by sowing the seeds in poor, exhausted soil containing no minerals. The trees also grow as such by seed dispersal.

Gum is collected by natives from 6–8 years old trees, twice a year, in dry weather in November or in February–March. Natives cut the lower thorny branches to facilitate the work. By means of an axe 2–3 ft long and 2–3 inches broad incision on the stem and branches is made. The bark is loosened by axe and removed taking care not to injure the cambium and xylem. Usually they leave a thin layer of bark on xylem. If xylem is exposed, white ants enter the plant and gum is not produced. After injury in winter gum exudes after 6–8 weeks, while in summer after 3–4 weeks. It is believed that bacteria finding their way through the incision are more active in summer and gum is produced quickly. The exuded gum is scraped off, collected in leather bags and sent to El-Obeid where it is cleaned by separating debris of bark and wood and separating sand, etc. by sieving.

Gum is dried in the sun by keeping it in trays in thin layers for about three weeks when bleaching takes place and it becomes whiter. This results in uneven contraction and cracks and fissures are formed on its outer surface and as a result original transparent gum becomes opaque. This process is called ripening of the gum.

Chemical Constituents

Acacia gum contains mainly arabin, which is a mixture of calcium, magnesium and potassium salts of arabic acid. Arabic acid on complete hydrolysis produces D-glucouronic acid, L-arabinose, L-galactose and L-rhamnose. Besides, gum contains an enzyme oxydase. Moisture is about 15% in the drug.

Uses

Gum acacia is demulcent. It is used as an emulsifying agent and suspending agent for volatile oils and resins and as binding agent for pills and tablets. Gum acacia solution has consistency similar to blood and is administered intravenously in haemolysis.

It is used in the manufacture of adhesives and ink, and as a binding material for marbling colours. The gum is considered as a gum of choice due to its compatibility with plant hydrocolloids, starches and carbohydrates.

Its use dates back about 5000 years by Egyptians as the oldest and best known natural gum including as an agent in the mummification process.

INDIAN ACACIA

Babul or Kikar Gond (Hindi)

Botanical Source
Indian acacia is the dried gummy exudation from the stem and branches of *Acacia arabica*.

Family
Leguminosae.

Geographical Source
India.

Characters
The gum is similar to gum acacia. Its solution is dextrorotatory. It does not yield xylose on hydrolysis. It is considered inferior and used in the same way as gum acacia.

Adulterant
Ghatti Gum, Indian Gum.

INDIAN GUM

Botanical Source
Indian gum is the exudation obtained from the stem of *Anogeissus latifolia*.

Family
Combretaceae

Geographical Source
This plant is native of India and Ceylon. In India the gum is collected especially in Western Ghats.

The gum occurs in vermiform or round tears and is white in colour. Inferior gum may be yellow to brown in colour. Outer surface is dull and without cracks. Fracture is uniform and glassy. The solution of ghatti gum shows only slight precipitate with lead subacetate compared to acacia. Its solution has greater viscosity than acacia solution.

Chemical Constituents
These are similar to acacia. It also contains oxydase.

This gum shows excellent emulsifying properties.

TRAGACANTH

Gummi Tragacanthae, Gum Tragacanth, Gum Dragon Anjira (Hindi)

Botanical Source

Tragacanth is the dried gummy exudation obtained from the stem of *Astragalus gummifer* and other *Astragalus* species.

Family

Leguminosae.

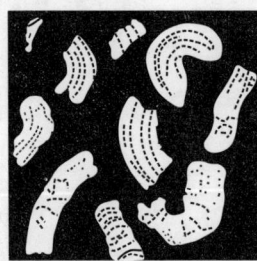

Fig. 3.11. Tragacanth pieces in black background.

Geographical Source

Iran and North Syria supply Persian tragacanth. Tragacanth is also produced in Anatolia in Asiatic Turkey and exported from Smyrna Port and is known as Smyrna tragacanth.

Plant Habit

The plant of tragacanth is a thorny shrub, about 1 metre in height and found in mountainous regions at 1350 to 3500 metres altitude. By some process, which is not known, the cells of medullary rays and pith undergo changes in their cell walls and the gum is produced in them. This gum absorbs water from the soil, swells and exerts pressure on the stem. If the stem is incised or undergoes injury the gum exudes with great speed.

Collection

It is collected by natives from two years old shrubs. Gum collected in the first year is of inferior quality. Soil is removed at the base and a vertical incision is made two inches above the soil and wedge-shaped piece of wood inserted and kept for 12–24 hours to widen the incision. The piece of wood is removed. Gum exudes with great speed and its shape depends on the type of incision. If the incision is straight, exudation is flat and ribbon-shaped and if round, shape of the gum is vermiform.

Gum is collected two days after the incision. Exudation of gum takes place regularly at intervals and on the ribbons definite concentric ridges indicating periodic exudation are seen. Rarely drastic method like burning the leaves and branches at the top of the shrub is employed. By this method large quantity of the gum is produced. Sometimes the shock is much greater and the tree dies. The gum obtained in this way is inferior, dirty and red-coloured.

Chemical Constituents

Tragacanth contains about 60–70% bassorin, the water-insoluble fraction, containing methoxy groups, which are responsihle for the swelling and gelatinizing properties of the drug. The water-soluble part is called tragacanthin and is about 30%. Tragacanthin contains tragacanthic acid and a polysaccharide. Tragacanthic acid on hydrolysis yields galactouronic acid, xylose, fructose and galactose. The polysaccharide arabino-galactose yields on hydrolysis arabinose and galactose.

Persian tragacanth contains scattered starch grains while Smyrna tragacanth contains more starch and both the gums can be identified with iodine test.

Uses

Tragacanth is used as demulcent and suspending agent for insoluble substanes and binding agent in pills and tablets. It is used as emulsifying agent for fixed oils, volatile oils and resins and in calico printing. Because of swelling properties it is used as bulk laxative (3 g powdered tragacanth with about 300 ml of liquid) and in confectionery. Swelling of tragacanth is 43% in neutral, 37% in alkaline, and 13% in acidic media.

GUAR GUM

Guar gum, Guaran guar flour, Jaguar gum

Botanical Source

Guar gum is obtained from the endosperm of the seeds of *Cyamopsis tetragonoloba*.

Family

Leguminosae.

Geographical Source

The plant is cultivated in India and Pakistan, and in USA for the production of gum.

The Plant

Guar gum or cluster bean is a drought-tolerant annual legume that was introduced into the United States from India in 1903. The commercial production of guar in the United States began in the early 1950s and has been undertaken mostly in Northern Texas and South-Western Oklahoma.

The major world suppliers are India, Pakistan and the United States, with smaller acreages in Australia and Africa.

Production

The plant is cultivated in India and Pakistan and in USA for the production of gum. Guar gum is the primary marketable product of the plant. India and Pakistan export much of their guar crop to the United States and other countries in the form of partially processed endosperm material. World demand for guar has increased in recent years leading to crop introduction in several countries.

The fruits are used as vegetable and seeds as cattle food especially for buffaloes in their native lands.

Constituents

Even though called gum, it belongs to Leguminosae mucilage, present in the endosperm of the seed and it is galacto-mannan and consists of a linear chain of 1,4-β-glycosidal mannose. 1,6-α-glycoside galactose is combined in the side chain of mannose. Guar gum consists of 60–65% mannose and 35% galactose. The gum also contains fatty acids, both free and esters, as per GLC-MS analysis.

Uses

Guar gum is used in pharmaceuticals as a thickening agent, binder and disintegrating agent for tablets. It is largely used in food processing and paper industries. It is used as appetite suppressant, bulk laxative and in the treatment of peptic ulcer.

Guar gum has recently been considered as a possible oral hypoglycemic drug. It is said to produce changes in gastric emptying and in the gastro-intestinal transition time and this can delay absorption of sugars and oligo-saccharides from the gut. Guar gum also lowers cholesterol levels possibly by binding bile salts in the gut. However, this contribution of guar gum in diabetic control remains unproven.

In the United States the food processing and paper industries are the largest users of guar gum. An important propriety product has been Gentlax®.

PECTIN
Pectins

Botanical Source

Pectins are polyuronoids and consist of mixtures of pectic substances like protopectin, pectin, pectinic acid and calcium pectate. Pectins are present in middle lamella and in walls of parenchyma.

Pectin is obtained from the dilute acid extract of inner portions of the rind of citric fruits or from apple pomace. In addition to citrus fruits (*C. aurantium, C. limon,* Family Rutaceae) a large number of other fruits, e.g. papaya, mango, guava. apples, etc. also form the sources of pectines.

Pharmaceutical pectin differs from commercial pectins, as the former is pure pectin, having no addition of sugars, organic acid, etc.

Geographical Source

Pectin is produced on large scale in India and USA. In USA commercially large amounts of pectin is obtained as a by-product of citrus canning industries.

Description

Pectin occurs as a coarse or fine powder. It is yellowish-white or cream-coloured and almost an odourless powder having mucilaginous taste. Twenty parts of water completely dissolve the pectin powder, yielding a viscous, opalescent, colloidal solution, which is acidic to litmus. One part of pectin if heated with nine parts of water should give a stiff gel.

Constituents

Pectins are linear polymers of α-1,4-glycosidally combined galactouronic acid, which is partially methylated. They are hydrocolloids and form colloidal solutions with water. Protopectin is the parent substance (of pectins), which on restricted hydrolysis gives rise to pectinic acids.

Pectins of different sources show variations in their complete constitution. These are accompanied by small amounts of neutral arabinans and galactans.

Pectinic acid

Uses

Pectins are used as emulsifying and thickening agents, plasma substitutes and in preparation of jellies. Pectin is protective and absorbs toxins because of colloidal nature and is used in digestive disturbances like diarrhoea, gastroenteritis and ulcer. Pectins are haemostyptic and are used in the treatment of wound healing. Pectins dampen the taste of other medicines and are used in improving the taste. Thus apples and lemons taste less sour because of pectins than their acid content. Fruit juices containing less pectin or no pectin are sourer than those containing pectin. Pectins are cementing substances in middle lamella and by boiling with potassium hydroxide solution hydrolysis takes place and cells are separated. In pharmacognosy this method is used for isolation of elements such as vittae of Umbelliferous fruits, laticiferous vessels and different phloem elements.

SODIUM ALGINATE

Botanical Source

Sodium alginate is obtained by alkaline extraction of *Laminaria* species (Laminariaceae) known as Kelp, of *Fucus* species (Fucaceae), and of *Macrocystis pyrifera* and other *Macrocystis* species (Lesoniaceae). Brown seaweeds belong to Phaeophyceae. The brown colour of the algae is due to carotenoid pigment fucoxanthin, which masks other pigments.

Geographical Source

Alginic acid is present in the cell wall. Brown seaweeds are found on coasts of Atlantic and Pacific Oceans. They are also found on coasts of Saurashtra in India. Alginic acid is obtained by treatment with sulphuric acid from sodium alginate.

Characters

Sodium alginate is tasteless and odourless and occurs as a coarse or fine powder. It is yellowish-white in colour. With water it forms viscous colloidal solution. It is insoluble in alcohol, ether and chloroform.

Constituents

Alginic acid is straight chain glycoside of 1,4-β-glycosidal linkage of D-mannuronic acid and L-guluronic acid residues.

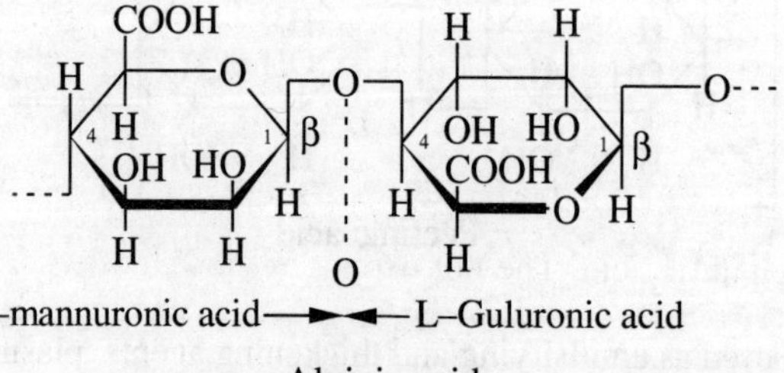

D–mannuronic acid ⟶ ⟵ L–Guluronic acid

Alginic acid

Uses

Alginates are used as stabilising, thickening, emulsifying and suspending, gelling and film and filament forming agents in pharmaceutical formulations and industries. It is used as a disintegrating agent in tablets, in cosmetics, in food industries, in the manufacture of jellies and ice creams, in textiles, inflammation of skin, dental preparation and externally as haemostatic. Besides sodium alginate, calcium, aluminium and potassium salts of alginic acid have many medicinal uses.

AGAR

Agar-agar, Japanese isinglass

Botanical Source

Agar is the dried gelatinous substance obtained by extraction with water, concentration and drying of red algae from various species of *Gelidium*, *Gracilaria* and *Pterocladia*.

Order

Rhodophyceae.

Geographical Source

Japan – *Gelidium amansii* and other *Gelidium* species; Australia – *Gracilaria confervoides*; New Zealand – *Pterocladia lucida* and other allied species. Agar is produced in USA also on Atlantic Coast area and in countries of Pacific Coast and in India. Before the Second World War Japan was the only country producing agar but it is now produced in other countries as mentioned above.

Collection

Red algae grow in rocks in shallow water and are collected by diving or by rakes with long handles. Algae are also grown on bamboos by placing them in the sea near the coast. The bamboos are taken out and algae stripped off. Collection is usually made in summer in July or August. Algae are kept in thin layers in trays in sunlight when partial drying and bleaching takes place. They are then beaten with sticks and shaken by which sand and shells attached to them are removed. After washing with water they are bleached completely by keeping them in trays in the sunlight, sprinkling water and rotating them periodically. It is then converted into agar by heating one part of algae with 30 parts of water acidified with acetic acid or dilute sulphuric acid. The hot extract is subjected to coarse filtration, again heated and then subjected to fine filtration when both large and small impurities are removed. The extract on cooling forms a jelly-like mass. This mass is cut into bars which are forced through screw press when strips of agar are obtained. Water is present in these strips and to remove this water advantage is taken of special climatic conditions prevailing in Japan. During this season in Japan, days are warm and nights are very cool, having temperature below $0°$. The strips of agar are put into trays of wire nets. During nights water in strips in converted to ice and during days ice is converted into water which trickles down. After keeping them for few days water is removed and they are again dried in the sunlight in trays.

Modern Method

In California agar is prepared utilizing recent development of techology. The algae are washed well in running water for about 24 hours and then extracted in steam-heated digester first with dilute acid and then with water for about 30 hours. This hot solution is cooled and put into an ice machine (deep freezer). Water in agar is converted into ice. Masses of agar-ice weighing about 300 lb. are powdered, melted and filtered in rotary vacuum filter. Moist flakes are put into tall cylinders and dried with dry air. Dried agar can also be obtained as a powder.

Constituents

Agar is a complex heterosaccharide and contains two polysaccharides agarose and agaropectin. Agarose is neutral galactose polymer and is mainly responsible for the gel property of agar. The structure of agaropectin is not fully known but it is sulphonated polysaccharide in which galactose and uronic acid are partly esterified with sulphuric acid.

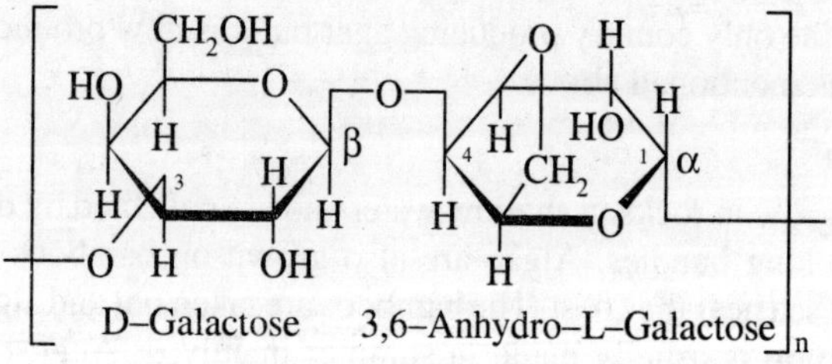

D–Galactose   3,6–Anhydro–L–Galactose

Agarose

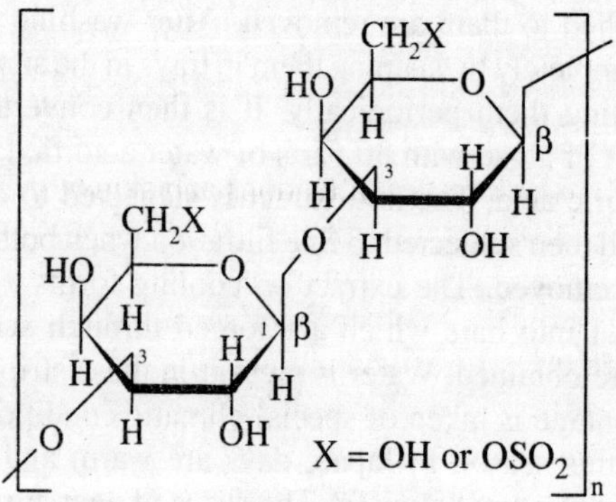

$X = OH$ or OSO_2

Agaropectin

Uses

Agar is an important material in many ways. Its uses in short are outlined below.

- It has been used as a laxative in chronic constipation (4–15 g once or twice daily in milk, fruit juice or water) and as an appetite suppressant.
- Agar can be used as an excipient for the manufacture of emulsions and fat-free ointment bases. Agar jellies are excellent nutritional support for the cultures of microorganisms; as a solid substrate to contain culture medium for microbiological work.
- In the food industry agar is an important gelling material. As such it is used as an ingredient in desserts, vegetarian gelatin substitute, a thickener for soups and ice cream.

Note: Agar, as a drug, does not practically occur as a special proprietary medicinal product. It is comparatively costly and is mostly substituted by other gelators (for detailed uses see Pharmacognosy by the same author).

GELATIN
Gelatinum

Biological Source

Gelatin is the protein derivative obtained after purifying and evoporating the aqueous extract of skin, bones and tendons of animals. The skin and bones of ox and sheep are used in the preparation.

Family

Bovidae.

Skin and bones contain a scleroprotein ossessin. Ossessin (in hide) on reaction with tannins produces leather but on boiling with water it is partially hydrolyzed and protein, gelatin, is obtained. Besides ossessin, other chemical constituents of skin and bones are different. So different methods of preparation for each are employed.

Skin Gelatin: Small pieces of tendons and skin which are not suitable for manufacture of leather are utilized. These pieces are immersed in a mixture of milk of lime and aqueous caustic soda solution for 10–30 days. As a result fat present in the material is saponified or emulsified, partial bleaching of skin takes place and putrefaction is prevented. The material is taken out, washed with water and treated with sulphurous acid when bleaching takes place. This soft and bleached skin is washed, put into a cloth bag and extracted with water by heating on water-bath at a temperature not exceeding 85°C as direct heating and higher temperature affect the quality of gelatin. After heating for few hours gelatin solution is taken out and the material again heated as above. In the first extraction about 20% and in second extraction about 12% gelatin is obtained. Both the solutions are combined and purified and made colourless as follows.

The solution is allowed to stand for some period when many impurities settle below by sedimentation. The upper clear solution is decanted and heated again after adding alum, egg-albumin, or animal blood. Many of the impuirities like albumin, mucin and mineral matter are precipitated and filtered. The solution is decolorized with animal charcoal. Gelatin solution is then concentrated in multiple-effect evaporator at as low a temperature as possible and at reduced pressure. Concentrated solution is chilled in metal trays or dried in thin films on wire nets and it solidifies. Solid mass is cut into strips and dried in vacuum by keeping on frames or in well-ventilated rooms at a temparature below 20°C very carefully. Gelatin if kept at higher temperature loses its jellying power. If it contains more moisture, it becomes flexible and deteriorates during storage.

Bone Gelatin: Bones, in addition to ossessin, contain 12–18% fat, and 50% mineral matter consisting of calcium and magnesium phosphate and calcium carbonate. So at first fat and mineral matters are separated. Bones are washed, cracked and extracted in soxhlet with lipid solvents like ether or light petroleum. The defatted bones are treated with dilute hydrochloric acid and mineral matter is removed. Bones are removed, washed well and extracted by keeping them in cloth bag. The extracted solution is purified. It is decolorized, concentrated and dried as in skin gelatin.

Chemical Constituents

Gelatin contains protein glutin which on hydrolysis yields non-essential amino acids (see description on proteins).

Uses

Gelatin is used in the manufacture of capsules and suppositories and also for coating of pills and tablets. It is used as a culture medium in bacteriology and as a substitute of blood plasma. In nutritional experiments it is used as a protein, containing non-essential amino acids.

ARACHIS OIL

Earth-nut oil, Peanut oil, Groundnut oil, Fool Sudani oil (Arab.)

Botanical Source

Arachis oil is the fixed oil obtained by expression from the seeds of *Arachis hypogaea*.

Family

Leguminosae (Papilionaceae).

Geographical Source

The peanut plant is a native of Brazil and is cultivated in India, tropical Africa, Brazil and South America. Groundnut is the third largest source of fixed oil in the world.

The plant is a low annual herb. After fruiting the small, immature, yellow gynophore extends and penetrates into the soil and it ripens, therefore buried underground. The fruit is yellow, reticulate, indehiscent legume and contains 1–3 (mostly 2, sometimes 4) red to brown seeds. Kernels contain 40–50% fixed oil. Kernels are expressed in hydraulic press at ordinary temperature. For pharmaceutical and medicinal purposes only the cold expressed oil is used. The oil cake is expressed at higher temperature and after that remaining oil is obtained by solvent extraction. The oil cake forms a rich cattle food. India's share in total world's production of oil amounts to 45%.

Characters

Arachis oil is a pale yellow or greenish-yellow oily liquid. It has a characteristic nut-like smell and taste.

Physical and Chemical Characteristics

Specific Gravity: 0.916–0.920. Refractive Index: at 40°, 1.4625–1.4645. Riechert Meissl No. 0.2–1. Saponification Value: 188–196. Iodine Value: 85–95. Acid Value: Mot more than 4. Solubility: Almost insoluble in alcohol, miscible with carbon disulphide, chloroform, ether and light petroleum.

Chemical Constituents

Peanut oil contains glycerides of oleic acid (50–60%) and of linoleic acid (18–30%). The remaining 10–12% acids are palmitic acid, stearic acid, arachidic acid, behenic acid and lignoceric acid. Seed coat contains catechol and leucoanthocyanide with vitamin properties. Seeds further contain thiamine and protein. Protein is rich in essential amino acids like threonine, methionine and tryptophan. Upon saponification with alcoholic potassium hydroxide crystals of the impure potassium arachidate are formed.

The melting point of arachidic acid is high and is 77°C and so the presence of groundnut oil as an adulterant in other oils can be detected by hydrolysis, separating arachidic acid and determining the melting point.

Identification Tests

Boil 1 g sample of oil under reflux for 5 minutes with 5 ml acetic acid and 50 ml alcohol. Warm until the solution is clear. Cool slowly and note the temperature at which turbidity appears. This should not be lower than 37°C for a good arachis oil.

Uses

Peanut oil is used mainly as an article of food in the form of cooking oil and as margarine. It is also used in India for preparation of hydrogenated fat. The properties of arachis oil are similar to olive oil and hence it is also used as a solvent for drugs and in preparation of liniments and plasters and as a vehicle for ointments. The oil is used in the manufacture of soaps.

OLIVE OIL

Sweet oil, Salad oil, Olea oliva

Botanical Source

Olive oil is the fixed oil expressed from the ripe fruit of *Olea europoea*.

Family

Oleaceae.

Geographical Source

The plant is a native of Palestine and has been largely cultivated in the Mediterranean countries for centuries. It is cultivated in the United States and some other subtropical localities. Spain olive and olive oil are highly esteemed worldwide.

Description

The tree is a short evergreen tree, grows up to 10 metres in height and attains a long age. Cultivation has resulted in a large number of varieties of olive fruits, which show various sizes, colours and different yields in oil. The drupaceous fruit is normally of purple colour when ripe. Large quantities of mature fruits are pickled and used very popularly as condiment.

Characters

Olive oil has several grades of purity. An important variety is virgin oil which is produced by lightly pressing the peeled pulp devoid of endocarp. Olive oil is pale yellow or light greenish yellow oily liquid which has faint but characteristic odour. It has a bland to slightly acrid taste. The oil is miscible with ether, carbon disulphide and chloroform. It is only slightly soluble in alcohol. For further physical and chemical characteristics see the Chapter 6 of book of Pharmacognosy, 12th ed. by J.S. Qadry.

Constituents

The composition of olive oil seems to vary rather widely due the reasons mentioned above. Two major kinds can be easily distinguished depending upon the relative concentrations of the component acids of the glycosides. The Turkish variety contains 75% of oleic acid, 10% of palmitic acid and

9% of linoleic acid, with lesser amounts of stearic, myristic, hexadecenoic and arachidic acids. The Italian variety contains only about 65% of oleic acid, 15% each of palmitic and linoleic acids, and other minor component acids. There are some other minor components like squalene, phytosterol, tocopherols, etc.

Uses

Olive oil is an important edible oil and a pharmaceutical aid. Its use in dentistry as a setting retardant material for dental cements is highly valued. It is used in the preparation of soaps, plasters and liniments. It is also esteemed as a demulcent, an emollient, and a laxative. The consumption of olives as such and olive oil as a nutrient, as a salad oil, now globally, has made the oil most outstanding amongst the fixed oils. It is now regularly used for cooking food.

BEESWAX

White and Yellow Beeswax, Cera Alba and Cera Flava, Shamah Al Nahl (Arabic)

Zoological Source

Beeswax is the purified wax obainted from honeycomb of *Apis mellifica* and other species of *Apis*.

Family

Apidae.

Order

Hymenoptera.

Geographical Source

Jamaica, East and West Africa, India, France and Italy. Also in countries where honey is produced.

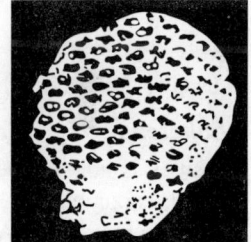

Fig. 3.12. Honey comb.

Preparation

The worker bee prepares wax in the last four segments of abdomen on the ventral surface which comes out through the pores in chitinous exoskeleton. This wax is utilized by the worker bee for preparation of honeycomb as well as for capping the honey cells. Wax forms about 1/8th part of the honeycomb. After removal of honey, honeycomb mainly consists of wax. It is put into water and water is heated. Remains of honey dissolve in water and other imputrities settle below. On cooling melted wax gets solidified and floats on the surface of water and is separated. For further purification wax is melted and kept in a long cylindrical vessel and in this condition the remaining impurities settle below and wax is removed. Wax so obtained is yellow beeswax.

Beeswax is a by-product of bee-keeping in most areas.

White Beeswax: White beeswax is obtained by the action of charcoal, potassium permanganate, chromic acid or chlorine on yellow beeswax. It is also obtained by bleaching by the action of sunlight, moisture and air. Melted yellow beeswax is placed onto revolving wet cylinders when strips similar to ribbon are obtained. These are placed on cloth in thin layers in sunlight and periodically rotating them and moistened by sprinking water and kept till the outer layer becomes white. Thus white beeswax is produced.

Characters

Wax is white, yellow or yellowish-brown solid having pleasant smell of honey. It breaks with granular fracture. It is insoluble in water but slightly soluble in alcohol but soluble in chloroform, ether, fixed oil and volatile oils including turpentine oil. Specific gravity is 0.958–0.970. Melting point 62–64°C and refractive index at 80°C is 1.4380–1.4420.

Chemical Constituents

Beeswax contains about 80% myricin which is myricyl palmitate $C_{15}H_{31}.COO.C_{30}H_{61}$. Free cerotic acid $C_{26}H_{53}COOH$ about 15% myricyl and ceryl alcohol and higher hydrocarbons are also present.

Uses

Beeswax is used in the preparation of plasters, ointments and polishes. It is used for hardening the soft ointment.

Adulterants

Beeswax is adulterated by a number of adulterants like solid paraffin, ceresin, caranuba wax, Japan wax (fat obtained from the fruits of *Rhus* species belonging to Anacardiaceae), stearic acid, colophony and other fats and waxes.

Adulteration can be detected by the following two tests:

1. If wax is heated with aqueous sodium hydroxide, cooled and acidified, turbidity should not be produced. Wax is not hydrolyzed by aqueous alkali and cerotic acid present in it does not form water-soluble soap. Japan wax, other fats, fatty acids and colophony form with aqueous alkali water-soluble soaps which on acidification give free fatty acids, or resin acids which are precipitated. Thus adulteration of the above substances can be detected.

2. Wax is hydrolyzed by heating with alcoholic potassium hydroxide. If the reaction-liquid is cooled stirring continuously it should become cloudy between 59–61°C and not above 61°C. The substances obtained

on hydrolysis are alcohol-soluble. Upto 61°C they remain dissolved in alcohol and below 61°C they get precipitated. Hard paraffin and ceresin are very little soluble and they get precipitated above 61°C.

LANOLIN

Wool fat, Adeps Lanae, Soof Al Kharoof (Arabic)

Biological Source

Lanolin is purified wax prepared from the wool of sheep, *Ovis aries*.

Family

Bovidae.

Preparation

Wool fat is secreted in the glands on the skin of the sheep and passes into the wool. Wool is cut and washed with detergents such as soap, alkali or sulphonated alcohols. As a result an emulsion of wool fat, known as wool grease and water takes place. The emulsion is cracked with sulphuric acid and the wool grease forms the upper layer. The fatty acid is separated from the lower layer.

The neutralization of these free acids is carried out with sodium hydroxide or sodium carbonate in the presence of solvent like benzene. The lower aqueous layer of acids is separated and from the upper wool fat-containing layer benzene is distilled off and wool fat is obtained. Lanolin so obtained is purified by treatment with sodium peroxide or other suitable bleaching agents.

Characters

Wool fat is a pale yellow tenacious solid with a characteristic smell. It is insoluble in water but a high proportion of water may be incorporated in it by melting and stirring. Its melting points is 36–43°C.

Chemical Constituents

Wool fat consists of esters of cholesterol and isocholesterol with lanoceric, lanopalmitic, caranubic, myristic and oleic acids. These acids also occur free. Chemically wool fat is not a fat but wax and its correct name should be "wool wax".

Uses

Wool fat has capacity of absorbing water and is used as a base in water-absorbable ointments. It increases the absorption of the drug from the skin. It is used also as an emollient.

MISCELLANEOUS DRUGS

Under section (u) of **Chapter 5** of the P.C.I. Syllabus there are nine drugs which are not placed under any category of therapeutic efficacy or any other technical virtue. Hence, these drugs are considered as **miscellaneous drugs**. Miscellaneous is a word, an adjective, meaning here "consisting of a variety of ingredients or parts having diverse characteristics, abilities or appearances". Its equivalent other words or synonyms are assorted, mixed, motley or sundry. The drugs are: Liquorice, Garlic, Picrorhiza, Dioscorea, Linseed, Shatavari, Shankpushpi, Pyrethrum and Tobacco.

Their description below, one by one, will make the above fact rather more clear to show that no two of these drugs have similar or allied phytochemicals, no generic relationship and no pronounsed therapeutic uses close to each other. Hence, the name miscellaneous to this section.

LIQUORICE
Licorice

Licuorice root, Radix Glycyrrhiza, Sweet root, Mulethi (Hindi), Jethi Madh (Guj.), Yastimadhu (Sanskrit), Asalassus (Arab. and Pers.)

Botanical Source

Licorice consists of peeled and/or unpeeled roots and stolon (and subterranean stems) of the plant *Glycyrrhiza glabra* and other species of *Glycyrrhiza*. The drug is now mostly avaliable as unpeeled, even through the pharmacopoeias have been requiring it as a peeled drug.

Geographical Source

The main supplies of the drug come from Spain, Iran, Iraq, Sicily, Russia, Greece and Asia Minor (Anatolia), Afghanistan, India and Pakistan. The licorice plant is a perennial plant attaining a height of about 1 metre. It is cultivated in Spain and Italy. Russia and Iran get the drug from wild plants.

There are some varieties or subspecies which supply the drug. They are:

1. *G. glabra* var. *typica*: This variety has purplish blue flowers and is cultivated mainly in Spain and Italy and southern France. This forms the so called Spanish licorice of the market and represents the underground long roots, stolons and rhizomes.

2. *G. glabra* var. *glandulifera*: The fruit of this variety has glands and hence the name. It grows wild in central and southern Russia. It has no stolons.

3. *G. glabra* var. *violacea*: This variety has violet-coloured flowers and gives the so called Persian licorice. It grows wild in Iran and Iraq.

Chemical Constituents

Glycyrrhiza contains 2.5–7% glycyrrhizin, a very sweet water-soluble substance which is 50 times sweeter than sucrose. Glycyrrhizin is a mixture of potassium and calcium salts of glycyrrhetic acid. Glycyrrhizinic acid is a glycoside and on hydrolysis 18-β-glycyrrhetinic acid and 2 mols of glucouronic acid are obtained. Glycyrrhizinic acid is a triterpenoid saponin having β-amyrine structure. It shows esepecially in alkaline solution frothing but it has very weak haemolytic property. Medicinal activity is atributed to 18β-structure. 11-α-isomer has very little medicinal action. Glycyrrhiza also contains 18-OH-glycyrrhetic acid or glabrin acid. The yellow colour of the drug is due to chalcone glycoside isoliquiritin. During drying isoliquiritin is converted partially into flavone glycoside liquiritin and is present in the drug. Isoliquiritin also undergoes hydrolysis and produces isoliquiritingenin, which has spasmolytic action. Glycyrrhizin probably prevents inactivation of glucocorticoid in the liver and has glucocorticoid action like loss of potassium, retention of sodium and causes oedema. As a result, in USA use of glycyrrhiza in candies and other preparations is not permitted. It also contains glucose, sucrose, asparagine, β-sitosterol and probably estradiol and estrol.

18-β-glycyrrhetinic acid

Saponins increase the absorption of other constituents and this potentiating action of saponin can be illustrated by a simple experiment. Magnesium salts given orally to frogs in whatever great doses will cause only purgation but no hypnosis. If magnesium salts are administered by injection they will cause hypnosis. If magnesium salts and saponin are given orally to frog, absorption will increase and hypnosis will be produced. Similarly the lethal dose of strophanthin or digitoxin will be produced nearly one-tenth when combined with saponin.

Chemical Test

Section or powder of the drug shows with 80% sulphuric acid orange yellow colour. This test is due to transformation of flavone glycoside liquiritin to chalcone glycoside isoliquiritin.

Uses

Glycyrrhiza is used as a sweetening agent and expectorant but it is recently used as antispasmodic, anti-ulcer, antiinflammatory and estrogenic drug. Glycyrrhiza is used as a sweetening agent for improving the taste of bitter medicines like quinine, aloe and ammonium chloride and others. For this purpose ammoniated glycyrrhizin is also used in tobacco industries and confectionery as a sweetening and flavouring agent. Because of the irritant property of saponins, glycyrrihiza is used as an expectorant and diuretic. 18β-glycyrrhetic acid possesses anti-inflammatory property. Therefore, it is used for helping stomach and intestinal ulcer like peptic ulcer. Isoliquiritigenin possesses ½ papaverin-like spasmolytic action and contribute to above healing. Isoliquritin glycoside has ¼ papaverin action while liquiritin has no such action. Succus of glycyrrhiza possesses greater spasmolytic property. Glycyrrhiza has no laxative action but it potentiates the laxative action of senna.

Glycyrrhiza is used in Addison's disease because of glucocorticoid action. It causes oedema and glycyrrhizin-free preparations are available. Glycyrrhetic acid is used in skin diseases because of anti-inflammatory action. Because of the frothing property it is used as fire extinguisher. Stick or block licorice is used in cough and bronchitis as tablets or lozenges.

GARLIC

Garlic, Lasum (Sanskrit), Lasun (Hindi), Lasan (Guj.), Assom (Arab.)

Botanical Source

Garlic consists of ripe bulbs of *Allium sativum* and contains not less than 0.1% allicin.

Family

Liliaceae.

Geographical Source

Garlic is cultivated in India and in many other countries of the world, like southern Russia, S.E. Europe, Italy, USA, etc.

Characters

The fresh bulb consists of an ovate main bulb and 6–15 secondary bulbs. Both are surrounded by common white dry leafy membranes.

Chemical Constituents

The active priniciple **allicin** is active bacteriostatic and volatile with steam, with a typical garlic smell. Allicin is produced during crushing or distillation of garlic from bacteriostatic inactive, odourless, water-soluble ester **allin**

$$2CH_2=CH-CH_2-\underset{\underset{O}{\|}}{S}-CH_2-\underset{\underset{NH_2}{|}}{CH}-COOH$$

Allin

$$H_2O \downarrow Enzyme$$

$$CH-CH_2-\underset{\underset{O}{\|}}{S}-CH_2CH=CH_2 + 2CH_3CO-COOH + 2NH_3$$

Allicin   Pyruvic acid

by the action of the enzyme **allin-lyase**. Thereby further pyruvic acid and ammonia are also produced.

Allicin is unstable and by distillation or in the presence of water and oxygen it is decomposed into polysulphides, which are responsible for the unpleasant smell of valatile oil. The same degradation occurs in the organism and imparts smell to the exhaled breath.

Uses

Garlic is popularly used as a spice. Allicin is active in dilution 1 : 100000 against pathogenic gram-positive and gram-negative bacteria. 1 mg of allicin corresponds to 15 I.U. of pencillin (= 10 mg) and thus surpasses phenol and sublimate. Garlic pressed juice is active against interdigital mycosis. Garlic is antibacterial and its standardized preparations are used in fermentative dyspepsia and chronic intestinal infections and other digestive disturbances. Garlic is found useful in respiratory diseases such as chronic bronchitis, bronchial asthma, whooping cough and tuberculosis. It is used in high blood pressure and atherosclerosis. It is also recommended is rheumatism and arthritis. At present in the market dehydrated garlic is available.

PICRORHIZA

Katuki (Sanskrit), Kutki (Hindi), Kadu (Guj.), Katuki (Beng.)

Botanical Source
Picrorhiza consists of dried stolons and rhizomes of *Picrorhiza kurroa*.

Family
Scrophulariaceae.

Geographical Source
Plant is distributed in alpine Himalayas from Kashmir to Sikkim at an altitude of 2790–5000 metres. It is a low, more or less hairy herb with a perennial woody rootstock. The drug is collected in Kashmir.

Chemical Constituents

The drug contains picroside I and II and kutkoside. Picroside and kutkoside are C_9 monoterpene iridoid glycosides and contain an epoxy oxide in the ring. They have similar ring structures except that *trans*-cinnamoyl moiety in picroside I and vanilloyl in picroside II and in kutkoside are at different carbon atoms. The glycosides are considered responsible for the activity. The drug further contains apocyanin. Apocyanin is 4-hydroxy-5-methoxy acetophenone and has cholagogue action.

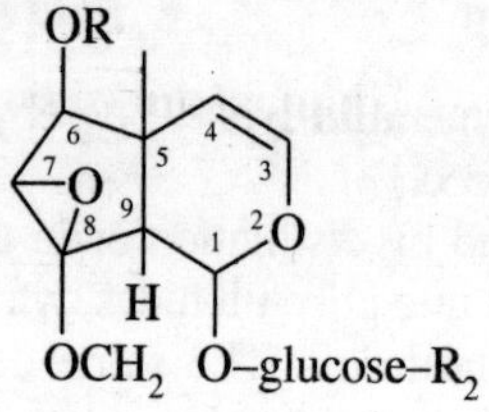

	R	R_1	R_2
Picroside I	H	H	*trans*-Cinnamoyl
Picroside II	Vanilloyl	H	H
Kutkoside	H	Vanilloyl	H

Uses

The drug is popularly used in India as a bitter tonic, cathartic, stomachic and febrifuge including as antimalarial. In recent clinical investigations the drug was found useful in different types of jaundice and especially useful in hepatitis. It has cholagogue and choleretic action and is useful in infective and amoebic type of inflammation in liver. **Kutkin**, a stable mixture of glycosides, has weak diuretic activity, about one-sixth of chlorthiazide.

DIOSCOREA

Yam, Mexican Yam

Botanical Source

Dioscorea consists of tubers of several species of the genus *Dioscorea*, such as *D. floribunda*, *D. spiculiflora* and *D. villosa*. In India, however, *D. deltoida*, *D. prareri*, *D. bulbifera* and *D. bellophyla* are found.

Family

Dioscoreaceae.

Geographical Source

Different species of *Dioscorea* have been found growing and successfully cultivated in different countries like Mexico and Central America, Guatemala, China, Japan, India and Pakistan. *D. deltoida* is being successfully cultivated in Jammu & Kashmir, Tamil Nadu, Karnataka; Bengal and Maharashtra.

D. floribunda is also now cultivated in India, while *D. bellophylla* in Pakistan.

Constituents

Diosgenin ($C_{27}H_{42}O_3$) is the **sapogenin** obtained on hyrolysis of the steroidal glycoside, dioscin. Diosin is present in yams and is obtained commercially from the roots and rhizomes of *Dioscorea* species.

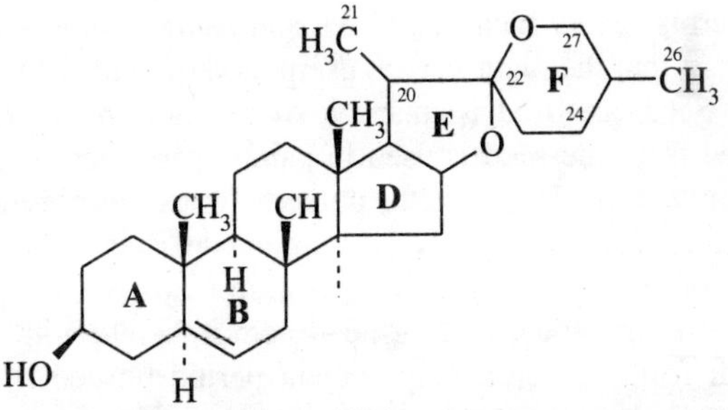

Diosgenin (Δ^5,25α-Spirosten-3-β-ol)

Diosgenin was isolated from the Mexican yam is 1970 and as such was the first and the only source for the manufacture of steroidal contraceptives. Later, sources like **hecongenin** for corticosteroids and other diosgenin sources and steroidal alkaloids of Solanum were exploited. Small quantity of hecogenin, with a keto group at position 12 in diosgenin, is also present in dioscorea.

Uses

Diosgenin and other related steroidal sapogenins are used as starting materials for the production of steroidal drugs. The natural steroids may be grouped into androgen (male sex hormones), esterogens and progestogens (female sex hormones), and corticosteroids. The steroid drugs are employed for a variety of chemical syndromes, for example, as anti-inflammatory agents and as anticancer agents, in the treatment of hormone deficiency disorders, as oral contraceptives and as diuretics.

Some species of *Dioscorea* because of good quantity of starch present in them like *D. batatas* (Chinese potato) and very minute quantity of diosgenin are used as food especially in eastern countries. Some species of *Dioscorea* also contain alkaloids.

LINSEED

Flax Seed, Semen Lini, Alasi (Hindi), Bizra Al Kattan (Arab.)

Botanical Source

Linseed consists of the dried ripe seeds of *Linum usitatissimum* Linn.

Family

Linaceae.

Geographical Source

Argentina, India, Russia, Canada, USA.

Characters of Plant

The Latin terms *Linum* meaning fibres and *usitatissimum* meaning very useful, suggest that the plant is very useful and of considerable economic importance. Seeds are used as an article of food and in medicine. Linseed oil expressed from the seed is used in paints, varnishes, etc. Oil cake is used as a cattle feed. In the stem, phloem fibres are present which are called flax fibres and they are used in surgical dressings and for articles of cloth. Straw of the stem is used in paper pulp industry.

Flax plant is an annual herb of 30–40 cm in height with blue flowers and capsular fruits. Since a very ancient period linseed is obtained by cultivation only. If cultivation is carried out in cold countires, fixed oil contains more percentage of unsaturated acids while in tropical countries more saturated acids are found in the oil. The oil with saturated acids is less perferred.

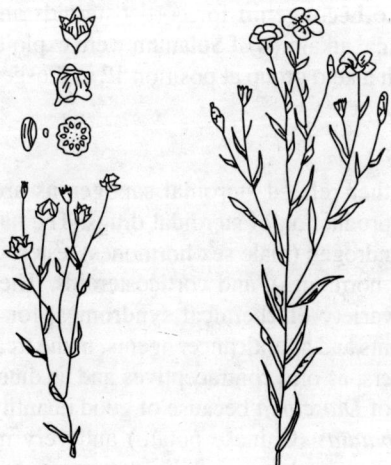

Fig. 3.13. Linseed, *Linum usitatissimum.*

Chemical Constituents

About 6% mucilage is present only in ripe seeds in the epidermis, the outermost tissue of seed coat. Unripe seeds contain starch which proves that mucilage is formed from starch of calcium salt, which on hydrolysis yields xylose, galactose, rhamnose, arabinose and galactouronic acid. Mucilage swells with water and gives red colour with ruthenium red. **Linseed oil** (30–40%) is drying oil and consists of glycerides of linoleic acid, linolenic acid, oleic acid and saturated acids. **Linamarin**, a cyano-genetic glycoside, on hydrolysis yields acetone, hydrocyanic acid and glucose. Linamarin is identical with **phaseolunatin**, a glycoside isolated earlier from *Phaseolus lunatus*. About 20% protein is also present in linseed.

Uses

Mucilage has demulcent or soothing action on skin or mucous membrane and so linseed is used in cough and bronchitis as a haustus. It is used as a poultice as mucilage is bad conductor of heat. Because of anaesthetic action of hydrocyanic acid, linamarin may contribute in the above action. Because of swelling property, it is sometimes used as a bulk laxative. Linseed oil being a drying oil is used in paints and varnishes. Linseed is also used as an article of food for people and cattle in some countries.

SHATAVARI

Shatavar, Shahakul Satavari (Hindi); Satavar (Guj.); Safaid Musli (Unani)

Botanical Source

The drug, Shatavari, consists of the dried tubers or tuberous roots of the plant *Asparagus racemosus*. (The correct botanical identity of the roots of Shatavari continues to be disputed, in spite of the fact that the literature mentions it to be derived from *A. racemosus*.)

Family

Liliaceae.

Geographical Source

The plant is a perennial climber that grows in many parts of India, especially in the northern part of India, more commonly in Himalayan and sub-Himalayan regions.

Constituents

Shatavari contains four steroidal saponins, Shatavarin I–IV. Shatavarin I is the main active glycoside of sarsapogenin with sugar moieties of 3 glucose and 1 rhamnose. Shatavarin IV is structurally related to shatavarin I and has 2 glucose and 1 rhamnose. Shatavarin I has been found to possess anti-oxytocic activity. The drug also contains starch.

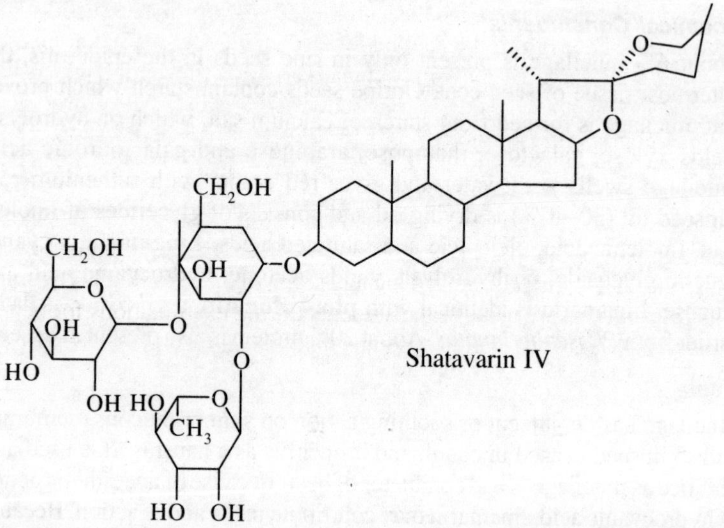

Shatavarin IV

Uses

The drug is very much esteemed in indigenous Ayurvedic and Unani systems of medicine. Total saponins mixture from Shatavari is pharmacologically active, showing uterine blocking activity. Thus its use in Ayurveda in threatened abortion and for safe delivery is justified. The drug also has galactogogue property. Its petroleum ether exract has shown diuretic activity. Shatavari has great reputation in Ayurveda in uterine diseases and as an antacid and tonic. In Unani system it is considered antidiarrhoeal, demulcent, etc.

SHANKHPUSHPI

Shankhpushpi (Hindi), Vishnukaranti (Sanskrit), Shankhvalli (Marathi)

Botanical Source

Shankhpushpi consists of the dried herb of *Convolvulus pluricaulis* (Syn. *Convolvulus microphyllus*) and herb of *Evolvulus alsinoides*.

Family

Convolvulaceae.

Geographical Source

Both the plants are found as wild in India.

Chemical Constituents

The drug contains an alkaloid shankhpushpine $C_{17}H_{25}NO_2$, melting point 162–164°C. Fresh plant contains volatile oil. According to recent work

C. micropyllus contains *n*-tricontane, higher aliphatic primary alcohols and phytosterols. Later, from the alcohol extract of defatted plant, kampherol and its 3D-glucoside, 3,4-dihydroxy cinnamic acid, β-sitosterol D-glucoside and glucose, rhamnose, sucrose and starch were isolated. The drug also contains potassium chloride.

Uses

The drug is used in hypertension and as tranquilizer. It potentiates barbitone hypnosis; leaves possess maximum activity. The drug has reputation as brain tonic and is used for improving and strengthening memory. The drug or its preparations are used by the students during examinations for better memory. In Ayurveda it is used in mental diseases like insanity and epilepsy.

EVOLVULUS ALSINOIDES

Vishnukranta (Sanskrit)

Chemical Constituents

It contains **betaine** and a water-soluble base, melting point 60–61°C. An alkaloid **evolvine** has also been isolated.

Uses

It is used as a brain tonic. It is sedative and increases sleep. It increases the activity of metrazole but has no action on strychnine activity. It decreases the hallucinogenic activity of mescaline.

Adulterants

In some parts of the country entire plant and juice of *Canscora decussata* are used as Shakhpushpi. Family is Gentianaceae.

In Kerala *Clitoria ternatea* (Family Papilionaceae) because of blue flowers is considered as Shankhpushpi.

PYRETHRUM

Pyrethrum flowers, Insect flowers, Flores Pyrethri

Botanical Source

Pyrethrum consists of dried flower heads of *Chrysanthemum cinerarifolium* and many other species of the genus *Chrysanthemum* e.g. *C. roseus*.

Family

Compositae.

Geographical Source

The plant is a native of Dalmatia (Yugoslavia – Balkans) and is now widely cultivated in Kenya, East Central Africa, Japan, Yugoslavia, Brazil, Ecuador and India.

Pyrethrum is a perennial herb about 1 metre in height. The plant is cultivated by planting seeds and transplanting in calcareous soil. The plant grows better in warm dry climate in sunny position.

Chemical Constituents

Pyrethrum flowers contain 1–2% esters known as pyrethrins. Pyrethrins are a mixture of **pyrethrin I**, **jasmoline I** and **cinerine I** esters of **chrysanthemic acid** (chrysanthemum monocarboxylic acid) and **pyrethrin II**, **jasmoline II** and **cinerine II** esters of **pyrethric acid** (monomethyl ester of chrysanthemum dicarboxylic acid). The corresponding alcohols of pyrethrins are keto alcohols, **pyrethrolone**, **cinerolone** and **jasmolone**.

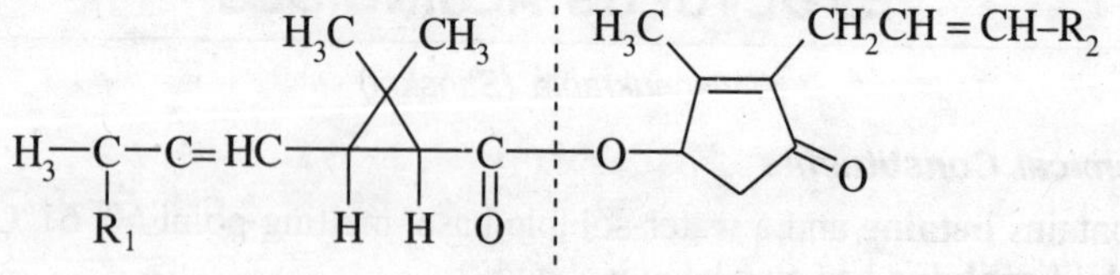

	R_1	R_2
Pyrethrin I	CH_3	$-CH=CH_2$
Pyrethrin II	$COOCH_3$	$-CH=CH_2$
Cinerine I	CH_3	$-CH_3$
Cinerine II	$COOCH_3$	$-CH_3$
Jasmoline I	CH_3	$-CH_2-CH_3$
Jasmoline II	$COOCH_3$	$-CH_2-CH_3$

All the esters are yellowish oily liquids and unstable to air and light because of unsaturation especially of pyrethrins I and II which contain two double bonds in the side chain of the alcohol. As esters they are unstable in alkali. They are insoluble in water but soluble in all organic solvents including petroleum ether from which pyrethrins have maximum insecticial properties.

Uses

Pyrethrum flowers and pyrethrins are contact insecticides. They are quite harmless to warm-blooded animals like humans but are contact poisons and poisonous to cold-blooded animals and kill insects like cockroaches, lice, bugs, flies, mosquitoes, etc.

Pyrethrins and pyrethrum extract are known for their quick 'knock down effect' of flying insects, particularly flies and mosquitoes.

The activity of pyrethrins is increased by combining with synergists like **piperonyl butoxide** and **sesamin**, containing dioxymethylene group and by DDT and thus positive 'Kill' effect is obtained.

TOBACCO

Tambaku, Tamaku (Hindi, Beng., Guj., Urdu)

Botanical Source

The drug, Tobacco, consists of the dried leaves of *Nicotiana tabacum*. Of the other species of the genus *Nicotiana*, *N. rustica* also forms the source of tobacco.

Family

Solanaceae.

Geographical Source

The plants grow in many parts of India and are cultivated.

Constituents

The leaves of tobacco contain many alkaloids, such as nicotine, nicotyrine, nicotinamine, nornicotine, etc. Nicotine is, however, the best known and the important most alkaloid as far as the drug under consideration is concerned. There are other species of the genus *Nicotiana*, like *N. rustica*, *N. glauca*, and *N. glutinosa* which contain similar alkaloids belonging to the pyridine group. Nicotine contains both the pyridine and pyrrolidine rings and is a colourless liquid. The leaves of tobacco show variable composition of nicotine, the lower ones showing more percentage of nicotine. Thus the percentage of nicotine in *N. tabacum* varies from 4–6%. *N. rustica* contains more nicotine, which may be as high as up to 8%. Tobacco leaves also contain carbohydrates, mostly reducing sugars, starch, sucrose and pentose.

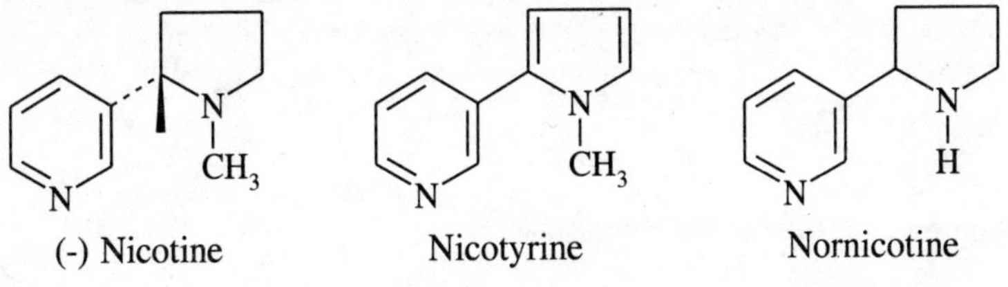

(-) Nicotine   Nicotyrine   Nornicotine

Uses

Tobacco is primarily produced in India for smoking purposes in cigarettes, pipes, cigars and in snuffs. It is also chewed as such or in beetle leaves.

Nicotine is a toxic alkaloid and 40 mg is fatal to human beings. Nicotine exerts action on all transient stimulation leading to depression and thereafter paralysis. It has a paralytic action on the skeletal muscles and manifests other physiological alterations and/or secondary effects which are extremely complex. Although nicotine has been used as an insecticide in agriculture in the form of 40% solution of nicotine sulphate in various formulations, its use has now been replaced by other chemicals.

SECTION 2

Applied Work
Practical Course

- Morphological and Anatomical Description of Plant Organs
- Study of Individual Drugs in Practical Classes
- Study of Fibres and Surgical Dressings

Morphological and Anatomical Description of Plant Organs

Pharmacopoeias of most of the countries including Indian Pharmacopoeia and the Ayurvedic Pharmacopoeia of India give detailed morphological and anatomical description of the plant drugs, included in the syllabus of pharmacy courses, in their monographs. Thus as a consequence to this understanding and especially in the light of the fact that the PCI syllabus deals with morphology and gross anatomical studies of the drugs, it becomes expedient to follow the chapter three (3) with this chapter four (4) dealing with morphological and anatomical studies of plant and its parts, which comprise a large number of drugs included in the syllabus.

Besides, this chapter is written here due to the following additional reasons:

1. To refresh the knowledge of students in different botanical aspects and consolidate it in the direction of pharmacognostic botany, followed by collection, preparation, storage, etc.
2. To enable the teachers and students to start the practical work right from day one following the commencement of pharmacognosy teaching.
3. To let the students have continuity in practicals from the point of view of the importance of drug evaluation in the practicals as per pharmacopoeial standards (Part I, Chapter 7).

1. PARTS OF PLANTS AS DRUGS

The plant consists of several parts. They may be classified according to their functions e.g. (a) vegetative parts, and (b) reproductive parts.

Vegetative parts are responsible for carrying out the activities of maintenance, growth and repair of the plant. Leaves, stems and roots are vegetative parts. Reproductive parts are responsible for production of new plants and maintenance of species. Flowers, fruits and seeds are reproductive parts.

2. LEAVES

Leaves may be (a) cotyledon or seed leaves situated on hypocotyl of the embryo; (b) scale leaves found on subterranean stems or sometimes on stems above ground; (c) bracteal leaves; and (d) foliage leaves. Usually, under leaves, foliage leaves are understood and the same will be considered here.

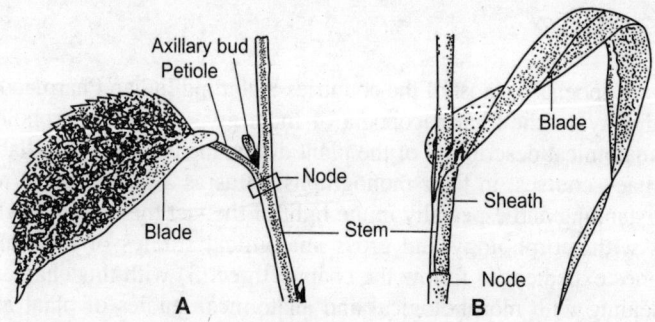

Fig. 4.1. Stems with leaf attached.

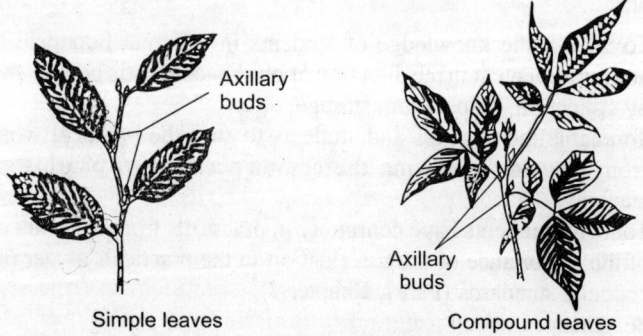

Fig. 4.2. Simple and compound leaves showing parts and types of venations.

Leaves are lateral appendages of the stem. They are green-coloured because of the presence of chlorophyll, which by using energy of the sun, carbon dioxide and water perform the important activity of photosynthesis. The flattened and thin nature of leaves is suited for maximum activity of photosynthesis as rays of sun fall on a greater area. Leaves have veins in their entire lamina which perform the function of conduction and support.

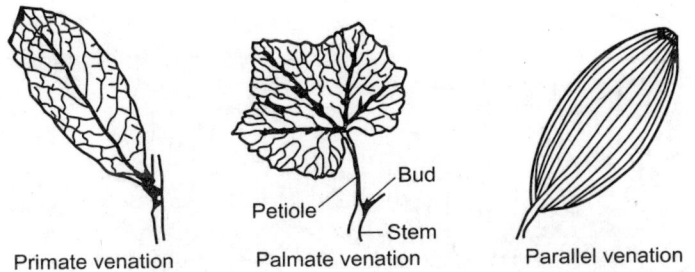

Fig. 4.3. Simple leaves. Venation types: Primate venation, Palmate venation, and Parallel venation.

Leaf Anatomy

The leaf is the primary photosynthetic organ of the plant. It consists of a flattened portion, called the blade, which is attached to the plant by a structure called the petiole. The histology of leaf is given below.

The outer surface of the leaf has a thin waxy covering called the cuticle. The primary function of this layer is to prevent water loss from the leaf. Below the cuticle is the outer layer of cells called the epidermis. The vascular tissue, xylem and phloem are found within the veins of the leaf. Veins are actually extensions that run from tips of the roots all the way up to the edges of the leaves. The outer layer of the vein is made of cells called bundle sheath cells, and they may encircle the xylem and the phloem. Picture shows xylem as the upper layer of cells and is shaded a little lighter than the lower layer of cells, the phloem (Fig. 4.4).

Within the leaf is mesophyll. Mesophyll can be divided into two layers, the palisade layer and the spongy layer. Palisade cells are more column-like and lie just under the epidermis. The spongy cells are more loosely packed and lie between the palisade layer and the lower epidermis. The air spaces between the spongy cells allow for gas exchange. Mesophyll cells (both palisade and spongy) are packed with chloroplasts, and this is where photosynthesis actually occurs.

Epidermis is also present on the lower surface of the leaf, also covered by the cuticle. Within the epidermis are present stomata, more on the lower side. Changes within water pressure cause the stoma to open or close.

Leaves are collected from the plants during the flowering period, as in this season plant is very active, the sap movement and photosynthetic activity are maximum and leaves contain maximum percentage of active constituents. As the moisture decreases their constituents, they are collected in dry weather.

Method of collection of leaf drugs is characteristic of each drug. Thus digitalis, Indian senna and tea leaves are picked up individually from the plant. In case of Alexandrian senna and buchu leaves, on the other hand,

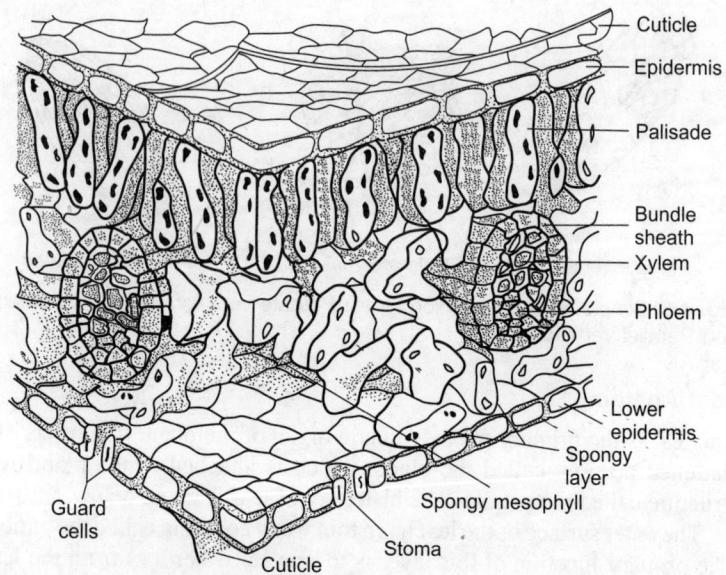

Fig. 4.4. Leaf anatomy. Three-dimensional view.

leafy shoots are cut and after drying the leaves are separated by beating. In solanaceous plants like belladonna, hyoscyamus, leaves with flowering tops are collected.

Fresh leaves contain about 50–60% water and they are dried after collection. Leaf drugs are dried at low temperature and as quickly as possible. In tropical countries leaves may be dried in shade to maintain their green colour but sheds with heating arrangements and cross ventilation are also used for drying.

During drying, because of loss of moisture, shrinkage or contraction occurs and some leaves like belladonna become crumpled. Small leaves like buchu or senna or succulent leaves like digitalis are not affected much by drying and they maintain their shape. Thus the condition of the dried leaves may be different according to the method of preparation, drying and their nature. Leaves are packed and stored in air-tight containers at low temperature and protected from light and moisture.

3. BARKS

Barks consist of the external tissues of stem or root of dicotyledon plants lying outside the cambium. The tissues present in the bark looking from outside are: cork (phellem), phellogen and phelloderm, collectively called periderm, cortex, pericycle, primary phloem, usually crushed or obliterated and secondary phloem.

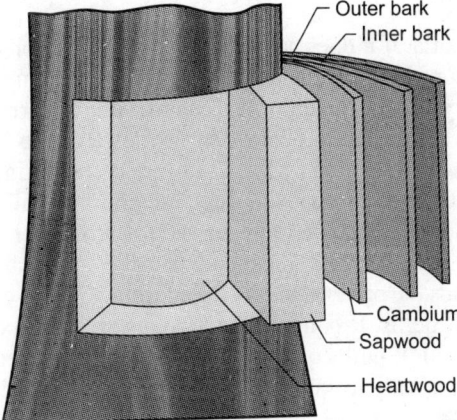

Fig. 4.5. Bark and wood. A view of a trunk/stem showing layers of a pharmacognostic bark and wood. Outer bark: consisting of cork, cork cambium (phellogen) and phelloderm (secondary cortex). Inner bark: consisting of primary cortex (mostly crushed), primary phloem, endodermis (visible, if not crushed) and secondary phloem. Cambium separating the bark from the wood, which in older stem can be distinguished in **sapwood** and **heartwood**, as shown.

Formation of bark

The stem of the dicotyledon plant, in which no secondary growth has taken place, contains the tissues in the following order: epidermis, primary cortex, pericycle, primary phloem, cambium, primary xylem and pith. As the plant becomes older it requires additional conducting tissues. For this purpose vascular cambium lying between the primary phloem and primary xylem in the stem starts its activity. This cambium produces on its inner side secondary xylem and on its outer side secondary phloem. Gradually, more and more secondary phloem is produced on outer side and it pushes and exerts pressure on the primary tissues. As a result primary phloem usually gets crushed or obliterated and epidermis which is thin-walled gets ruptured and peeled off. The plant requires new protective tissues. At this stage, phellogen or cork cambium starts its activity usually in the sub-epidermal tissue or in the cortex. Phellogen produces on its outer side cork or phellem and on its inner side phelloderm. Cell walls of cork cells are suberized and because of the fatty nature do not allow moisture and air to pass and thus give protection to the plant.

Diagnostic characters

Barks show important diagnostic characters like shape, nature of outer and inner surfaces and fracture which help in distinguishing them. We will consider these characters now one by one.

Shape

Shape of bark is flat if it does not undergo any contraction during drying. Quillaia and arjuna bark are flat as they are collected from main trunk and being thick they do not undergo any contraction. If during drying both sides of the bark are slightly bent or curved towards the inner side, it is called curved, e.g. **wild cherry bark**. In rare cases, as in **kurchi bark**, curvature is outside or in opposite direction and it is called recurred. If both sides of the bark become more curved towards inner side forming a channel, as in **cassia bark**, it is called channelled. If during contraction, one edge overlaps the other edge it is called **quill**. **Ceylon cinnamon** bark is in the form of quills. If both edges curve inwards, as in **cinchona**, it is called double quill. If quills of smaller diameter are inserted into quills of larger diameter, usually to save space, it is called compound quill.

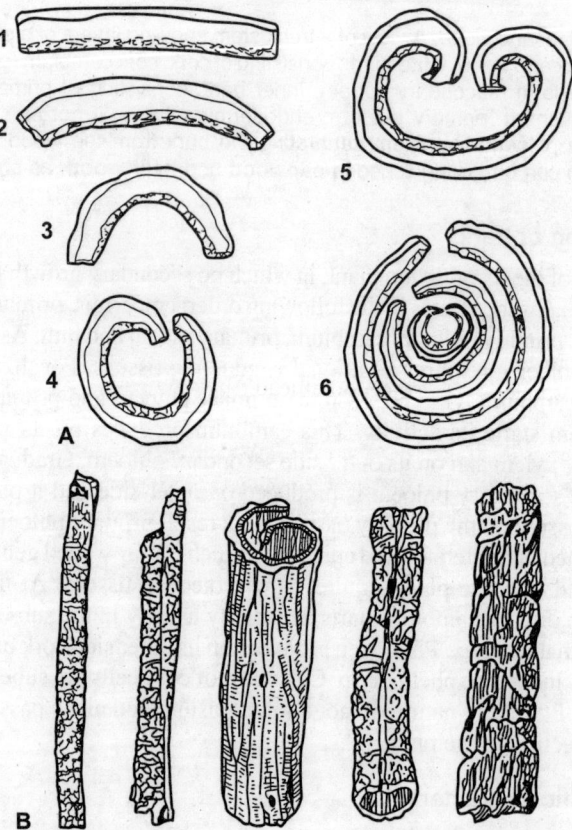

Fig. 4.6. (A) Shapes of barks: 1, flat; 2, curved; 3, channelled; 4, single quill; 5, double quill; 6; compound quill. (B) Pieces of barks showing their appearances with internal and external markings, striations, wrinkles and cracks.

Outer Surface

Bark is surrounded externally by cork and the nature and properties of cork usually impart characteristics to the outer surface of the bark. Outer surface of bark is called smooth if cork formation is regular and uniform as in arjuna bark. Cork is a dead tissue and its cells are non-elastic. It completely encloses the bark. Because of the lateral pressure of secondary tissues from within, transversely elongated holes, called **lenticels**, are formed on the outer surface as in wild cherry, cascara and young alstonia barks. Gaseous exchange of the plant with external atmosphere can take place through lenticels. Because of increase in diameter, cracks and fissures are formed on the outer surface. Their occurrence and arrangement are characteristic. Sometimes, small circular patches, called corky warts, are found in older barks, e.g. in *Cinchona succirubra* and ashoka barks. During drying, because of more shrinkage of softer tissues, longitudinal wrinkles are seen. If the troughs between wrinkles are wide, they are called furrows.

Older, outer cork of bark often exfoliates or flakes off exposing sometimes small or large areas of inner bark. This exfoliation is not uniform and in some barks at one place cork is seen while at the remaining place inner bark is exposed. Exfoliation takes place in wild cherry bark.

Rhytidoma: It is a composite dead tissue consisting of alternate layers of cork layers and cortical and/or phloem layers. Rhytidoma is formed as a result of the activity of phellogen successively in deeper and deeper layers. Phellogen starts its activity in the cortex and forms in the outer side cork and in inner side phelloderm. As the cork is a dead tissue, tissues lying outside the cork do not remain more in contact with the plant and die. Again phellogen starts its activity successively in deeper layer and tissues surrounded by cork become dead. In some cases, phellogen may start its activity still deeper in phloem and encloses some phloem tissue which becomes dead. Rhytidoma formation takes place in quilaia bark but it is removed during peeling. Rhytidoma is also formed in *Terminalia tomentosa* bark and in old cinchona bark.

Epiphytes like moss, lichen and liverworts are sometimes present on the bark. They are of diagnostic importance as in cascara bark.

Inner Surface

Because of contraction on the inner surface, parallel longitudinal ridges are formed, They are called striations. These striations may be fine or coarse. In some cases, as in cascara, parallel transverse ridges, called corrugations, are seen on the inner surface. The colour of inner surface is usually lighter.

Fracture

If the bark is broken, the nature of the exposed surface is called fracture. If the exposed surface is smooth and even, fracture is said to be short. Fracture is called granular if the exposed surface shows grain-like minute prominences. If the exposed surface shows uneven projecting points, fracture is splintery; if fibres are seen, it is known as fibrous; and if it separates into parallel tangential layers, as in mica, fracture is said to be laminated. In some cases, outer and inner parts of bark show different fractures.

Histology

Sometimes, epidermis cells may be present in the bark but usually these are replaced by cork. Cork cells in transverse section are tabular and usually radially arranged and tangentially elongated. They are polygonal in surface view. Cork cells may be thin-walled and lighter in colour or thick-walled and darker. A drug contains either thin-walled or thick-walled cells or both may be present in alternate rows. Cork cells are suberized but sometimes may be lignified as in cassia. **Suberin** is the glyceride ester of fatty acids and gives red colour with Sudan red III on heating and is unaffected by concentrated sulphuric acid. Phellogen cells are thin-walled, meristematic and rectangular in transverse section. Phelloderm formation is usually less than cork but in some barks, e.g. kurchi bark, wide phelloderm with stone cells is present. Phelloderm is a living tissue. Its cells are made up of thin-walled cellulosic parenchyma and are arranged in radial rows. Sometimes, the cells are also collenchymatous. Function of phelloderm is photo-synthesis and storage of starch. Primary cortex consists of an outer collenchymatous and an inner parenchymatous zone. Cortex may contain starch, calcium oxalate, oil cells, mucilage, latex or stone cells. Cork, phellogen, phelloderm and primary cortex may be present or absent. They

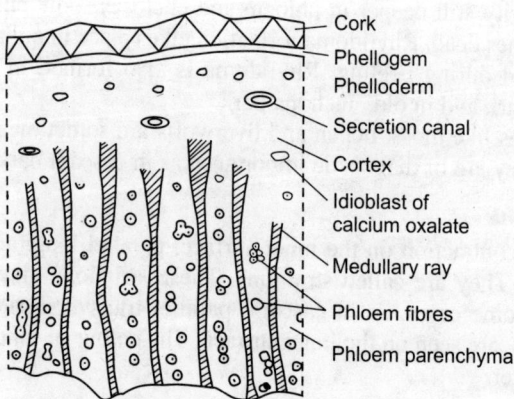

Fig. 4.7. T.S. of bark showing typical arrangement of cellular layers from outer to the innermost regions with special tissues like medullary rays, secretary canals, idioblasts, etc.

may be absent because of exfoliation or might have been removed during peeling. Pericycle is an outermost stelar tissue and is usually parenchymatous but sometimes it is sclerenchymatous, as in cinnamon and cassia barks, and consists of band of stone cells and fibres. Primary phloem is usually obliterated and is known as ceratenchyma and has translucent horny appearance. In **cascara** and **arjuna** sometimes crushed primary phloem is seen. Secondary phloem is an important tissue of bark and consists of sieve tubes, companion cells, phloem parenchyma and usually phloem fibres and stone cells. Phloem fibres and stone cells are of diagnostic importance in identifying the barks. Some barks, like cinchona, contain only phloem fibres; while **kurchi** contains only stone cells. **Cinnamon** and cascara barks contain both phloem fibres as well as stone cells. In cinchona, phloem fibres are isolated, in radial rows; while in cinnamon they are either isolated or in tangential rows. Their measurements, nature of thickening, lignification of cell walls and lumen are important in distinguishing different barks. **Sclereids** or **stone cells** may be present in any part of the bark like cork, phelloderm, cortex, pericycle or phloem. Stone cells are dead and may be present as isolated cells or in small groups or may be in continuous band. Stone cells are rounded, polyhedral or prismatic and their lumen may be narrow or large. In wild cherry bark stone cells are branched. Stone cells may contain inclusions like starch or calcium oxalate. Stone cells and fibres have mechanical functions and impart strength or rigidity. **Medullary rays** run radially and are usually made up of living cells. They may be one or more than one cell wide and may be straight or wavy. In cascara bark medullary rays contain active constituents, the anthracene derivatives.

Collection

Bark is usually collected in the spring or early summer by making suitable longitudinal and transverse incisions on the stem or root of the plant. In this season cambium is very active and since its cell walls are very thin, bark gets easily separated at cambium. In some cases bark is collected in other seasons. **Wild cherry bark** is collected in autumn because in this season it contains maximum percentage of active constituents, while cinchona bark is collected in rainy season because during that period it gets easily separated.

Methods of collection of bark from plants are different and are as follows:

1. **Felling:** This is a very primitive method of collection. The tree is felled at the base by an axe and bark is stripped off by making longitudinal and transverse incisions. In South America, cinchona bark in the beginning was collected by this method. By this method roots remain in the soil and root bark cannot be utilized and because of presence of roots, soil becomes unfit for further use.

2. **Uprooting:** Stems of trees of definite age and diameter are cut down and then the roots are dug out from the soil. Bark is then stripped off from stem, branches and roots and collected in the usual way. In Java cinchona bark is collected by this method.

3. **Coppicing:** In this method, stems of plants of definite age and diameter are cut at a certain distance above the ground and bark is collected in the usual way. From the stumps, remaining above the soil, new shoots arise. These shoots bear leaves, flowers and fruits. Birds and animals eat fruits and seed dispersal takes place and new plants are produced. Bark is collected from the shoots or branches of the plants produced in this way. Cascara bark and Ceylon cinnamon bark are collected by this method.

Drying

Barks are dried in tropical countries by keeping them in open air in sunlight. In other countries they are dried in drying sheds. Sometimes, bark is first dried in open air and then by artificial heat. During drying bark undergoes contraction because of loss of moisture. Contraction usually takes place in the transverse direction. The bark contains mechanical tissues like fibres in longitudinal direction and this prevents its contraction in that direction.

4. SEEDS

The seed is derived from a fertilized ovule. Seeds are *albuminous or endospermic* and *exalbuminonus or non-endospermic*. Further the seed shows certain characteristics like **hilum**, **raphe**, etc. To understand the development of seed, knowledge about the ovule from which it is formed is necessary.

Ovule contains parenchymatous tissue called **nucellus**. The ovule is surrounded on its outer surface by a single layer or a coat called **testa**. In some cases there are two coats when the outer one is called *testa* and inner one *tegument*. The coat or coats do not completely enclose the nucellus but have a small hole or opening at the apex called *micropyle* through which the pollen cells pass during fertilization. Nucellus encloses in itself a large cell called *embryo sac* which contains on its upper part an egg or ovum with synergids, in the centre secondary nucleus and in the lower part three antipodal cells.

Fertilization

During fertilization two pollen cells enter the embryo sac through the style and produce any of three types of seeds as described below:

1. **Exalbuminous or non-endospermic seed:** In this type one pollen cell combines with egg or ovum and forms a gamete from which embryo is

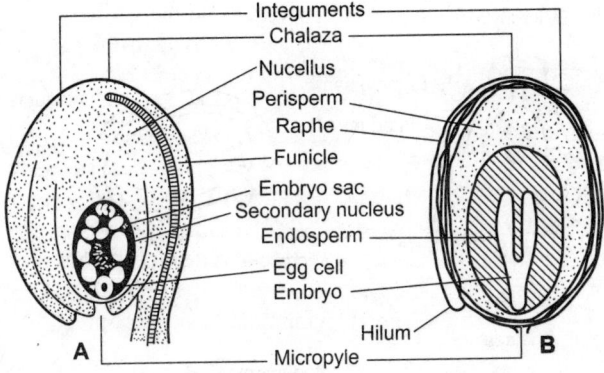

Fig. 4.8. Development of seeds. (A) Diagrammatic longitudinal section of anatropous ovule. (B) The same developing into seed.

produced and synergids help in the process. The activity during formation of embryo is intense and all the other cells of nucellus are absorbed. This type of seed contains only embryo surrounded by seed coat. Almond, groundnut, soyabean are exalbuminous seeds.

2. **Albuminous or endospermic seed:** In this type two pollen cells enter embryo sac and one pollen cell combines with egg and forms embryo as above and second pollen cell combines with secondary nucleus and forms endosperm. Endosperm usually contains protein albumin as reserve material and so these seeds are called albuminous while non-endospermic seeds are called exalbuminous. This process is called double fertilization and is also active and absorbs all cells outside embryo sac. These types of seeds contain embryo, endosperm and seed coat. Linseed and strophanthus are albuminous or endospermic seeds.

3. **Perisperm-containing seeds:** In this type embryo and endosperm are formed as a result of double fertilization. However, the activity is not much and some activity takes place in the nucellus mass outside embryo sac. As a result, tissue called perisperm is formed and these seeds have embryo, endosperm, perisperm and seed coat. **Cardamom and nutmeg** seeds have perisperm.

Ovules

There are four types of ovules named according to their position and from which, after fertilization, four different types of seeds are formed. They are as follows:

1. Atropous or orthotropous;
2. Campylotropous;
3. Anatropous; and
4. Amphitropous.

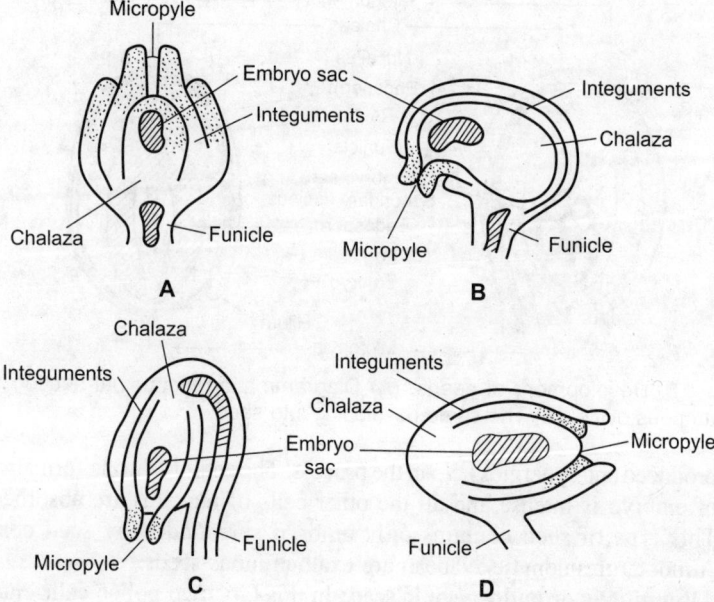

Fig. 4.9. Types of ovules. (A) Atropous; (B) Campylotropous; (C) Anatropous; and (D) Amphitropous.

1. **Atropous ovule:** In this ovule nucellus is in a straight line and micropyle and hilum are opposite to each other and they remain opposite also after fertilization in the seeds. Seeds developed from this ovule are not very common and are met with in species of Piperaceae and Polygonaceae.

2. **Campylotropous ovule:** In this ovule nucellus is curved or bent like a horseshoe. Micropyle and hilum are brought near the chalaza and there is no raphe. Seeds of Solanaceae and nux vomica belong to this type.

3. **Anatropous ovule:** This ovule is inverted at an angle of 180° over funicle or stalk of ovule because of rapid growth. Thus micropyle and hilum are brought near each other. During the fertilization funicle fuses with the mass of the seed and forms raphe. Micropyle and hilum are adjacent to each other with chalaza which is the base of the nucellus from which vascular strands start. Seeds from this ovule like strophanthus and linseed are found extensively.

4. **Amphitropous ovule:** In this type nucellus is straight and funicle is perpendicular or at an angle of 90° to the nucellus. During the development micropyle and hilum are separated in amphitropous ovule. Colchicum seed belongs to this group.

Appendages of the seed

These appendages or outgrowths are external to seed coat and partly or completely surround the seed coat. They arise from micropyle, hilum or raphe. Aril or arillus is a fleshly covering which originates from hilum and completely encloses the seed. Mace surrounding nutmeg is an example of aril. Arillode is a covering similar to aril but arises from micropyle as in cardamon. Aril and arillode are sometimes loosely used for each other. Caruncle is the localized fleshy outgrowth at the apex of seeds, as in castor seed and the other seeds of Euphorbiaceae. Strophiole is the parenchymatous growth along the raphe as seen in colchicum seed. Plume of hairs or awn consists of a stalk and crown and is found in seeds belonging to Asclepiadaceae and Apocynaceae. Awn is present in strophanthus seed.

Reserve material of seeds

Seeds contain as reserve materials starch, fixed oil and protein. Reserve materials supply nutrition during germination of the seeds. In some seeds in nux vomicà as cell walls are thick-walled because of reserve carbohydrate, hemicellulose. Protein consists mostly of aleurone grains. Aleurone grains consist of amorphous bed of protein and may contain as inclusions crystalloids, globoids, fixed oil and sometimes crystals of calcium oxalate. Crystalloids are well-formed crystals of proteins while globoids are spherical crystals of calcium or magnesium salts of organophosphoric acid. By difference in solubility behaviours and chemical tests aleurone grains and their inclusions can be identified. Aleurone grains give yellow colour with iodine solution and they are present only in seeds and their presence in powdered drugs helps in identifying seed drugs.

5. SUBTERRANEAN PARTS

Subterranean (underground) parts are roots or modifications of stems and roots. Roots may be true roots or adventitious or tuberous roots. Some of the drugs known as root drugs, e.g. gentian root, are partly or entirely rhizomes. Liquorice, though mostly consisting of stolons and rhizomes, is known as root. Generally, subterranean drugs are mixtures of both roots and rhizomes.

Rhizome

It is a subterranean stem and may grow in vertical, horizontal or oblique direction. Surface of the rhizome bears scale leaves and sometimes buds may be present in their axils. Rhizomes also show encircling scars of aerial leaves as seen in orris rhizome. Rhizome has nodes and internodes and its lateral and lower surface bears thin adventitious roots as seen in podophyllum and valerian rhizomes.

Rhizome may be monopodial or sympodial. In monopodial rhizome there is the same growing point and every year from the same point new flowering shoots arise and rhizome develops. Male fern is a monopodial rhizome. Ginger is a sympodial rhizome and this rhizome has apical bud as well as lateral buds. In first season from the apical bud a flowering stem is produced. Then the rhizome develops by the lateral bud which next year becomes the apical bud. The flowering stalk arises from the newly formed apical bud. In this way rhizome develops and shows the scars of flowering stems of previous years. Vertical rhizome grows vertically straight in the soil and is known as rootstock. The diameter of rootstock is nearly the same as that of the main root or tap root. Rootstock has short internodes and on its outer surface ring-shaped leaf scars and transverse wrinkles are seen. Stolon is a subterranean stem similar to runner. Stolon is however thick and it runs near or under the soil. Glycyrrhiza mostly consists of stolons.

Rhizome shows a central parenchymatous pith. Rhizomes never show central solid lignified xylem similar to roots and thus can be distinguished from roots. Rhizomes contain starch as the reserve material. Starch is present in rhubarb, ginger, etc. Inulin, sugars and other reserve materials are also found in rhizomes.

Root

The axis of the plant going vertically downwards in the soil is known as root. In some drugs primary roots persist and develop more than lateral roots. These roots are called tap roots. Roots of aconite and belladonna are tap roots. Lateral roots are produced endogenously from the primary root. The structure of lateral roots is the same as in tap root. Leaves and buds are absent in roots and no leaf scars are found on the surface of roots.

Small roots when they go downwards in the soil meet obstacles and they turn hither and thither. Thus roots available in commerce are rarely straight but to a lesser or greater extent tortuous. Ipecac and rauwolfia roots are tortuous. Some roots like aconite, jalap and calumba become fleshy or tuber-like because of storage of starch in them. These roots are called tuberous roots or tubercles.

There are a number of drugs which belong to the subterranean class of drugs as mentioned above and in the following paragraphs and these will be discussed at their appropriate places.

Corm

It is a short, thickened, fleshy, subterranean stem and contains buds, e.g. colchicum corm.

Bulb

It is a subterranean bud whose surrounding scale leaves have become fleshy. Scilla and onion are bulbs.

Collection and Drying

Subterranean drugs are usually collected in autumn. In this season plant is inactive. Its vegetative processes have ceased and thus it contains maximum percentage of active constituents. Sometimes subterranean drugs are collected in winter before the vegetative processes have started. The roots or rhizomes are dug out from the soil and cleaned by removing the adhering soil by shaking and washing. Then the aerial and other parts are separated. If the roots or rhizomes are big, transverse or longitudinal slices or small pieces are made to facilitate drying. Drug is dried directly in sunlight by putting on concrete floors or trays. Because of natural heat currents, the drug gets dried. In unfavourable climate drug is dried by artificial heat. If the temperature is more during drying the starch present in the drugs gets gelatinized. It is important to dry the drugs completely. Fungus, mould and other microorganisms grow and fermentation takes place if moisture is present in the drug. After drying it is stored in airtight containers.

WOOD

Wood consists of tissues of stem or root of dicotyledon plants lying internal to cambium and contains secondary xylem and primary xylem. Wood obtained from the stem also contains pith. Wood available in the commerce is of two types: (1) heartwood or duraman, and (2) sapwood or alburnum.

Heartwood is the inner, non-functioning, non-living part of the wood and is darker in colour because of the presence of resin, gums, tannins or colouring matter. In heartwood tyloses are produced in the vessels and thus vessels cannot carry out conduction and as a result lose their activity and become non-living. Sandalwood is an example of heartwood. **Sapwood** is the outer functional wood and is lighter in colour. Quassia wood is sapwood. The specific gravity of the mass of wood is 1.5 and thus wood is heavier than water. However wood floats in water because air is present in the cells of wood which makes it lighter. If we look in the transection of the wood, concentric annual or growth rings, which are arranged radially, are seen. Each growth ring consists of springwood and summerwood. Growth rings of wood are more prominent in temperate countries where there is wide difference between winter and summer temperatures. In tropical countries because of less difference in temperature, these rings are less conspicuous. Medullary rays are present at right angles to the rings. They may be uniseriate, biseriate or multiseriate. In each wood number of rays per mm is constant and their number in series and number per mm are of diagnostic importance. Xylem vessels can be seen as pores in the wood with naked eye or with magnifying lens. If the vessels are single or in small groups scattered more or less uniformly throughout the wood, the wood is called diffuse porous wood, e.g. quassia. The wood in which vessels are formed in the early springwood and from concentric rings is called ring porous wood. Woods of oak and ash are ring porous woods. Associated with the vessels is xylem parenchyma, which may be present in small patches or in large band and is usually paler in colour. If parenchyma is scattered uniformly throughout the wood it is called diffuse parenchyma. Tracheids are present in some woods, and do the function of local condition. Each tracheid is a single cell. In gymnosperm woods tracheid is the only conducting element. The remainder of the wood consists of fibres which impart strength and rigidity to the wood and as a result wood becomes hard. If the fibres are straight and arranged parallel, the wood breaks easily with smooth and uniform fracture and wood is called straight-grained. If the fibres in the wood are arranged at 30°, wood does not break easily and the fractured surface is irregular and splintery, it is called interlocked grained. Wood can be studied in longitudinal sections like radial or tangential, longitudinal sections. In radial section medullary rays are at right angles and in tangential section vessels and fibres appear more elongated and medullary rays appear in a lenticular cavity.

Lignin is present in the middle lamella and secondary cell walls and also gives strength to the wood. Wood shows characteristic red colour with phloroglucinol and hydrochloric acid because of lignin.

Examples of wood drugs which are included are only few and they will be described under the therapeutic principles they contain.

5

Study of Individual Drugs in Practical Classes

LAXATIVE DRUGS

ALOES

Aloe, Ghritkumari, Aliyo (Guj.)

The drug aloe is the dried residue left from the cell juice of the fleshy leaves of xerophytes, the *Aloe* species [dried juice of different species of *Aloe* (see Part 2)].

Botanical Source

Aloe is the dried juice collected by incision from the bases of the leaves of various species of *Aloe*.

Family

Liliaceae.

Geographical Source

There are about 160 species of aloe distributed in African countries, West Indies and India.

Characters

Curacao aloe is opaque and is yellow-brown to chocolate-brown in colour. Inferior overheated drug is nearly black. The fracture is waxy. Cape aloe is glassy, bark chocolate or green-chocolate in colour. Small pieces are reddish-brown or yellow-coloured or amber. Odour is characteristic sour and taste unpleasant and bitter. Socotrine aloe occurs in masses of different shapes and sizes and is yellow-brown to dark-brown and opaque. Fracture is irregular and porous and taste is bitter. Zanzibar aloe is opaque, more firm than Socotrine and livery brown in colour. Fracture is smooth as wax. Odour is considered pleasant but taste is bitter.

Chemical Tests

For carrying out the tests a clear solution of aloe is prepared as follows:

Boil 1 gm with 100 ml of water, allow it to cool; add 1 gm kieselguhr, stir well and filter through filter paper.

General Tests (for all aloes)

1. **Borax Test:** Take 10 ml of solution and add 0.5 gm of borax and heat. Green-coloured flourescence is seen which is due to aloe-emodin anthranol. This test becomes more sensitive if 5 to 10 drops of this reaction mixture are taken in a test tube and filled with water.

2. **Bromine Test:** Add equal volume of bromine solution to solution of aloe. Bulky yellow precipitate of tetrabromaloin is formed.

3. **Modified Anthraquinone Test:** Take 0.1 gm of drug and add 5 ml of 5% solution of ferric chloride and 5 ml dilute hydrochloric acid and heat on boiling water-bath for 5 minutes, cool the solution and shake gently with an organic solvent like benzene. Separate the organic solvent layer and add an equal volume of dilute ammonia. A pinkish-red colour is formed in ammoniacal layer. This test is of C. glycoside.

The following two tests Nos. (4) and (5) due to isobarbaloin are strongly positive in Curacao aloe and faint in Cape aloe and negative in Zanzibar and Socotrine aloes.

4. **Cupraloin Test:** Dilute 4 ml of the solution of aloe to 10 ml with water and add to it 1 drop of copper sulphate solution. Bright yellow colour is produced. Add 10 drops of saturated solution of sodium chloride. Colour changes to purplish. Add 20 drops of 90% alcohol, the purplish colour persists.

5. **Nitrous Acid Test:** Add few small crystals of sodium nitrite and few drops of dilute acetic acid to 5 ml of solution of aloe. Pink or purplish colour is produced.

6. **Nitric Acid Test:** Different aloes show different colours with nitric acid. To 5 ml of solution of aloe add 2 ml of concentrated nitric acid.

   (a) Curacao aloe   Deep reddish-brown
   (b) Socotrine aloe   Pale yellow-brown
   (c) Zanzibar aloe   Yellow-brown
   (d) Cape aloe   First brown, changing to green later.

Nitric acid test can be performed by taking little coarse drug on white porcelain tile and adding nitric acid to it.

RHUBARBS

The drug rhubarb consists of mainly the peeled pieces of dried rhizomes and roots of *Rheum palmatum* and *Rheum officinale* or from hybrids of both the species (and other species of *Rheum*), but not the rhizome and roots of *Rheum rhaponticum*. The drugs are called medicinal rhubarbs. Five- to seven-year-old plants give the drug roots and rhizomes.

Family

Polygonaceae.

Geographical Source

China, Tibet.

Indian Rhubarb

Indian Rhubarb, Revandchini

Botanical Source

Indian rhubarb consists of dried rhizome of *Rheum emodi* and *R. webbianum* and other species of *Rheum*.

Rhapontic Rhubarb

The drug contains undesirable chemical constituent rhaponticine (see Part 2).

Test

Rhaponticine and rhapontigenin give intense bright blue fluorescence in UV-light. This helps detect the rhapontic rhubarb, which is considered as an adulterant and hence is not official in pharmacopoeias.

RHUBARB

Rhizoma Rhei, Rhubarb Rhizome, Rheum, Rhei Radix, Revanchini (Hindi)

Botanical Source

Rhubarb consists of the peeled dried rhizomes and roots of *Rheum palmatum* Linn., *Rheum officinale* and other species of rhubarb, excepting *Rheum rhaponticum*.

Morphology

- **General appearance:** Rounds, flats or high-dried drug.
- **Size and Shape:** Round—5–12 cm long, 3–8 cm diameter, cylindrical, conical, barrel-shaped; Flat—Upto 15 cm long, and upto 5 cm thick, planoconvex.

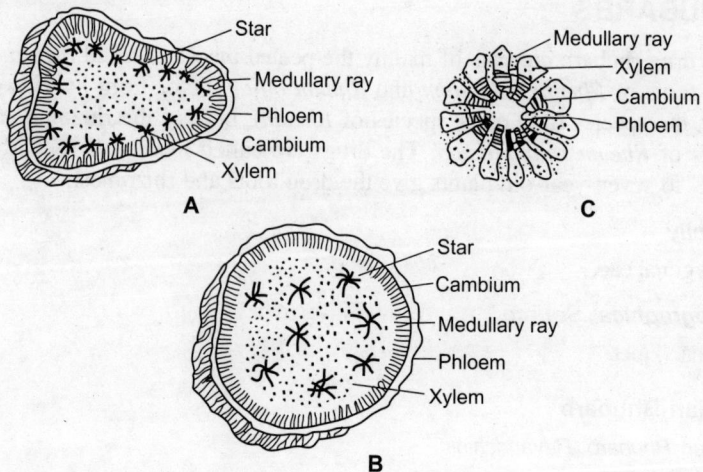

Fig. 5.1. Rhubarb, *Rheum* species. (A) Transverse section of *R. palmatum* (diagrammatic), (B) Transverse section of *R. officinale* (diagrammatic), (C) Single star spot.

- **Surface:** Smooth, pale brown to reddish and mottled due to reddish-brown network of medullary rays in white parenchyma of phloem or xylem. Abnormal or accessory vascular bundles known as star spots, and drying holes are seen. Most of the surface is covered with yellow powder.
- **Fracture:** Irregular, granular. Drug with pink fracture is considered of good quality.
- **Fractured surface:** It shows on the outer region a distinct and continuous cambium with external phloem and internal radial, non-lignified secondary xylem with reddish-orange medullary rays and a wide pith.
- **Odour:** Characteristic, slightly aromatic.
- **Taste:** Bitter, slightly astringent, gritty.
- **Star spots:** Within the cambium star spots or abnormal vascular bundles are present. They are in a continuous ring in palmatum type and irregularly scattered in officinale type. The star spots have internal phloem, cambium, radiate or star-shaped medullary rays (hence the name star spots) and external xylem.

Chemical Tests

1. Microsublimation.
2. With ammonia pink colour.
3. With 5% potassium hydroxide blood-red colour.

INDIAN RHUBARB

Indian Rhubarb, Revandchini

Indian rhubarb consists of the dried rhizome of *Rheum emodi* Wall. and *Rheum webbianum* Royle and other species of *Rheum*.

Morphology

It is compact, firm and occurs in subcylindrical, conical or barrel-shaped planoconvex pieces. These pieces are 2–20 cm in length, 1.5–8 cm in diameter. Outer suface is yellowish-brown to purplish-brown. It is longitudinally wrinkled, furrowed or ridged.

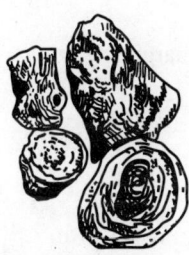

Cork
Cortex
Phloem
Cambium
Xylem
Medullary ray
Pith

Fig. 5.2. Pieces of rhizomes of *Rheum emodi*.

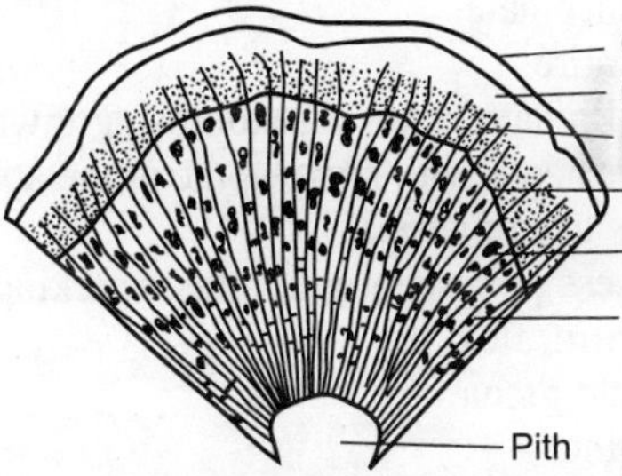

Fig. 5.3. Indian Rhubarb, *R. emodi* and *R. webbianum* (T.S. of Rhizome ×150).

Uses

A well-known purgative.

SENNA LEAVES

Tinnevelley Senna Leaves, Senna Indica, Indian Senna

Botanical Source

Tinnevelley senna consist of dried compound leaflets of *Cassia angustifolia* Vahl.

Family

Leguminosae.

Geographical Source

South India, Tinnevelley district and its adjoining areas.

Morphology

• General appearance: Entire and less broken.
• Size: 2.5–6 cm long, 7–8 mm wide.

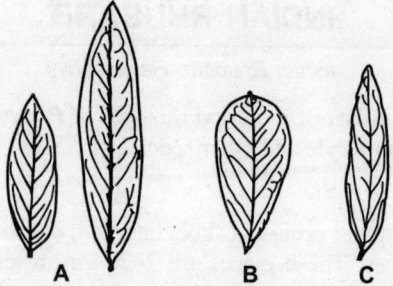

Fig. 5.4. (A) Indian senna; (B) Dog senna; (C) Palthe senna.

- Shape: Lanceolate.
- Margin: Entire.
- Venation: Pinnate, veins anastomosing towards margin.
- Apex: Less acute with sharp spine at the apex.
- Base: Less asymmetrical.
- Surface: Less pubescent with press markings.
- Texture: Firm, flexible.
- Colour: Pale green.
- Odour: Faint.
- Taste: Mucilaginous and slightly bitter.

Histology

The leaf shows characteristic epidermal trichomes which are unicellular, conical, thick-walled and with a warty cuticle. These trichomes are curved near the base. The lamina is isobilateral with a single layer of palisade beneath each epidermis. The anastomosing veins are accompanied by prisms of calcium oxalate. The paracytic stomata are present on the both the surfaces.

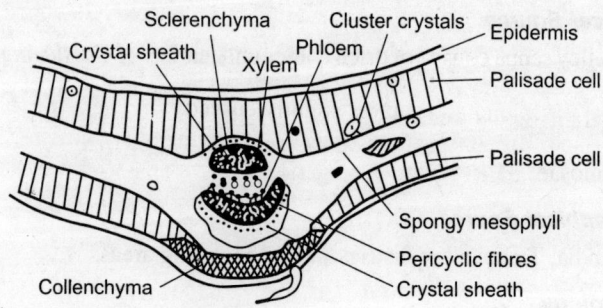

Fig. 5.5. T.S. of Senna leaf.

Chemical Test

Borntrager's test for anthraquinones: Boil few leaves with dilute sulphuric acid, filter and to the filtrate add organic solvent like benzene, ether or chloroform and shake. Separate the organic solvent layer by pipette and add ammonia. The ammoniacal layer becomes pink to red. Senna pods, rhubarb and cascara contain anthraquinone derivatives and show the above test.

SENNA PODS

Sennae Fructus, Senna Legumes, Senna Fruits

Botanical Source

Senna pods are the dried ripe fruits of *Cassia angustifolia* Vahl known as Tinnevelley senna pods.

Family

Leguminosae.

Geographical Source

Upper Nile territories, South India.

Morphology

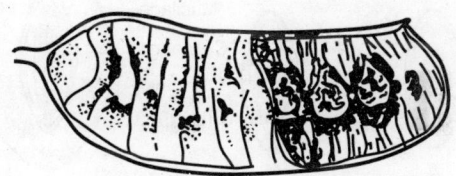

Fig. 5.6. Tinnevelley Senna pods.

- General appearance: Superior, unilocular, laterally flattened, dehiscing by both sutures.
- Size: About 5 cm long and 1.5–2 cm broad.
- Shape: Oblong and sutures slightly curved.
- Surface: Brownish-green, veins less prominent and less regular.
- Apex: Rounded on the ventral surface, remains of the style distinct.
- Seeds: 5–8 attached to the ventral surface by fanicle. Seeds of both pods are similar.

Chemical Test

Borntrager's test can also be performed like the one performed for the senna leaflets.

Uses

Senna pods are used like senna leaflets. The action takes place after 6–8 hours after taking the drug or preparation made from anthraquinone-containing drugs.

ISPAGHULA

Ispaghula, Ispagol, Ishabgula, Isabgol

Botanical Source

Ispaghula consists of dried seeds of *Plantago ovata* Forssk.

Family

Plantaginaceae.

Geographical Source

The plant grows wild in Punjab, Sind and Persia. It is cultivated in North Gujarat around Siddhpur and to some extent in south Rajasthan.

Morphology

Ispaghula seeds are derived from amphitropous ovules.

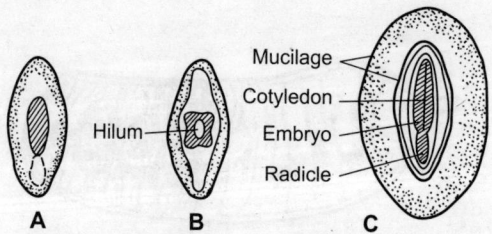

Fig. 5.7. Ispaghula seed. (A) Dorsal surface; (B) Ventral surface; (C) Soaked in water.

- Size: 2–3.5 mm long, 1–1.75 mm broad.
- Shape: Ovate, cymbiform.
- Outer surface: Hard translucent, smooth. On the dorsal or convex surface there is a small elongated glossy reddish-brown spot in the centre; on the ventral or concave surface there is a cavity having hilum covered with a thin whitish membrane.
- Colour: Pinkish grey to brown.
- Odour: None.
- Taste: Bland, mucilaginous.

Chemical Tests

1. Ispaghula seeds with ruthenium red show red colour because of mucilage.
2. Take few seeds on slide and add water. Mucilage comes out and forms zone surrounding the seeds.
3. Swelling factor: Seeds containing mucilage absorb water and swell. Swelling can be determined quantitatively by swelling factor. 1 gm of the drug is put in a measuring cylinder of 25 ml capacity and 20 ml water is added. It is shaken periodically during first 23 hours and kept for one more hour. The volume occupied by the drug is called swelling factor. Swelling factor of ispaghula seeds is 10–13.

The demulcent property of mucilage can be shown by following simple experiments.

1. Take a reflex frog and dip one leg into dilute hydrochloric acid. There will be movement because of irritation. Add mucilage to the acid and dip. There will be no movement.
2. If on a cut on a finger 5% sodium chloride solution is put there will be smarting pain. If mucilage is added to the salt solution and put on finger no pain will be felt.

ISPAGHULA HUSK

Ispghulae Testa, Sat Isobgulo

Ispaghula husk consists of the dried seed coats of *Plantago ovata*. Husk is thin, boat-shaped, white or translucent, 2–3 mm long and 0.5–1.0 mm wide. Swelling factor is 20. According to Atal and his co-workers the value mentioned in I.P. is low and 0.5 gm. gives the same value.

Uses

As a mild laxative (see Part 2). This is the best mucilage-containing drug.

CASTOR OIL

Castor Oil, Oleum Ricini

Botanical Source

Castor oil is the fixed oil obtained by expression of the seeds of *Ricinus communis* Linn.

Family

Euphorbiaceae.

Geographical Source

India and other tropical and subtropical countries.

Characters

Medicinal castor oil is colourless or slightly yellow-coloured viscid liquid. Odour is slight and taste slightly acrid. Castor oil is soluble in absolute alcohol in all proportions. The solubility is attributed to OH group of ricinoleic acid present in castor oil.

Chemical Tests

5 ml of light petroleum (50° to 60°) with 10 ml of castor oil at 15.5° shows a clear solution. If light petroleum is increased to 15 ml the mixture becomes turbid. Other oils do not show this test and their adulteration can be detected by this test.

Uses

It is a mild purgative and has other properties and uses (see Part 2).

CARDIOTONIC DRUGS

DIGITALIS LEAVES

Foxglove Leaves, Folia Digitalis

Botanical Sources

Digitalis consists of dried leaves of *Digitalis purpurea*. After collection leaves are dried immediaely at temperature below 60° and they contain not more than 5% moisture. After drying leaves are stored in moisture-proof containers.

Family

Scrophulariaceae.

Geographical Sources

European countries, England, Germany, France, North America, Kashmir.

Morphology

- General Appearance: Usually broken and crumpled.
- Shape: Ovate-lanceolate.
- Size: 10–40 cm long and 3–10 cm wide.
- Margin: Crenate to dentate.
- Apex: Obtuse or rounded.
- Base: Tapering, decurrent.
- Upper surface: Slightly pubescent, dark green, little wrinkled, one water pore present near each tooth.
- Lower surface: Greyish-green, very pubescent.

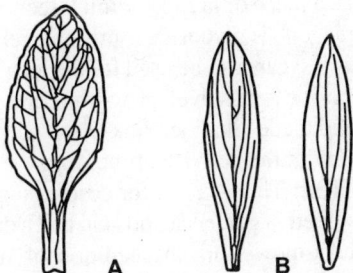

Fig. 5.8. Morphological comparison of the leaf of *Digitalis purpurea* (A) with *D. lanata* (B).

- Venation: Pinnate, mid-rib, lateral veins, veinlets and still smaller veinlets prominent on the under-surface; lateral veins leave the mid-rib at an acute angle and anastomose on the margin.
- Petiole: Winged, 2.5–10 cm long.
- Odour: Characteristic.
- Taste: Bitter.

Histology

Digitalis is dorsiventral and can be easily identified due to the presence of characteristic simple covering and glandular trichomes. The covering trichomes are uniseriate, usually three to four cells long, having collapsed cells, acute apex and finely warty cuticle. The glandular trichomes have a short unicellular stalk and bicellular or rarely unicellular head. These glandular trichomes are usually located over the veins. Further anomocytic (ranunculaceous) type of stomata are also present mainly on the lower surface.

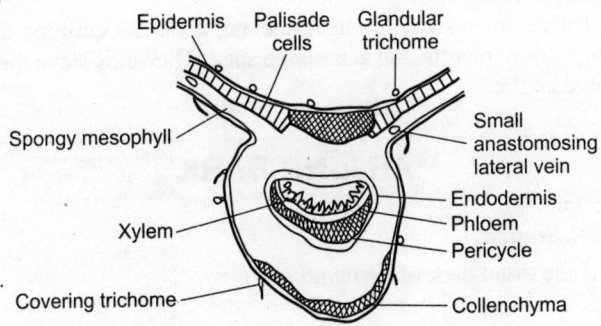

Fig. 5.9. *Digitalis purpurea.* T.S. of mid-rib.

Chemical Tests

Digitalis glycosides having five-membered lactone ring are C_{23} glycosides. These glycosides show the following tests which are due to the intact lactone (see also Part 3).

1. **Baljet Test:** Take a piece of lamina or thick section of the leaf and add sodium picrate reagent. If glycoside is present, yellow to orange colour will be seen. This test can also be used for the localization of glycoside.
2. **Legal Test:** Glycoside is dissolved in pyridine and sodium nitroprusside solution added and made alkaline. Pink to red colour is produced. This test runs parallel with the activity of the drug.
3. **Keller-Killiani Test:** This is a test for desoxy sugar. Digitoxose or its glycoside is dissolved in glacial acetic acid and a drop of ferric chloride solution is added followed by the addition of sulphuric acid which forms the lower layer. A reddish-brown colour is seen at the junction of two liquids and the upper layer becomes bluish-green.

Uses

As a cardiotonic used to increase the activity and efficiency of heart. Used in congestive heart failure.

DIGITALIS LANATA LEAF

Botanical Source

The drug consists of the dried leaves of *Digitalis lanata*.

Family

Scrophulariaceae.

Geographical Source

This species grows in the region adjacent to the Danube in Central Europe. It has been cultivated in England and in the USA. It is also cultivated in India. The plant is biennial.

The leaves are sessile, linear-lanceolate, about 30 cm long and 4 cm broad with entire margin and acuminate apex. The veins leave the mid-rib at an acute angle.

ARJUNA BARK

Botanical Source

Arjuna is the dried bark of *Terminalia arjuna*.

Family

Combretaceae.

Members of this family are characterized by the presence of tannins and are used as tanning agents. Myrobalans (Haritaki or Harde) and beleric fruits belong to this family.

Geographical Source

India. Trees are found in North Gujarat at Balaram, a picnic place.

Morphology

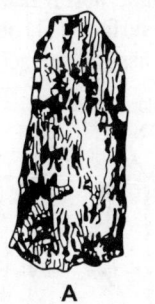 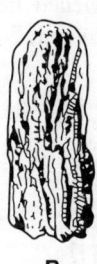

A   B

Fig. 5.10. (A) Outer surface of *T. arjuna*; (B) Inner surface of *T. arjuna*.

- Size: Pieces of varying sizes upto 15 cm or more in length, 10 cm or more in width and 3 mm to 1 cm thick.
- Shape: Flat or slightly curved.
- Outer surface: Smooth and grey-coloured.
- Inner surface: Finely striated, brown.
- Fracture: Short, revealing stratified nature of the bark.
- Odour: None.
- Taste: Astringent.

Uses

The bark is popularly used as a cardiotonic drug.

CARMINATIVES AND G.I. REGULATORS

These are those drugs which lead to eructation (belching) reflex. A number of volatile oils containing drugs are said to show this action. Hence they are included in this category of drugs. Their action takes place in stomach and partly in gastrointestinal tract.

Since a number of such drugs belonging to the Family Umbelliferae are fruits, it is considered logical to describe their common morphological and microscopical characters before actually taking up the individual fruit, called the umbelliferous fruit.

Umbelliferous fruits (Family Umbelliferae) show common characteristics as morphological and microscopical characters. Even their chemical constituents and method of cultivation and collection show similarities in one way or the other. The drugs belonging to this family which are going to be studied are Fennel, Coriander, Caraway, Anise, Cumin, Dill, Asafoetida, Hemlock, Majus and Visnaga.

A mericarp shows at its apex stylopod and it has a base, the point at which the pedicel is attached. It has two surfaces: (1) outer, dorsal or curved surface; and (2) inner, ventral or commissural surface.

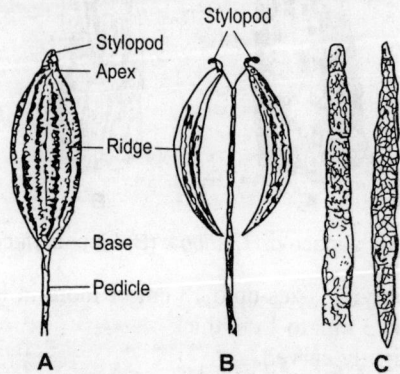

Fig. 5.11. (A) A cremocarp; (B) A fruit of caraway showing the two mericarps attached to the carpophore; (C) Isolated vittae.

The pericarp consists of three parts:

1. The outer layer, called epicarp, forms the skin of the fruit.
2. The middle layer, called mesocarp (like pulp in mango), encloses other well-defined tissues e.g. vascular bindles, vittae, fibres, etc.
3. The inner part, called endocarp, is often thin and single-layered.

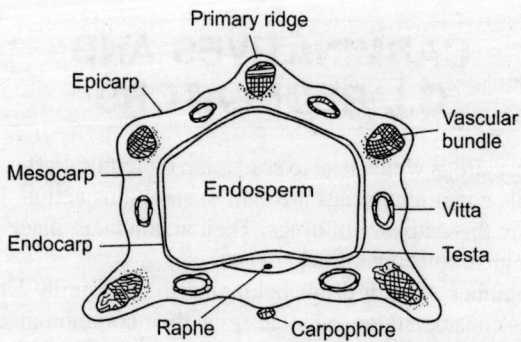

Fig. 5.12. A typical mericarp in T.S. showing different sides and anatomical parts.

The seed is composed of testa (seed coat), endosperm embryo. Some fruits show epicarp with covering trichomes of different shapes and sizes.

CORIANDER

Fructus Coriandri, Coriander Fruits, Dhaniya (Hindi),
Dhana (Guj.), Kazbara (Arabic)

Botanical Source
Coriander consists of dried ripe fruits of *Coriandrum sativum* Linn.

Family
Umbelliferae.

Geographical Source
Cultivated in many countries of Central and Eastern Europe, especially Russia and Thuringia, Mediterranean countries, Morocco and India.

Morphology

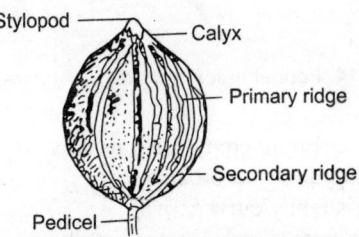

Fig. 5.13. A cremocarp of coriander fruit, *Coriandrum sativum.*

- General appearance: Entire cremocarps.
- Size: 3–4 mm in diameter.
- Shape: Sub-spherical.
- Surface: A short stylopod with 5 small calyx teeth present at the apex. Ten inconspicuous wavy primary ridges alternating with 8 prominent straight secondary ridges present.
- Colour: Yellowish-brown.
- Odour: Aromatic.
- Taste: Spicy, aromatic.

Uses
Aromatic, carminative and flavouring agent.

FENNEL

Fructus foeniculii, Fennel fruit, Badi saunph (Hindi), Variyali (Guj.)

Botanical Source
Fennel consists of the dried ripe fruits of *Foeniculum vulgar* Miller obtained by cultivation.

Family

Umbelliferae.

Geographical Source

Indigenous to Mediterranean countries and Asia. Cultivated in many countries of Central and Eastern Europe, India and Japan.

Morphology

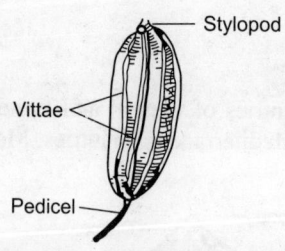

Fig. 5.14. Fennel fruit (cremocarp) – lateral view.

- General appearance: Entire cremocarps usually with pedicels.
- Size: 5–10 mm long, 2–4 mm broad.
- Shape: Straight or slightly curved, oval.
- Surface: Glabrous with 5 straight prominent straw-coloured primary ridges and bifid stylopod at the apex.
- Colour: Greenish-brown.

Microscopy

- Epicarp: It consists of outer epidermis; cells of epidermis in transection tabular and tangentially elongated. Cuticle unstriated. Trichomes absent.

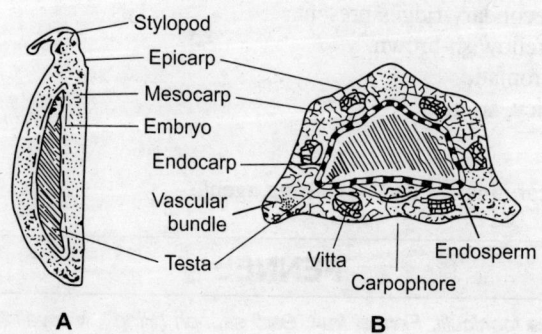

Fig. 5.15. Sections of fennel: (A) Longitudinal section of a single fennel fruit (mericarp); (B) Transverse section of a single fennel fruit (mericarp).

- Mesocarp: Five bicollateral vascular bundles with lateral phloem are present below each ridge tangentially elongated. Reticulate parenchyma present above and below the vascular bundles. Four vittae are present on dorsal surface and two vittae on ventral surface.
- Endocarp or inner epidermis: Shows parquetry arrangement; a group of 4–5 cells parallel are placed at acute angles with groups of similar cells. These cells appear tangentially elongated is transection.
- Testa: Narrow, having tangentially elongated cells with brownish granular contents.
- Endosperm: Consists of wide polyhedral thick-walled cells. Cells contain fixed oil and aleurone grains with globoids and minute rosette crystals of calcium oxalate as inclusions.
- Embryo: Present in upper 1/3 area at the apex.

Uses

Aromatic, carminative and flavouring agent. Also used as a respiratory stimulant and expectorant.

AJOWAN

Ajwan Fruits, Ajowain (Hindi), Ajwain (Urdu)

Botanical Source

Ajwan consists of the dried ripe fruits of *Trachyspermum ammi* (L.) Sprague (Syn. *Carum copticum*; *Ptychotis ajowan*).

Family

Umbelliferae.

Geographical Source

Cultivated mainly in India.

Morphology

- General appearance: It occurs mostly as carps.
- Size: About 2 mm long; compressed.
- Shape: Ovoid.
- Surface: Bears short pale coloured protuberances, six vitrae, five primary ridges pale in colour.
- Colour: Greyish-brown.
- Odour: Thymol-like odour.
- Taste: Aromatic spicy.

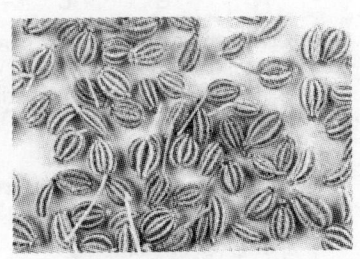

Fig. 5.16. Ajowan fruit.

Uses

Spice and a source of thymol.

CARDAMOM

Cardamom fruit, Cardamom seed, Ilayachi (Hindi and Guj.)

Botanical Source

Cardamom consists of the dried ripe seeds of *Elettaria cardamomum* var. *minuscula*. Seeds are removed from fruits when required for use.

Family

Zingiberaceae.

Geographical Source

Cultivated in Mysore and Kerala States in South India and Guatemala and Sri Lanka.

Mysore and Malabar varieties though originally obtained from Mysore and Malabar respectively are at present cultivated in Ceylon from Mysore-type and Malabar-type plants and do not refer to the present geographical source and hence are called Ceylon-Mysore and Ceylon-Malabar. Mysore or Ceylon-Mysore fruits are smooth, ovoid, bleached and have cream colour. Malabar or Ceylon-Malabar fruits are smaller, darker and less smooth than Mysore fruits. **Mangalore cardamoms** are more globular and more rough and resemble Malabar fruits. Aleppy cardamoms are green-coloured, narrower, similar in size and shape to Malabar with striated pericarp.

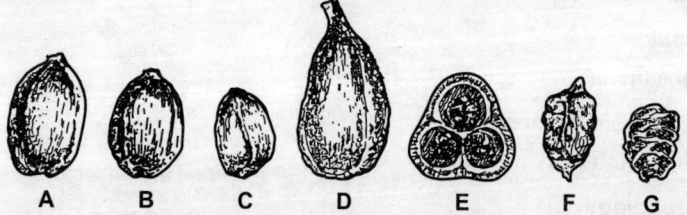

Fig. 5.17. Cardamom, *Elettaria cardamomum*. (A–D) Different varieties of the fruit. (A) Mysore; (B) Mangalore; (C) Malabar; (D) Wild; (E) T.S. of fruit showing the seeds; (F) Seed covered by arillus; (G) Seed without arillus.

Morphology

- General appearance: Inferior trilocular 3-angled capsule.
- Size: 1–2 cm long.
- Shape: Ovoid or oblong.
- Apex: Beaked.
- Base: Rounded with remains of stalk.
- Surface: Smooth or longitudinally striated.
- Colour: Pale buff.

- Seeds: Seeds are derived from anatropous ovules. They are 5–12 in each capsule, and attached in double rows with axile placentation in each of three cells of the capsule and are surrounded by arillus.
  - Size: Upto 4 mm in length and 3 mm in width.
  - Shape: Irregularly angular.
  - Colour: Dark reddish-brown.

Uses

As an aromatic stimulant, carminative and flavouring agent.

CLOVE

Caryophylli, Clove buds. Clove flowers, Lovang (Hindi), Laving (Guj.)

Botanical Source

Clove consists of the dried flower buds of *Eugenia caryophyllus* Spreng and contains not more than 5% of its stalks and not more than 1% other organic matter.

Family

Myrtaceae.

Geographical Source

Plant native of Molucca Islands (Indonesia). It is cultivated mainly in Islands of Zanzibar, Pemba, Amboiana and Sumatra. It is also found in Madagascar, Penang, Mauritius, West Indies and Ceylon.

Morphology

- Clove: It is reddish-brown, plump, heavy, about 16–20 mm long and consists of lower solid stalk-like portion called hypanthium and upper crown or cap.
- Hypanthium: It is sub-cylindrical, slightly flattened and tapering below. It is 10–13 mm long, 4 mm wide and 2 mm thick. Numerous shizolysigenous oil glands are found in the hypodermis. Inferior bilocular ovary is seen at its upper part.
- Crown: It consists of calyx, corolla, stamens and style. Calyx consists of four thick, spreading projecting sepals. Corolla is dome-shaped and is made up of four pale yellow-coloured, imbricate, immature, membranous petals and is also called head, crown, cap or dome. Numerous, free, introse and tetradelphous stamens are enclosed in the crown. Gynaecium consists of inferior bilocular ovary containing numerous ovules with axile placentation. A single erect, firm style reaching nearly upto corolla is seen. At the base of style a nectar disc or nectary is present.
- Odour: Strong, spicy and aromatic.
- Taste: Pungent and aromatic.

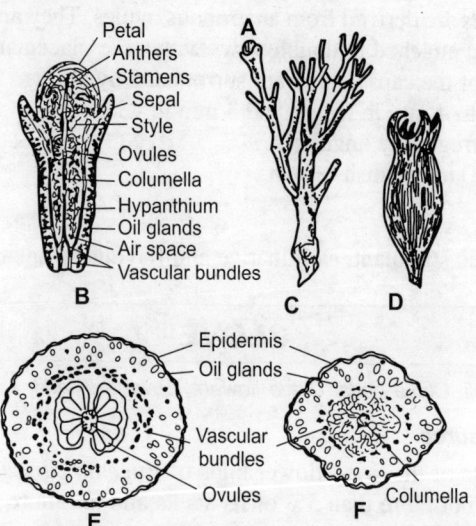

Fig. 5.18. Clove, *Eugenia caryophyllus.* (A) Single clove attached to the clove stalks; (B) Clove cut longitudinally; (C) Trichotomous stalks of clove; (D) Clove fruit (mother clove); (E) T.S. of hypanthium in the region of the ovary; (F) T.S. of hypanthiurn in the middle part.

- Test: Clove when indented with fingernail exudes volatile oil and when put into freshly boiled and cooled water it sinks.

For detailed anatomical description consult the advanced pharmacognosy book by the same author (J.S. Qadry).

Tests

1. Treat a thick section of hypanthium of clove with 50% potassium hydroxide solution. Needle-shaped crystals of potassium eugenate are seen.
2. Place a drop of chloroform extract of clove or clove oil or eugenol on a slide and add to it a drop of 30% aqueous solution of sodium hydroxide saturated with sodium bromide. Needle- and pear-shaped crystals of sodium eugenate arranged in rosette are seen almost immediately.
3. Dissolve a drop of clove oil in 5 ml of alcohol and add a drop of ferric chloride solution. Blue colour is seen because of phenolic OH group of eugenol.
4. Prepare a decoction of clove and add to it ferric chloride solution. Blue-black colour is formed because of the tannins.

Uses

As a carminative and a flavouring agent. Also used as an antiseptic and aromatic stimulant (see Part 2).

NUTMEG

Semen myristicae, Myristica, Jayfal (Guj.)

Botanical Source

Nutmeg is the kernel of the dried ripe seed of *Myristica fragrans* Houtten, deprived of its arillus and seed coat and with or without a thin coating of lime.

Family

Myristicaceae.

Geographical Source

A native of Mollucca islands in Indonesia and at present cultivated in West Indies and other tropical countries.

Morphology

- General appearance: Kernels consist of outer and inner perisperm, endosperm and embryo.
- Size: 2–3 cm long, 1.5–2 cm wide or in diameter.
- Shape: Ovoid or broadly elongated.
- Outer Surface: Outer surface consists of external perisperm and is rough, dark-brown, with reticulate furrows, which are the vascular bundles. At one end of the kernel there is small projection in the centre of which is the position of micropyle and slightly by its side is the position of hilum. Chalaza is indicated near the other end by slight depression. From chalaza to hilum there is a distinct furrow indicating the position of raphe.
- A longitudinal preparation shows perisperm, the inner part of which penetrates the endosperm showing a ruminated appearance and a small shrunken embryo at the micropylar end.

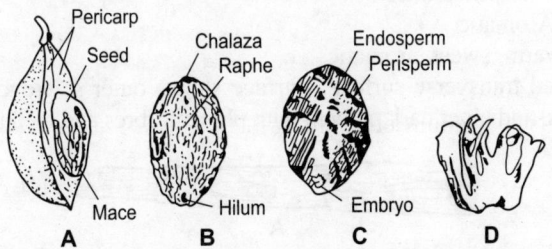

Fig. 5.19. Myristica seed, *Myristica fragrans.* (A) Seed in half of the pericarp; (B) Seed; (C) Longitudinal section of the seed; (D) Entire mace.

Uses

Aromatic, carminative and flavouring agent (see Part 2 for more uses).

MACE

Banda mace, Javantri, Jaypatri

Mace is the arillus of the seed of *M. fragrans*. Dried mace is of golden yellow colour. Mace gives yellow colour with alkali or concentrated sulphuric acid, while Bombay mace and Papua mace give dark red and cherry red colour respectively.

Mace has similar uses like that of nutmeg.

CINNAMON BARK

Cortex cinnamonni, Ceylon cinnamon, Ceylon Taj (Guj.), Dalchini (Hindi)

Botanical Source

Cinnamon is the dried inner bark of the coppiced shoots of *Cinnamomum zeylanicum* Nees.

Family

Lauraceae.

Geograpbical Source

Ceylon, Java, Sumatra, West Indies, Seychelles, Jamaica, Brazil.

Macroscopy

- General appearance: Single or double compound quills of about 30 pieces.
- Size: Length of quill upto 1 metre, 6–10 mm in diameter, 0.5 mm thick.
- Outer surface: Yellowish-brown, showing longitudinal wavy lines, pericyclic fibres and holes indicating the position of twigs.
- Inner aurface: Dark brown longitudinally striated.
- Fracture: Short, splintery.
- Odour: Aromatic.
- Taste: Warm, sweet, aromatic.
- Smoothed transverse surface: Surface shows outer sclerenchymatous pericycle and inner dark phloem with phloem fibres and medullary rays.

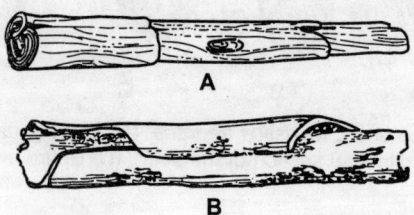

Fig. 5.20. Barks of Cassia and Cinnamon. (A) Cassia (quill); (B) Cinnamon (compound double quill).

Chemical Tests

1. One drop of volatile oil is dissolved in 5 ml of alcohol and a drop of ferric chloride solution is added. A pale green colour is produced. With ferric chloride cinnamic aldehyde gives brown colour and eugenol, because of phenolic OH gives blue colour and an intermediary green colour is obtained.
2. In cassia bark oil, brown colour is obtained as it contains only cinnamic aldehyde.
3. Prepare a chloroform extract by extracting few milligrams with 1 ml of chloroform on slide and to 2 drops of chloroform extract or of volatile oil add 2 drops of 10% aqueous solution of phenylhydrazin hydrochloride and cover with cover slip. Small rod-shaped crystals of the phenylhydrazone of cinnamic aldehyde are seen.

Uses

It is used as an aromatic carminative, flavouring agent, stomachic and antiseptic and mild astringent.

CASSIA BARK

Chinese cinnamon, Cassia lignea

Botanical Source

Cassia bark is obtained from *Cinnamomum cassia* Blume.

Family

Lauraceae.

Geographical Source

South-eastern provinces of China and Cochin.

Morphology

- Size: Upto 40 cm in length, 1–2 cm in width, 1–3 mm in thickness.
- Shape: Channelled to single quills.
- Outer surface: Dark reddish-brown, somewhat rough patches of gray cork.
- Inner surface: Finely striated.
- Fracture: Short.
- Odour: Less aromatic than Ceylon cinnamon.
- Taste: Aromatic, astringent, mucilaginous.
- Smoothed transection: Shows patches of greyish cork, cortex with sclereids and sclerenchymatous pericycle and phloem similar to Ceylon cinnamon bark.

Uses

It is a good substitute of cinnamon and is used similar to it.

GINGER

Rhizoma zingiberis, Zingiber; Ginger, Soonth (Guj.), Saunth (Hindi)

Botanical Source

Ginger consists of the rhizome of *Zingiber officinale* Roscoe, scraped and dried in the sun.

Family

Zingiberaceae.

Geographical Source

Jamaica, South India (Cochin), Africa, Japan.

Morphology

- General appearance: Sympodial branching, horizontal rhizome.
- Size: Length 5–15 cm, width (height) 3–6 cm, thickness 0.5–1.5 cm.
- Shape: Laterally flattened on the upper side with short flattened oblique, obovate branches or fingers. Each branch is 1–3 cm long and at its apex shows a depressed scar of the stem.
- Surface: Longitudinally striated with occasional projecting fibres.
- Fracture: Short, starchy, fibrous.
- Fractured surface: Shows a narrow bark, a well-marked endodennis and a wide stele, showing numerous scattered greyish points (fibrovascular bundles) and smaller yellowish points (secretion cells).
- Colour: Buff.
- Odour: Agreeable and aromatic.
- Taste: Agreeable and pungent.

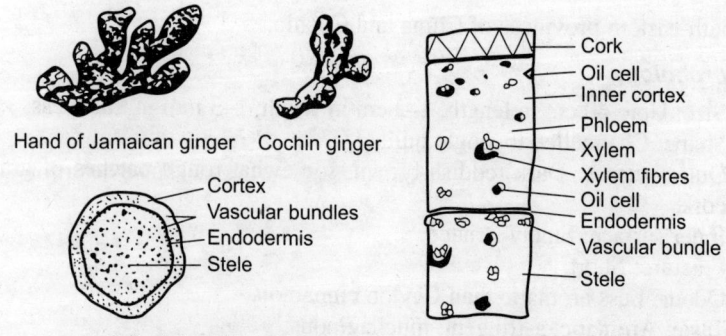

Fig. 5.21. Ginger, *Zingiber officinale*. (A) Hand of Jamaican ginger; (B) Cochin ginger; (C) T.S. of Jamaican ginger; (D) T.S. of ginger enlarged.

Microscopy

- Cork: Outer zone consists of irregularly arranged cells and inner zone consists of cells arranged in radial rows. Cork is absent in Jamaica ginger.
- Phellogen: Indistinct.
- Cortex: Cortex consists of thin-walled, cellulosic rounded parenchyma with intercellular spaces. These cells contain simple, ovate or sac-shaped starch grains with hilum at the pointed end. Cortex contains closed collateral fibrovascular bundles. Some cells contain yellow-brown oleo-resin.
- Endodermis: It is distinct and consists of tangentially elongated cells containing suberin in radial walls. Starch is absent.
- Stele: Below the endodermis is a ring of vascular bundles without fibres. The remaining tissue contains fibrovascular bundles, starch and oleo-resin cells similar to cortex.

Pharmacopoeial Standards

1. 90% alcohol-soluble extractive is not less than 4.5%.	Ginger exhausted with alcohol has 1.5% extractive. Water-exhausted ginger cannot be evaluated in this way.
2. Water-soluble extractive is not less than 10%.	Water-exhausted ginger has 6% extractive. Alcohol-exhausted ginger passes this standard.
3. Total ash is not more than 6%.	In ginger, not well-washed or limed, total ash is more.
4. Water-soluble ash is not less than 1.7%.	In water-extracted drug this ash is 0.5% and water-exhausted drug can be identified by this standard.

Adulteration of ginger by exhausted or not well prepared or limed drug can be determined by the above standards.

Sometimes, in exhausted ginger, capsicum or paradise grains are added to increase pungency. Paradise grains are the seeds of *Alframomum melegueta* (Zingiberaceae). Pungency of capsicum and paradise grains is not destroyed by boiling with alkali while it is destroyed in case of ginger. Adulteration of ginger by capsicum and paradise grains can be determined by this way.

Uses

Ginger is stomachic, stimulant and aromatic carminative. It is used more as a spice. Much of the ginger at present is used in manufacture of gingerale.

BLACK PEPPER

Kali Mirch, Golmirch

Botanical Sources

Pepper or Black pepper consists of the dried unripe or nearly ripe fruits of *Piper nigrum.*

Family

Piperaceae.

Geographical Source

Malaysia, Indonesia, India, South America and the West Indies.

Morphology

The black pepper fruits are irregularly round or globular, 3–6 mm in diameter. They are greyish brown or greyish-black on the outer surface, which is highly reticulated. The apex and the base are easily distinguishable as the apex shows the remains of the stigmas and the basal side shows a scar representing the points of attachment to the axis. Black pepper has distinct aromatic odour and strong pungent taste.

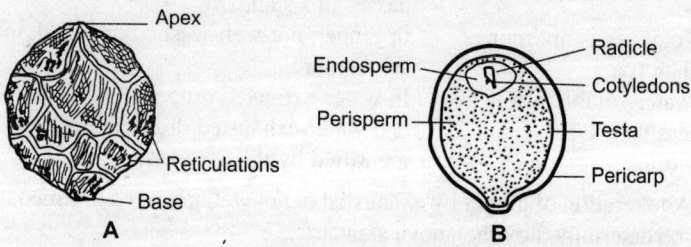

Fig. 5.22. *Piper nigrum* Fruit, whole and its longitudinal section. (A) A single black pepper showing reticulated pericarp surface and distinguishable apex and base. (B) L.S. of piper fruit showing single albuminous seed with various parts, including large perisperm.

The white pepper is devoid of the outer part of pericarp, but it shows about 16 vascular bundles running from the base to the apex.

There are, of course, a number of species of *Piper* and their fruits known as varieties in commerce also resemble the pepper. The powdered spice is usually a blend of these different species and varieties.

Uses

Used as a condiment and spice.

ASAFOETIDA

Asofoetida, Devil's dung, Hing (Hindi and Guj.)

Botanical Source

Asafoetida is an oleo-gum-resin obtained from the rhizome and root of *Ferula faetida* Regal, *F. rubricaulis* Boiss, *F. asafoetida* L. and other species of *Ferula*.

Family

Umbelliferae.

Geographical Source

Eastern Iran, Western Afghanistan.

Morphology

Asafoetida occurs in two forms: tears and mass. Tears consist of pure drug, while impurities are often present in mass. Tears are usually agglutinated though few are separate. Tears are rounded or flattened 0.5–3 cm in diameter. They are greyish-white or dull yellow or some becoming reddish-brown on keeping. Fresh tears are tough but when dried are hard and brittle. Tears are internally milky-white or yellowish translucent or opaque. Mass consists of agglutinated tears with foreign mass like stone, earth, pieces of roots, calcium salts and is of inferior quality. Odour is intense, penetrating, persistent, alliaceous and taste is bitter, acrid and alliaceous.

Chemical Test

1. When triturated with water it forms yellowish-orange emulsion.
2. To the fractured surface add sulphuric acid, a red or reddish-brown colour is produced. When washed with water, the colour changes to violet.
3. Add to the fractured surface 50% nitric acid. Green colour is produced.
4. Combined umbelliferone test: Boil 0.5 gm of the drug triturated with sand with 3 ml of hydrochloric acid and 3 ml of water for several minutes. Filter and to the filtrate add equal volume of alcohol and excess of strong solution of ammonia. A blue fluorescence is produced.

The above test performed without hydrochloric acid does not show blue fluorescence.

Asofoetida can be standardised by its ash value, which is not more than 15% and by its alcohol soluble extractive, which should not be less than 60%.

Uses

Used in gastric diseases (as flatulence) and as a carminative.

ASTRINGENTS

CATECHU

As stated in the theoretical part, there are two kinds of catechu, which though incidentally distinguish with simple adjectives, Pale Catechu and Black Catechu, are poles apart as far as their botanical sources with Families are concerned. Not only that their geographical sources, plant parts/organs used to prepare (method of preparation) them, are totally different. However, they show much resemblance in main chemical constituents. The difference in their secondary chemical constituents fortunately help us to distinguish them through chemical tests. They are:

- **Pale Catechu or Gambir:** It is the dried aqueous residue prepared from the leaves and shoots of *Uncaria gambier* (Family Rubiaceae).
- **Black Catechu or Cutch:** It is the dried aqueous extract prepared from the wood of *Acacia catechu* (Family Leguminosae).

Characters

Both kinds of catechus should be compared in their forms, size, colour and solubility and observation recorded.

The following tests are performed to identify and distinguish them from one another (see also Part 2).

Chemical Tests

1. Gambir-fluorescein test: Boil a little powdered drug with alcohol, filter and add sodium hydroxide solution to the filtrate, stir and add few ml of light petroleum. Petroleum layer shows green fluorescence. Black catechu does not show this test.

2. Heat about 0.5 gm powder with 5 ml chloroform on water-bath and filter in white porcelain dish and evaporate on water-bath. A greenish-yellow residue, because of chlorophyll present in the drug, is seen. In black catechu, as chlorophyll is absent, this test is negative.

3. Dip a matchstick in decoction of pale catechu, dry in the air and dip it in concentrated hydrochloric acid and warm it near the burner. Magenta or purple colour is produced. In this test, by the action of hydrochloric acid on catechins, or catechol tannins, phloroglucinol is produced which with lignin of the matchstick shows the above test.

4. Vanillin-hydrochloric acid test (Vanillin 1 : Alcohol 10 : dil. hydrochloric acid 10): Catechu shows pink or red colour. In this test also phloroglucinol is produced which with vanillin shows the above colour.

Tests at Nos. 3 and 4 are also positive in case of black catechu.

Uses

Catechu has astringent action and is used in diarrhoea and in lozenges. It is mainly used in dye and tanning industries. In the countries of its origin it is added to betel leaves.

DRUGS ACTING ON NERVOUS SYSTEM

Drugs acting on nervous system included in the syllabus are serially (coursewise) arranged below for practical classes.

HYOSCYAMUS

Folio hyoscyamus, Hyoscyamus herb, Hyoscyamus leaf, Henbane, Khorsani Ajma (Hindi)

Botanical Source

Hyoscyamus consists of the dried leaves and floweing tops of *Hyoscyamus niger* Linn. It contains not less than 0.05% alkaloids, calculated as hyoscyamine.

Family

Solanaceae.

Geographical Source

Native of Europe and west and north Asia.

Biennial plant is cultivated and obtained from England, Germany, Balkan countries, Poland, Russia and Kashmir.

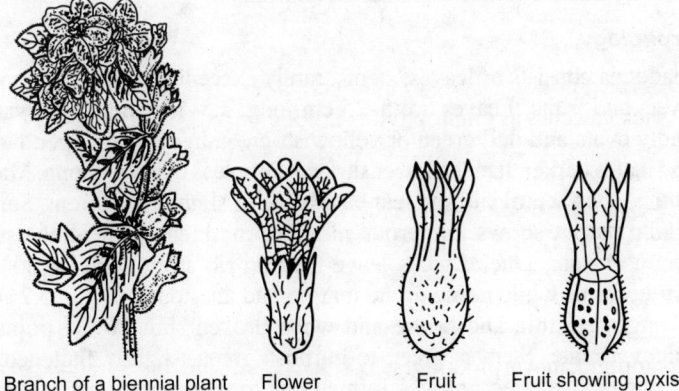

Branch of a biennial plant   Flower   Fruit   Fruit showing pyxis

Fig. 5.23. Hyoscyamus. Branch of a biennial plant.

Morphology

Drug found in commerce is pale greyish-green and consists of leaves and stem with flowering tops. Leaves are separate. or matted together. Stem is hairy and its diameter does not exceed 5 mm. Drug is sometimes viscid and resinous because of glandular trichomes. It has strong unpleasant smell and taste is bitter.

Standards

Total ash not more than 8–12%. In hyoscyamus, because of the glandular trichomes, clay sticks to the clammy leaves and total ash may be up to 22%. Higher quantity of clay can be determined by acid-insoluble ash.

Uses

See Part 2.

BELLADONNA

Folia belladonnae, Belladonna herb, Belladonna leaves, Deadly nightshade leaves, Sag-angur Patti (Hindi)

Botanical Source

Belladonna consists of dried leaves and other aerial parts of *Atropa belladonna* Linn. (known as European belladonna) or *Atropa acuminata* Royle ex Lindley (known as Indian belladonna). It contains not less than 0.3% of the alkaloids calculated as hyoscyamine.

Family

Solanaceae.

Geographical Source

Plant is a native of Central and Southern Europe. It is cultivated in England, Germany, Balkan countries, America and India.

Morphology

Belladonna consists of leaves, stems, rarely exceeding 5 mm in diameter, flowers and fruits. Leaves are 5–25 cm long, 2.5–12 cm broad, ovate to broadly ovate and dull green or yellowish-green in colour. Upper surface of the leaf is darker than the lower surface. Petiole is 0.5–4 cm long. Margin is entire, apex acuminate and leaf base acute or slightly decurrent. Surface is glabrous but shows numerous minute prominences of idioblasts of calcium oxalate. Lateral veins leave the mid-rib at an angle of 60° and curve upwards while going to the margin and anastomose (Fig. 5.24).

Leaves are thin and brittle and when broken show white points of calcium oxalate. Stem is green to purplish-green, slightly flattened and with one or two deep grooves formed due to contraction during drying. Leaf-scars are alternate.

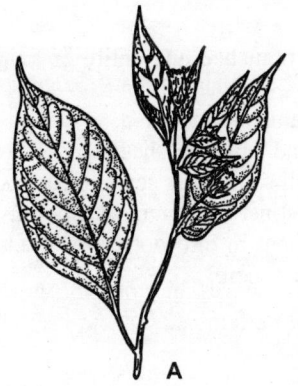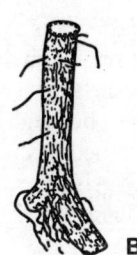

Fig. 5.24. Belladonna, *Atropa belladonna*. (A) A flowering shoot with leaves; (B) Root.

Flowers are small drooping about 2.5 cm long and pedicillate. Calyx is persistent five-lobed and campanulate Corolla is also five-lobed and campanulate and when fresh is dull purplish in colour but when dried becomes brown.

Fruits are small globular berries about 3–10 mm in diameter, surrounded by persistent calyx and green when unripe but dark purplish when ripe. Fruit is derived from superior bilocular ovary containing numerous ovules.

Seeds are small, sub-reniform with brown reticulations. In seeds alkaloid is present only in the tests.

Standard

Total ash not more than 14%, acid-insoluble ash not more than 3%.

Uses

All solanaceous drugs included here have similar uses (see Part 2).

BELLADONNA ROOT

Radix belladonnae

Botanical Source

Belladonna root consists of dried root and rootstocks of *Atropa belladonna*. It contains not less than 0.4% alkaloids calculated as hyoscyamine.

Family

Solanaceae.

Geographical Source

England, Germany and Balkan countries.

Morphology

- General appearance: Simple or branched and entire or longitudinally sliced roots.
- Size: Length from 10–30 cm, diameter upto 4 cm.
- Shape: Entire roots cylindrical and tapering; slices planoconvex.
- Surface: Longitudinally wrinkled; sometimes scars of roots seen.
- Fractured surface: It shows a distinct cambium with porous xylem in young roots but with radiate xylem in old roots. Fractured surface is white or sometimes brown if dried more.
- Colour: Greyish-brown.
- Odour: Characteristic.
- Taste: Bitter.

  Note: See diagram of root under Belladonna.

INDIAN BELLADONNA ROOTS I.P.

Botanical Source

Indian belladonna root consists of dried root and rootstock of *Atropa acuminata*.

Family

Solanaceae.

Geographical Source

India, Himalayas, Kashmir.

Morphology

Roots are pale brown to brownish-grey, cylindrical, longitudinally wrinkled and sometimes branched. The rootstock at the apex shows 4–12 aerial stem bases. The diameter of the rootstock at the apex is 3–12 cm. Rootstock and stem bases show pith in the centre. Pith in stem bases is hollow. Root and stem bases are also present.

STRAMONIUM

Botanical Source

Stramonium consists of the dried leaves and flowering tops of *Datura stramonium* Linn. and *Datura tatula* Linn.

Family

Solanaceae.

Geographical Source

Stramonium probably originated in Caspian Sea territories and from there spread to Europe in the first century. It is now found in Asia and Africa.

Morphology

The drug consists of stem, not exceeding 5 mm in diameter with leaves, flowers and fruits. Stem is flattened, curved or twisted and with transverse and longitudinal wrinkles. Dried leaves are greyish-green, thin, brittle and generally broken.

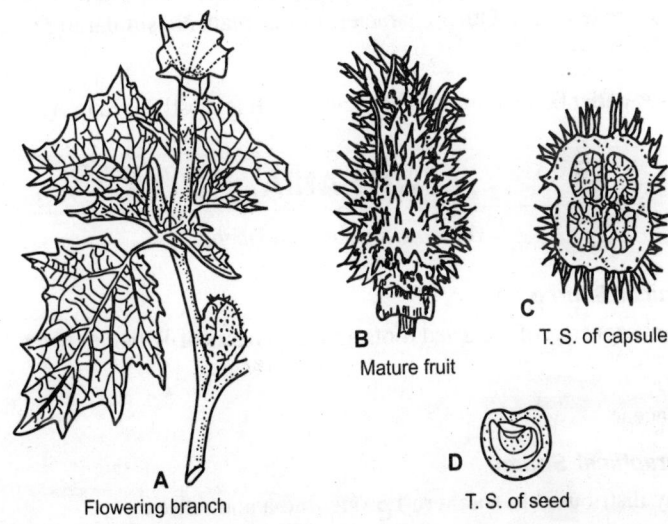

Fig. 5.25. Datura, *Datura stramonium*. (A) Upper part of a branch of the plant with leaves, flower and fruit; (B) Mature fruit; (C) Transverse section of capsule; (D) Transverse section of a seed with curved embryo.

Uses

Like belladonna, it is antispasmodic (see Part 2). It is smoked in cigarettes in asthma.

DATURA HERB I.P.

Botanical Sources

Datura herb consists of the dried leaves and flowering tops of *Datura metel* Linn. and *Datura metel* var. *fastuosa*.

Family

Solanaceae.

Geographical Source

India.

Morphology

- *Datura metel:* Stem is cylindrical, glabrous and shows leaf scars. Leaves are triangular and ovate. Apex is acute, base is asymmetrical and margin angular but sometimes entire.
- *D. metel* var. *fastusoa:* It is known in commerce as black datura. The stem, branches, main veins of leaves and flowers are purple-coloured. Corolla is double or triple. Outer corolla has five teeth and inner corolla has six to ten teeth. Other characters of this plant are similar to *D. metel.*

Uses

See uses under belladonna and hyoscyamus. It is mostly used in Ayurveda.

WITHANIA

Withania root, Ashwagandha

Botanical Source

Withania consists of the dried roots and stem bases of *Withania somnifera.*

Family

Solanaceae.

Geographical Source

Widely distributed in southern Europe, India and Africa.

Morphology

Withania shows variation in its different parts in India and hence in morphological characters of stem, root, flowers and fruits. The roots are used as the drug.

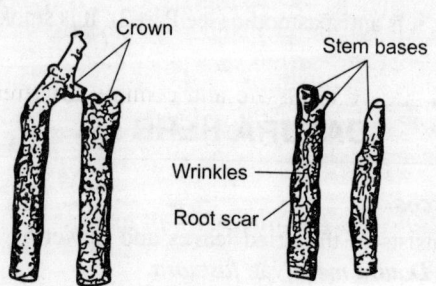

Fig. 5.26. *Withania somnifera* (Family Solanaceae). Roots showing crown, stem bases and longitudinal wrinkles.

Young roots are straight, unbranched and conical and in commerce occur in pieces of different lengths. The thickness varies according to age and is 5–12 mm below crown. Outer surface is buff to greyish yellow and longitudinally wrinkled. On the crown 2–6 remains of stem bases are seen. In the transverse surface of young roots small outer bark and in the centre soft solid parenchymatous mass with scattered vessels is seen. In the old and secondary roots, in the centre solid lignified ring of xylem is seen. Taste is mucilaginous and bitter.

Uses

Reputed to be tonic and aphrodisiac. Also used as a sedative in insomnia.

EPHEDRA

Ma-Huang, Ephedra

Botanical Source

Ephedra consists of the dried aerial parts of *Ephedra sinica* Stapf, *Ephedra equisetina* Bunge and other *Ephedra* species.

Family

Gnetaceae.

This family is considered transitional between gymnosperms and angiosperms and as such is very important to taxonomists. *Ephedra* species are grouped into Ephedraceae according to some authors.

Geographical Source

China, Pakistan and North West India.

Morphology

- General appearance: The stems of ephedra have on their outer surface numerous fine longitudinal ridges. The base of the old woody stem bears numerous small green or brown-coloured branches, showing a tufted appearance. At the nodes two but sometimes three or four small leaves are present. Leaves are decussate and connate. Different species of ephedra can be distinguished by thickness of the stem, length of internodes, number of ridges and number of leaves and their characters as teeth, sizes, etc.
- Stem: Stems of *Ephedra equisetina* are more woody and more branched.
- Size: *Ephedra sinica* – Thickness 4–7 mm of main stem and 1–2 mm of branches. Length up to 30 cm of branches and 3–6 cm of internodes. *Ephedra equisetina* – Thickness 1.5–2 mm. Length 25–200 cm of branches and 1–2.5 cm of internodes.

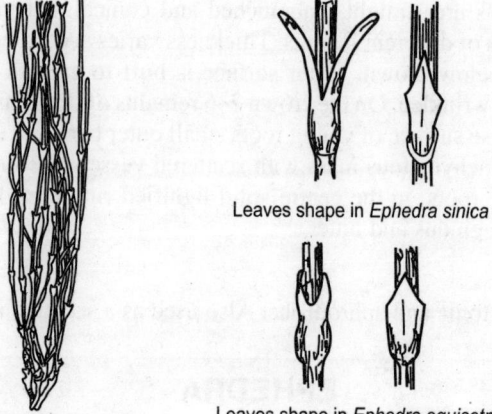

Leaves shape in *Ephedra sinica*

Leaves shape in *Ephedra equisetna*

Fig. 5.27. *Ephedra sinica.* Shape of leaves in *E. sinica* (A) and in *E. equisetna* (B).

- Outer surface: *Ephedra sinica* – Main stem brown because of cork with occasional silvery patches, branches green, rough, because of longitudinal ridges. *Ephedra equisetina* – Grey to pale green and smooth.
- Leaves: *Ephedra sinica* – A pair of sheathing leaves present at the nodes, encircling the stem and fused at the base. Leaves are 2–4 mm long, opposite, decussate and subulate. Leaf-base is reddish-brown, apex acute and recurved and lamina white in colour. *Ephedra equisetina* – Brown to purple, lower leaves black, apex short and not recurved.

Uses

The main alkaloid of the drug, ephedrine, is used in asthma, bronchitis and whooping cough.

ACONITE

Radix aconite, Aconite root, Monkshood, Wolfsbain, Vachhnag (Guj.)

Botanical Source

Aconite consists of the dried tubercles or tuberous roots of *Aconitum napellus* Linn. collected from wild or cultivated plants.

Family

Ranunculaceae.

Geographical Source

Mountainous regions of Europe and Himalayas. Obtained from wild plants from European and Asian countries.

Morphology

- Size: Length 4–10 cm, diameter 1–3 cm below the crown.
- Shape: Conical or obconical. tapering below.
- Surface: Slightly twisted, longitudinally ridged. In English aconite fibrous rootlets or their scars are seen. On the top of parent root remains of stem bases seen. This root is more shrivelled. At the apex of daughter root apical bud is present.
- Fracture: Short.
- Fractured surface: Starchy, with 5–8 angled satellite cambium and a pith in the centre.
- Colour: Brown to dark brown.
- Odour: Slight.
- Taste: At first sweetish, then tingling and later causing numbness on the tongue.

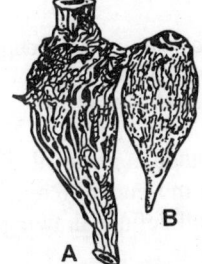

Fig. 5.28. Aconite, *Aconitum napellus*. (A) Parent root; (B) Daughter root.

Uses

Aconite, because of aconitine, is a poisonous plant. Rarely used internally except in homoeopathy. Externally used in neuralgia and rheumatism (see Part 2).

OPIUM

Afim (Hindi), Afin (Guj.)

Botanical Source

Opium is the dried latex obtained by incision from capsular fruits of *Papaver somniferum* Linn.

Family

Papaveraceae.

Geographical Source

Turkey, Yugoslavia (Macedonia), India, Pakistan, Iran, U.S.S.R. Lately Afghanistan is producing lot of opium for misuse.

Plant Habit

Opium is obtained from poppy plant. Poppy plant is an annual herb, about 1 metre in height and bears about 5–8 capsules.

Indian opium occurs in masses of various sizes, which are often soft and shiny and become hard and brittle after drying, usually moulded in masses of uniform size and shape, blackish-brown in colour and with strong characteristic odour.

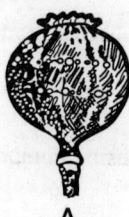 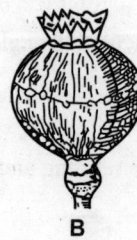 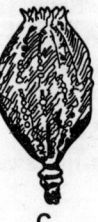

A   B   C

Fig. 5.29. Opium, *Papaver somniferum*. (A) Poppy capsule cut transversely in Turkish opium; (B) Capsule with one transverse incision in Macedonian opium; (C) Capsule cut longitudinally in Indian opium.

Usually opium is not studied in practical classes in India. However, an institution should have in its museum different types of capsule and opium products as such or their well defined drawings to show and acquaint the students.

Chemical Tests

1. Boil 0.1 gm of opium with 5 ml of water, filter and add to the filtrate few drops of ferric chloride solution. Deep reddish-purple colour is obtained. Add few drops of dilute hydrochloric acid. The colour persists. This test is due to meconic acid.
2. Morphine gives dark violet colour with concentrated sulphuric acid and formaldehyde and this test is used for identification of opium preparations.

Uses

Opium tharapeutically can be used in stomach cramps, colic and diarrhoea. It causes immobilization of the intestine.

CANNABIS

Indian hemp, Hashish, Bhang, Ganja, Charas, Cannabis indica, Marihuana

Botanical Source

Cannabis consists of dried flowering and fruiting tops of the pistillate plants of *Cannabis sativa* Linn.

Family

Cannabinaceae.

Geographical Source

North India, Maharashtra, Bengal, Africa and America.

Morphology

- Cannabis occurs in flattened cylindrical mass of a dull dusky green colour and consists of much branched upper portion of the stem. The stem bears bracts, bracteoles, flowers and fruits.
- Leaves are usually absent but if present they are few and broken. Because of the resin present in the drug and method of preparation cannabis mass appears matted and compact.
- Cannabis is uneven, rough, resinous and harsh to the touch. Length is 3–10 cm but sometimes upto 30 cm. Width is 5–10 cm.
- Stem is straight, cylindrical, longitudinally furrowed.
- Bracts are 1.5–2 cm long, simple or bilobed and bear two small subulate stipules. A pair of bracteoles is produced in the axil of bracts. Bracteoles have acute apex, are boat-shaped and incurved at the base and enclose flowers and fruits.
- Flowers are produced in the axil of bracteoles and are hairy and membranous.

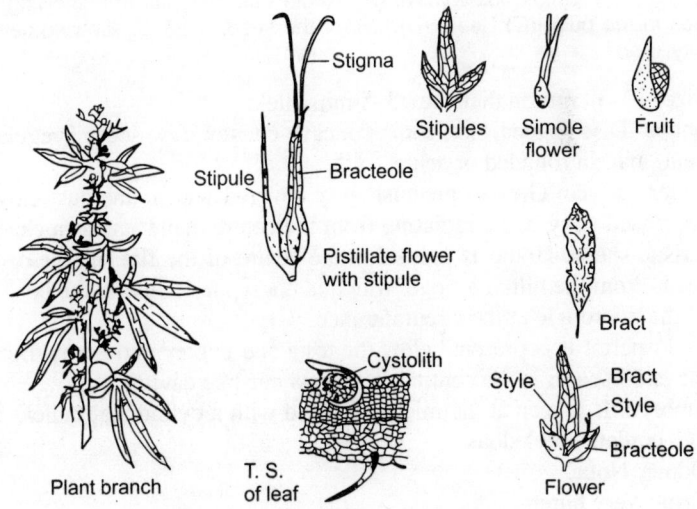

Fig. 5.30. Cannabis, *Cannabis sativa.*

Uses

Used as sedative, analgesic and narcotic. It has psychotropic properties and causes addiction.

NUX VOMICA

Semen strychni, Nux vomica seed, Kuchla (Hindi), Zer kachuro (Guj.)

Botanical Source

Nux vomica consists of the dried ripe seeds of *Strychnos nux-vomica* containing not less than 1.2% strychnine.

Family

Loganiaceae.

Geographical Source

South India, Malabar Coast, Kerala. Eastern Ghats, Bengal, Ceylon and North Australia.

Morphology

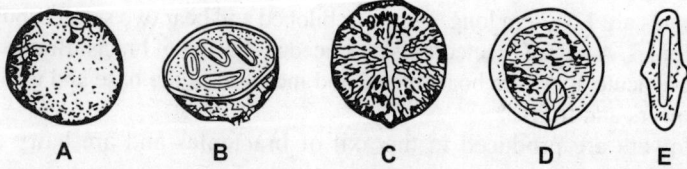

Fig. 5.31. *Strychnos nux-vomica.* (A) Whole fruit; (B) Half fruit showing the seeds in the pulp; (C) Seed; (D) L.S. of the seed; (E) T.S. showing central cavity.

- Size: 10–30 mm in diameter, 3–5 mm thick.
- Shape: Disc-shaped, flat, some concave-convex, few seeds irregularly bent, margin rounded or acute.
- Outer surface: Grey to greenish-grey covered with numerous, closely appressed silky hairs, radiating from the centre, hairs impart a characteristic sheen. Hilum is present in the centre of the flat surface of the seed. From the hilum a ridge, which is not raphe, connects the position of the micropyle at the circumference.
- Endosperm: It is present below the testa and is grey and horny. Below the endorsperm in the centre is a narrow slit-like cavity.
- Embryo: It is seen at the micropylar end with a cylindrical radicle and two cordate cotyledons.
- Odour: None.
- Taste: Very bitter.

Microscopy

Epidermis consists of thick-walled, bent and twisted lignified trichomes. The base of the trichome is large thick-walled with slit-like pits. The upper part of the trichome is nearly at right angle to the base and has wavy walls. A layer of collapsed cells is present below the epidermis.

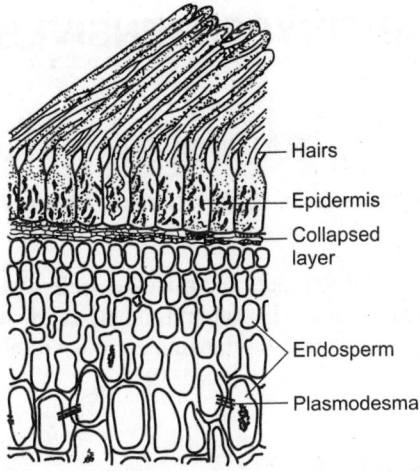

Fig. 5.32. Transverse section of outer part of Nux vomica seed.

Endosperm consists of thick-walled isodiametric cells consisting of hemicellulose which swells with water and contains plasmodesma. Endosperm and embryo contain fixed oil and aleurone grains.

Chemical Test

1. **Strychnos Test:** To a thick section of endosperm add ammonium vanadate and sulphuric acid. Middle portion of endosperm is stained purple because of strychnine.
2. Strychnine also gives violet colour with potassium dichromate and conc. sulphuric acid.
3. **Brucine Test:** To a thick section add concentrated nitric acid. Outer part of endosperm is stained yellow to orange because of brucine.

   The above tests can be used as localization tests.

4. **Hemicellulose Test:** To a thick section add iodine and sulphuric acid. The cell walls are stained blue.
5. **Organoleptic Test:** Put a little drug at the tip of the tongue. It tastes bitter.
6. **Biological Test:** 2 mg (2/1000 mg) of strychnine if injected into the tail of a two-week-old mouse will cause palpitation of the tail.

Uses

Strychnine has a stimulant action on spinal cord and increases the reflex movements. As a circulatory stimulant it is given in surgical shock. It is used in atonic dyspepsia. Brucine shows 1/50th of activity of strychnine. It is highly poisonous and is seldom used in medicine.

ANTIHYPERTENSIVES

RAUWOLFIA

Sarpagandha, Chhotachand, Pagla ki Jadibutti (Dawa), Rauwolfia roots

Botanical Source

Rauwolfia consists of dried roots and rhizomes of 3–4 years old plants of *Rauwolfia serpentina* collected in autumn and with bark intact and contains not less than 0.15% reserpine-rescinnamine groups of alkaloids.

Family

Apocynaceae.

Geographical Source

The plant is a small shrub, about 1 metre in height and occurs mainly In India, Pakistan, Burma, Thailand and Java.

Morphology

• External characters of roots and rhizomes are nearly similar but rhizomes can be distinguished by the presence of small central pith. In pieces of some rhizomes small pieces of aerial stems are attached. Drug consists of mostly pieces which are 2–15 cm long and 3–22 mm in diameter. Pieces are cylindrical, slightly tapering, tortuous and rarely branched.

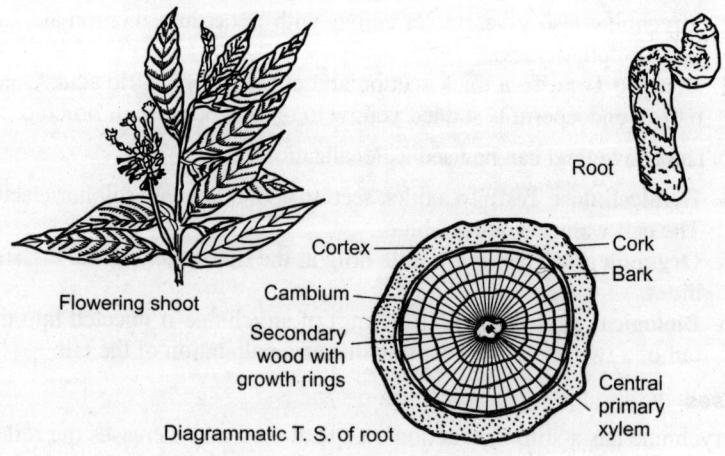

Fig. 5.33. *Rauwolfia serpentina*, Family Apocynaceae.

- Rootlets are rarely present and when present their diameter is 0.5–1 mm.
- Outer surface is grayish yellow, pale brown or brown. In young pieces wrinkles and in old pieces longitudinal ridges and sometimes scars of rootlets are seen. In pieces of especially old roots exfoliation of bark takes place at some places and patches of pale yellow to white wood are exposed.
- Root breaks easily compared to roots of other species of Rauwolfia because of absence of sclerenchyma and fracture is short.
- Smoothed transverse surface shows narrow yellow to brown bark and dense pale yellow radiate wood, with 2–8 growth rings occupying nearly three quarters of the diameter. Starch is abundant in bark and wood.
- Drug is odourless and its taste is bitter.

Uses

Hypotensive and tranquilizer.

ANTITUSSIVES

VASAKA LEAVES

Adhatoda, Vasaka folium, Adulasa, Ardushi, Sinhmukhi

Botanical Source

Vasaka consists of the fresh or dried leaves of *Adhatoda vasica* Nees.

Family

Acanthaceae.

Geographical Source

Plains of India and the Ranges of Himalaya,

Macroscopy

- General appearance: Fresh leaves entire, dried crumpled and in broken fragments.
- Size: 12–20 cm long, 2.5–6 cm broad.
- Shape: Ovate-lanceolate.
- Margin: Entire or slightly crenate.
- Venation: Pinnate, prominent midrib and 8–12 pairs of lateral veins.
- Apex: Acuminate.
- Base: Tapering.
- Surface: Glabrous, slightly pubescent.
- Texture: Thin and leathery.

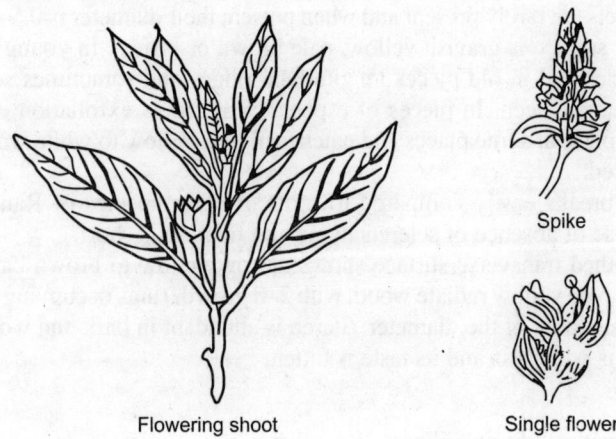

Flowering shoot

Spike

Single flower

Fig. 5.34. Vasaka, *Adhatoda vasica*, Family Acanthaceae.

- Petiole: 2–8 cm long, grooved.
- Colour: Light green.
- Odour: Characteristic.
- Taste: Bitter.

Uses

Vasaka is used as an expectorant and bronchodilator in cough and bronchitits.

BALSAM TOLU

Balsamum tolutanum, Balsam of Tolu, Tolu balsam

Botanical Source

Tolu balsam is obtained by incision on the stem of *Myroxylon balsamum* (*Myroxylon toluifera*).

Family

Leguminosae.

Geographical Source

Along the lower Magdalena river in Columbia, West Indies, Cuba and Venezuela.

Characters

- Fresh tolu balsam is soft, sticky, yellow, semisolid mass. Gradually it hardens and becomes brittle and brownish in colour. If a small quantity is heated, and the softened mass is put on slide and seen under microscope, crystals of cinnamic acid and amorphous vegetable debris are seen.

- Odour and taste are aromatic.
- Tolu balsam forms plastic mass when chewed.

Tests

1. Dissolve 1 gm of tolu balsam in 10 ml of alcohol by heating. The solution shows acidic reaction with litmus and the insoluble residue is not more than 4%.
2. Boil 1 gm of balsam with 5 ml water, filter and note the smell of filtrate. To the filtrate add 3 ml of 1% aqueous potassium permanganate solution and heat and smell. Cinnamic acid present in the balsam is oxidized to benzaldehyde giving bitter almond-like smell.
3. Add few drops of ferric chloride to alcoholic solution of tolu balsam. Green colour is seen because of tolu resinotannol.

Detection of Adulterants

1. **Exhausted Tolu balsam:** From tolu balsam cinnamic acid is removed by extraction. If a small quantity of this exhausted drug is heated, softened, put on side and seen under microscope, crystals of cinnamic acid are not seen.
2. **Calophony:** The adulteration of colophony can be detected as follows: Boil 5 gm of the drug with 25 ml of carbon disulphide on water-bath in a flask fitted with air condensor. Filter and evaporate the filtrate in a porcelain dish. Dissolve the residue in dish in 6 ml of light petroleum and add to it 10 ml of copper acetate solution and shake. Bright green colour of petroleum layer shows adulteration of colophony.

Uses

As an antitussive and expectorant.

TULSI

Surasa; Tulasi, Tulsi, Holy basil, Raihan

Botanical Source

Tulsi consists of the leaves of *Ocimum sanctum*.

Family

Labiatae.

Geographical Source

The plant is found throughout India and is considered sacred.

Macroscopy

- Annual herb 30–60 cm high, much branched, stems and branches usually purplish, sub-quadrangular, sometimes woody below and clothed with soft spreading hairs.

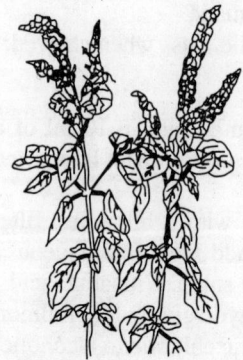

Fig. 5.35. Tulsi, *Ocimum sanctum* plant with leaves and inflorescence.

- Leaves are 2.5–5 cm long and 1.6–3.2 cm broad, elliptical, oblong, obtuse or acute, margin entire or serrate, surface pubescent on both sides, minutely gland-dotted, base obtuse or acute, petioles 1.3–2.5 cm long, slender, hairy.
- Inflorescence verticillate, flowers in recemes 15–20 cm long in close whorls. Bracts 3 mm, both long and broad, broadly ovate, calyx slender, pubescent, bilabiate, lower lip longer than upper. Corolla 4 mm long, purplish, bilabiate, upper lip pubescent on the back. Stamens exserted, filaments slender, the upper pair with a small branched appendage at the base.
- Nutlets 1.25 mm long, broadly ellipsoid, nearly smooth, yellow with small black markings.
- Seeds brownish, globose or sub-globose.
- Odour and taste aromatic and sharp.

Uses

Used as an expectorant, spasmolytic and in cold and cough (see Part 2).

ANTIRHEUMATICS

COLCHICUM SEED

Semen colchici, Autumn Crocus Seed,
Meadow Safftron Seed, European Colchicum Seed

Botanical Source

Colchicum consists of dried ripe seeds of *Colchicum autumnale* Linn. containing not less than 0.3% alkaloids calculated as colchicine.

Family
Liliaceae.

Geographical Source
Central and South Europe and England.

Morphology

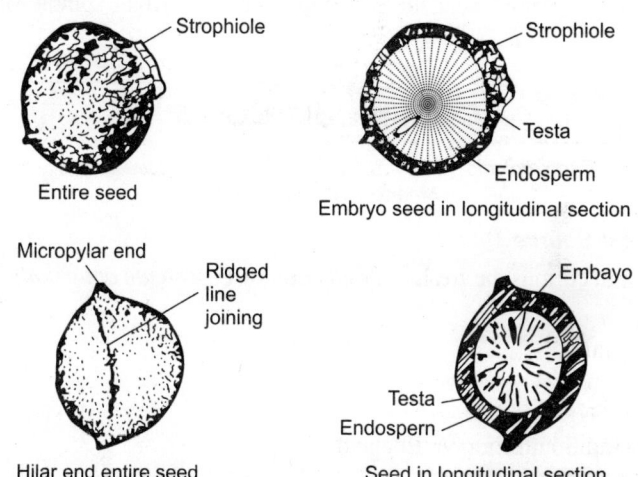

Fig. 5.36. Colchicum seed. (A & B) European colchicum, *Colchicum autumnale*; (C & D) Indian colchicum, *Colchicum luteum*.

- Size: 2–3 mm in diameter.
- Shape: Globular, with strophiole on one side which is the parenchymatous growth of the raphe.
- Outer surface: Dark reddish-brown, pitted, very hard.
- Endosperm: Large, very hard, oily.
- Embryo: Small, embedded at one end near the surface of the seed.
- Odour: None.
- Taste: Bitter and acrid.

INDIAN COLCHICUM SEED

Surinjan (Hindi)

Botanical Source
Colchicum consists of dry ripe seeds of *Colchicum luteum* Baker.

Geographical Source
The plant is found in the Northwest Himalayas and Kashmir, at an altitude of 4,000 to 7,000 ft. It is characterized by flowers of yellow colour.

Characters

Seeds (Fig. C & D) are 2–5 mm long and are oval but may become angular due to shrinkage. Testa is dark brown and finely pitted. There are two beaks, one at the hilar end, which is better developed, and another at the micropylar end. The two beaks are connected by a wavy somewhat feeble ridge. Endosperm forms the major portion of seed and contains fixed oil and aleurone grains. Near the micropylar end is a small spindle-shaped embryo.

COLCHICUM CORM

Radix colchici, Cormus colchici, Autumn Crocus Corm,
Meadow Saffron Corm

Botanical Source

Colchicum corm is the fresh or dried corm of *Colchicum autumnale* Linn.

Family

Liliaceae.

Geographical Source

Central and South Europe, England.

Fresh Corm

Fresh entire corm is conical about 4 cm long, 3 cm wide. One side of the corm is flat while the other side is convex. At the apex remains of last year's flowering stem is seen. At the base of flat side there is a cavity containing bud. From this bud next year new flowering stem and new corm are produced. At the base of the corm fibrous roots or their scars are seen. Inner surface is white and fleshly. Longitudinal slices resemble the corm, but their thickness is less than the entire.

Morphology

- General appearance: Dried transverse slices.
- Size: Length 3 cm, thickness 2–5 mm.
- Shape: Sub-reniform to ovate. A groove is seen on flat, or concave side because of contraction.
- Colour: Dark brown.
- Fracture: Short and starchy.
- Fractured surface: Numerous fibrovascular bundles are seen as grayish points in white mealy ground tissue.
- Odour: None.
- Taste: Bitter and acrid.

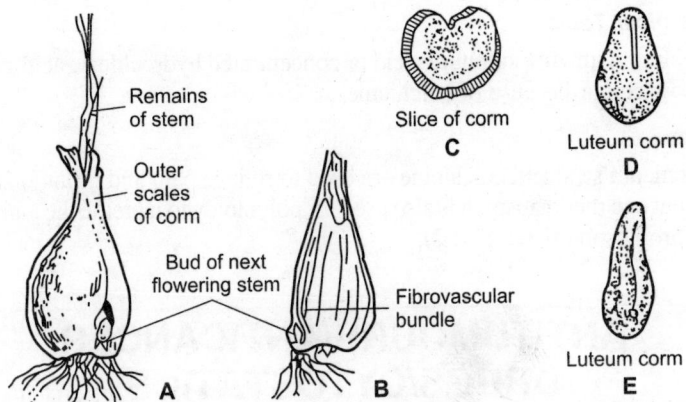

Fig. 5.37. Colchicum corm, *Colchicum autumnale* (A, B, C) and *C. luteum* (D, E). (A) Corm; (B) Longitudinally cut corm; (C) Slice of the corm; (D & E) *C. luteum* corm.

INDIAN COLCHICUM CORM

Surinjan

Botanical Source

Indian colchicum corm is the dried corm of *Colchicum luteum* Baker. The outer membraneous scales of the corm are removed after collection and the corm is dried.

Family

Liliaceae.

Geographical Source

India. Northwestern Himalaya 1,300–2,600 metres, Kashmir.

Morphology

The corm is yellow to brown in colour, ovoid, 3–6 cm long and 1.3–3 cm broad and tapering at the apex. There is distinct groove on one side. At the base of the groove is a bud. In addition to this bud, there is an accessory bud on the convex side. At the apex, a scar of flowering stem is seen. On the surface there are many transverse and longitudinal fissures. Fracture is horny and the fractured surface is similar to European colchicum corm. It is odourless and has a bitter taste. It contains an alkaloid colchicine which in the commercial drug is only 0.15% and its percentage is much less than the European drug. It is used similar to European colchicum corm (see figure above).

Chemical Tests

The drug with 70% sulphuric acid or concentrated hydrochloric acid gives yellow colour because of colchicine.

Uses

Colchicum seed and colchicine are used to relieve pain and inflammation of gout and rheumatism. It is also used for polyploidy to increase the number of chromosomes (see Part 2).

ANTITUMOURS/ANTICANCER DRUGS/CYTOSTATICS

CATHARANTHUS

Vinca, Madagascar periwinkle, Baramasi (Hindi & Gujarati)

Botanical Source

Catharanthus consists of the dried entire plant of *Catharanthus roseus* (*Vinca rosea*), belonging to the Family Apocynaceae.

Geographical Source

A native of Madagascar, the plant is growing in many tropical and sub-tropical countries, including India, Australia, South Africa and North and South America. The plant is cultivated in India.

Description of Plant

• The evergreen blooming plant, an undershrub, grows up to 100 cm high. The cultivated varieties bear flowers of violet, pink and white colours. The plants are easily available and the students should be able to see the entire plant with its different organs (Fig. 5.38).

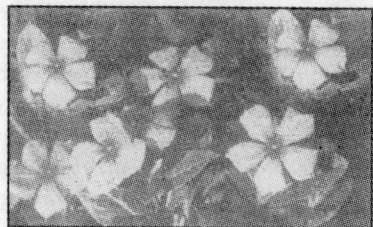 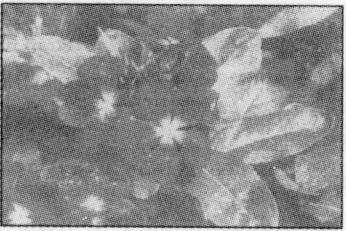

Fig. 5.38. (A) *Catharanthus roseus* (Apocynaceae), a wild form of the plant; (B) A cultivar form of *C. roseus*.

• The leaf, root and stem are anatomically well developed. The T.S. of root and T.S. of stem (Fig. 5.39) show the distribution of various tissues, clearly representing secondary cortex and the secondary xylem; the root devoid of central pith, while the stem showing the secondary xylem enclosing the central pith. Both the organs, i.e. root and stem, show the groups of unlignified patches of fibres.

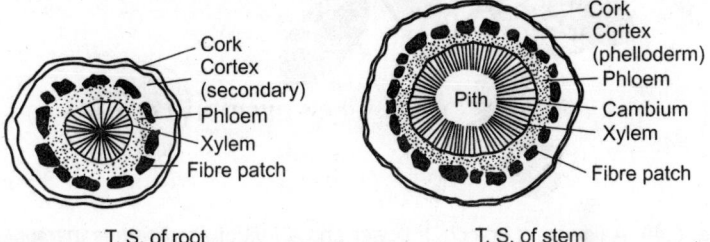

T. S. of root   T. S. of stem

Fig. 5.39. Periwinkle, *Catharanthus roseus* (*Vinca rosea*) showing transverse section (T.S.) of leaf, stem and root.

Uses

The drug and its alkaloids, vincristine and vinblastine, are antimitotic and are used in breast cancer, in childhood leukaemia and in Hodgkin's disease.

ANTIDIABETICS

PTEROCARPUS

Indian Kino Tree, Malabar Kino (Eng.), Vijasara, Bija (Hindi),
Biyo (Guj.), Bijasara (Sanskrit and Urdu)

Botanical Source

Pterocarpus consists of the heartwood of *Pterocarpus marsupium* (other parts of the plant, viz, kino gum. bark and leaves are also used).

Family

Leguminosae (Papilionaceae).

Geographical Source

The plant is found mainly throughout Gujarat, Madhya Pradesh, Bihar and Orissa.

Characters

The plant is a moderate to large-sized deciduous tree, upto about 90 feet high and with straight clear trunk. Bark gray, longitudinally cracked; leaves

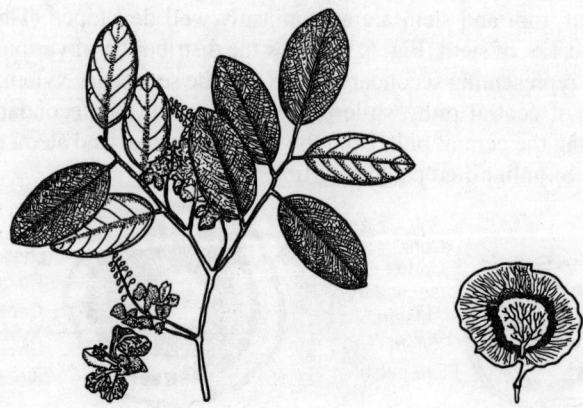

Fig. 5.40. A flowering branch, a flower and a fruit of *Pterocarpus marsupium*.

compound with 5–7 leaflets, elliptical with slight wavy margin; flowers yellow in dense bunches; fruit somewhat irregularly round, winged and with one seed.

Morphology

- Size and shape: Drug occurs as irregular pieces of variable size and thickness.
- Colour: Golden yellow brown with darker streaks.
- Texture: Strong, tough and very hard, moderately heavy.
- Fracture: Difficult to break (somewhat brittle).
- Odour: Characteristic.
- Taste: Astringent.

Test

On soaking with water gives yellow colour solution with blue florescence.

The bark yields a reddish gum, known as kino, which becomes brittle on hardening. The kino contains kino-tannic acid and is a strong astringent.

Uses

As an antidiabetic the drug shows hypoglycaemic action.

GYMNEMA SYLVESTRE

Meshasringi (Sanskrit and Bengali), Gurmar (Hindi),
Kharak (Arabic), Khar-e-khasak (Persian)

Botanical Source

Gymnema consists of the leaves of *Gymnema sylvestre* (Syn. *Asclepias geminata*).

Family

Asclepiadaceae.

Geographical Source

A climbing plant common in central and southern India, Western Ghats and in Goa.

Morphology

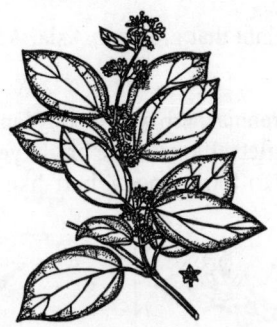

Fig. 5.41. A flowering branch of *Gymnema sylvestre*.

- General appearance: Leaves elliptic or ovate with both surfaces pubescent. The midrib has a central bulge.
- Size: Upto 2.0 × 1.5 inch.
- Shape: Lamina ovate, elliptic or ovate-lanceolate.
- Colour: Pale green.
- Odour: Characteristic, faintly aromatic.
- Taste: Almost tasteless.

Uses

It causes reduction in blood sugar by stimulating insulin secretion. It is also attributed uses like astringent, stomachic, tonic, refrigerant and diuretic (see Part 2).

DIURETICS

GOKHRU

Caltrop, Puncture vine, Cathead

Botanical Source

There are two plants of gokhru:

1. The fruits of *Tribulus terrestris* supplying small or chhota gokhru.
2. The fruits of *Pedalium murex* supplying large or bara gokhru.

TRIBULUS TERRESTRIS

Chhota gokhru consists of dried ripe fruits of *Tribulus terrestris*.

Family
Zygophyllaceae.

Geographical Source
Tribulus terrestris is a plant that grows in Asia, Africa and Australia.

Characters
The plant is annual or perennial herb with woody taproot. Leaves are pinnate with oblong to ovate leaflets. Flowers are bright yellow and solitary in the leaf axils. They mature to form woody, burr-like fruit with conspicuous sharp spines.

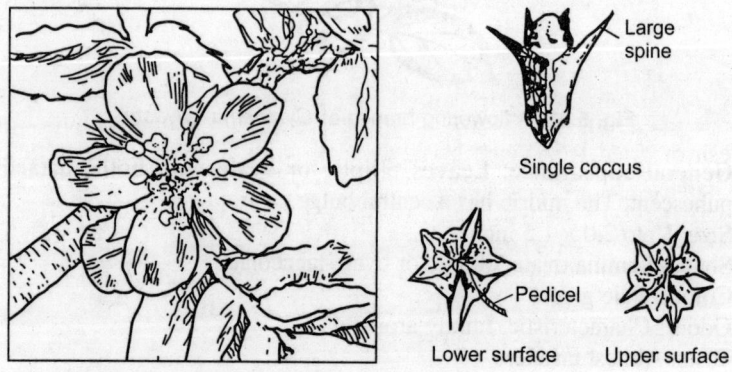

Fig. 5.42. *Tribulus terrestris* (Zygophyllaceae), herb and fruit.

Macroscopy
Fruit is globose, 0.5 inch in diameter and 1/3 inch in thickness. Fruit consists of five densely hairy, woody, often muricate cocci. Each coccus bears two large sharp, pointed, rigid spines directed towards the apex and two smaller, shorter spines directed downwards. Colour is yellowish-brown. Seeds several in each coccus with transverse partition.

Uses
Diuretic, aphrodisiac and tonic (see Part 2).

PEDALIUM MUREX

Botanical Source
Bara gokhru consists of dried ripe fruits of *Pedalium murex*.

Family
Pedaliaceae.

Geographical Source

The plant is found almost throughout India.

Characters

The plant is annual, diffuse, succulent herb, 15–20 cm high.

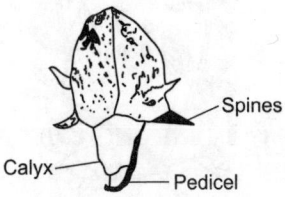

Fig. 5.43. *Pedalium murex* (bara gokhru) fruit.

Macroscopy

Fruit is 1.5–2 cm long, pyramidal ovoid, tapering at the base and apex, 4-sided with stout, sharp, conical horizontal four spines forming the four angles. At the base fruit abruptly tapers into a hollow cylindrical tube. The fresh or dried fruit when briskly shaken with cold water forms thick mucilage.

Uses

Demulcent, diuretic and tonic.

PUNARNAVA

Spreading Hogweed (Eng.) Godhaparna (Hindi),
Punarnava (Sanskrit and German)

Botanical Source

Punarnava consists of the herb of *Boerhavia diffusa*.

Family

Nyctaginaceae.

Geographical Source

The drug is found throughout India especially during the rains.

Macroscopy

- *B. diffusa* is diffusely branched, non-succulent herb. The whole plant of red flowers shows a slightly reddish tinge, while the white-flowered plant is absolutely green and is more robust.
- The root is fairly stout and fusiform having a woody rootstock. Many 1–3 ft. long slender prostrate stems arise from the crown of root.

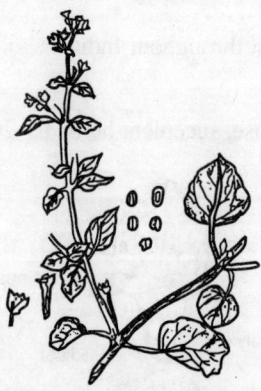

Fig. 5.44. Punarnava, *Boerhavia diffusa.*

- Leaves are slightly thick and opposite in unequal pairs at each node of the stem. Leaves vary in size being 0.5 × 0.75 inches. They are ovate or oblong having rounded apex. Margin is entire and pinkish. The petiole is about 0.5–1.0 inch long.
- There are tiny pedicillate pink-coloured flowers in small umbels of 5–10 forming long axillary and terminal panicles. There is about 2–2.5 mm long, funnel-shaped pink or red-coloured and five-lobed perianth tube. Stamens are 1–3 in number. The ovary is free with a single ovule. Style is filiform with a peltate stigma.
- The fruit is glandular, with ribs and 2–3 mm long.
- White variety is similar but more robust with white flowers and green stem.

Uses
Decoction is used as diuretic and in nephrotic syndrome.

ANTIDYSENTERICS

IPECACUANHA

*Radix ipecacuanhae, Ipecacuanhae Root,
Ipecac Rio, Brazilian or Johore Ipecac.*

Botanical Source
Ipecacuanha consists of the dried root or rhizome and roots of *Cephaelis ipecacuanha* (Rio or Brazilian ipecac) or of *Cephaelis acuminata* (Cartagena, Nicaragua or Panama ipecac).

Family

Rubiaceae.

Geographical Source

Brazil, Forests of Mattogrosso and Minas, Malaya States (Johore), Burma and Bengal in India.

Characters

The plant is a low straggling shrub of about 30 cm in height, growing wild in moist, swampy forests of Brazil. The rhizome is cylindrical and bears 4–5 adventitious roots, which are thickened because of the storage of starch.

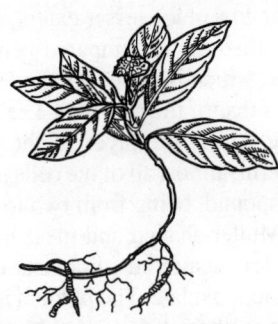

Fig. 5.45. *Cephaelis ipecacuanha* (Rubiaceae).

The roots of this small South American shrub are gathered throughout the year, although the Indians collect it when it is in flower during January and February.

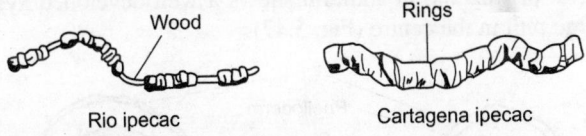

Fig. 5.46. Ipecacuanha. Rio ipecac, *Cephaelis ipecacuanha*; and Cartagena ipecac, *Cephaelis acuminata*.

Morphology

Rio Ipecac:
- Size: Length 5–15 cm; diameter 3–5 mm (usually 4 mm).
- Shape: Cylindrical, slightly tortuous.
- Surface: Annulated, each annulation or annulated ring encircles the root from the half to three quarters; annulations are broad and round; sometimes attached rhizome or its free pieces and lateral roots or their scars are seen.
- Colour: Brick red to brown.
- Odour: Slight, powder irritant and sternutatory.

- Taste: Bitter and acrid.
- Fracture: Short and starchy in the bark, splintery in the xylem.
- Fractured surface: Wide greyish bark occupying two-thirds diameter and central yellowish-white wood occupying one-third diameter.

Cartagena Ipecac:

- Root is greyish-brown up to 9 mm in diameter, uniformly thick, usually double than that of Rio. Annulations similar to Rio ipecac are absent, but it has transverse ridges which encircle about half the root. In the transverse section bark occupies about half the diameter.

Microscopy

Since the rhizome, though to a much lesser extent, also occurs in the drug, the structure of root and rhizome is compared here. The T.S. of the root shows outer layer of cork, which is rather thin and brownish in colour and this resembles the cork of that of the rhizome. The cork cells show brown granular material. Lying within the layer of the cork is a fairly broad parenchymatous phelloderm, almost all of the cells of which contain starch. The starch is mostly compound, being from two to eight components; the individual starch being Muller-shaped and measuring up to 20 m in diameter. Present are also few scattered idioblasts containing bundles of acicular rhaphides of calcium oxalate. The phloem is parenchymatous with sieve tubes embedded in it, there being no sclerenchymatous cells. The xylem occupies the centre as a compact mass of xylem tissue consisting of tracheidal vessels, tracheids and pitted xylem parenchyma, some of which get developed into substitute fibres. They and the medullary ray cells contain starch.

The T.S. of rhizome in addition shows a well developed xylem ring with a large pith in the centre (Fig. 5.47).

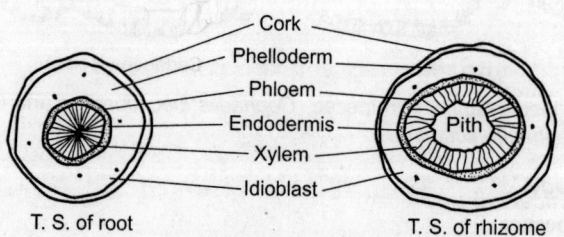

Cork
Phelloderm
Phloem
Endodermis — Pith
Xylem
Idioblast

T. S. of root   T. S. of rhizome

Fig. 5.47. Ipecacuanha.

Test for emetine

Add 5 ml of hydrochloric acid to 0.1 gm of powdered drug, heat and filter. To the filtrate add small crystals of potassium chlorate or chloramine T. The colour of the filtrate becomes yellow-orange and then red.

Uses

Ipecac is used in amoebic dysentery (see Part 2).

ANTISEPTICS AND DISINFECTANTS

BENZOIN

Benzoinum, Sumatra benzoin, Loban (Guj.)

Botanical Source

Benzoin is the balsamic resin obtained from the incised stem of *Styrax benzoin* and *Styrax paralleloneurus*.

Family

Styraceae.

Geographical Source

Sumatra.

Characters

- Benzoin consists of mass of brittle, opaque, hard, white or red tears. This mass is embedded in translucent, reddish-brown resinous matrix. Fractured surface is uneven.
- Odour is balsamic, aromatic and agreeable.
- The taste is slightly acrid.
- When heated irritating fumes of benzoic and cinnamic acids are produced.

SIAM BENZOIN

Botanical Source

Siam benzoin is the balsamic resin of *Styrax tonkinensis*. It is official in French and many European Pharmacopoeias.

Family

Styraceae.

Geographical Source

North Laos and north Vietnam at an altitude.

Characters

- Commercial drug occurs as tears or blocks of tears. Tears are hard, flattened or concavo-convex, brittle upto 5 cm in length and 1 cm wide. Outer surface is yellowish-brown or reddish-brown and inner surface is milky white and opaque. Blocks are made up of small tears. They are glassy, transparent, reddish-brown and embedded in matrix.
- Odour is vanilla-like and taste balsamic.

Chemical Test

1. Heat 5 gm of coarse Sumatra benzoin with 10 ml of 10% potassium permanganate solution in a test tube slowly. In Sumatra benzoin bitter almond smell of benzaldehyde is produced because of oxidation of cinnamic acid present in it. This test is negative in Siam benzoin because of very small quantity of cinnamic acid.
2. Digest 0.2 gm of coarse Sumatra benzoin with 5 ml ether for 5 minutes. Pour 1 ml of the ethereal solution in a porcelain dish containing 2–3 drops of sulphuric acid and rotate the dish. Sumatra benzoin shows reddish-brown colour without purplish tinge. Siam benzoin shows deep purplish-red colour by this test.

Uses

Antiseptic and expectorant. Externally as disinfectant.

MYRRH

Myrrh, Myrrha, Arabian Myrrh, Somali Myrrh, Hirabol (Guj.), Bol (Hindi)

Botanical Source

Myrrh is the oleo-gum-resin obtained by incision from the stem of *Commiphora molmol*, *C. abyssinica* and other species of *Commiphora*.

Family

Burseraceae.

Geographical Source

Somaliland (northeast Africa).

Characters

- Myrrh occurs in irregular agglutinated tears of masses. Its external surface is rough and reddish-brown, covered with yellowish dust. Pieces are brittle.
- Fractured surface is waxy granular and oily with whitish marks. Thin pieces are translucent or almost transparent.
- Odour is aromatic and taste aromatic, bitter and acrid.

Tests

1. When triturated with water it yields a yellowish-brown emulsion.
2. Ethereal solution of myrrh becomes reddish when treated with bromine vapour and purplish when moistened with nitric acid. The above tests are negative in case of bdellium.

Uses

Stimulant and antiseptic.

NIM LEAF

Nim, Nimba (Hindi and Punjabi), Margosa tree (Eng.),
Kohumba (Guj.), Neem (Unani)

Botanical Source

Nim consists of the dried leaves of *Azadirachta indica* (Syn. *Melia azadirachta*).

Family

Meliaceae.

Geographical Source

Throughout India and other countries of Southeast Asia.

Morphology

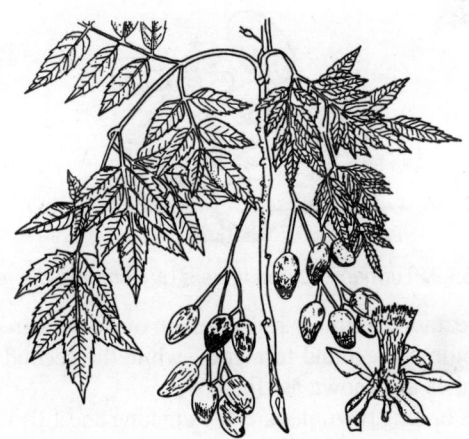

Fig. 5.48. Nim, *Azadirachta indica*. A branch with compound leaves showing opposite leaflets, two bunches of ripe fruits and a single flower.

- General appearance: Leaves compound, alternate, rachis upto 25 cm long, leaflets with oblique base, opposite and exstipulate.
- Size: 6–8 cm long and 1.0–1.6 cm wide.
- Shape: Lanceolate, acute and serrate.
- Colour: Slightly yellowish-green.
- Fracture: Brittle.
- Odour: Almost odourless.
- Taste: Bitter.

Uses

Different parts used as antiseptic, insecticidal, anthelmintic, emmenagogue and febrifuge (see Part 2).

CURCUMA

Turmeric (Eng.), Haldi (Hindi & Unani),
Zardchob (Pers.), Arqussofar (Arabic)

Botanical Source

Curcuma or turmeric consists of the dried rhizomes of *Curcuma domestica* (Syn. *C. longa*).

Family

Zingiberaceae.

Geographical Source

Tropical Asia and Africa, especially India, Pakistan, China and Malaysia.

Morphology

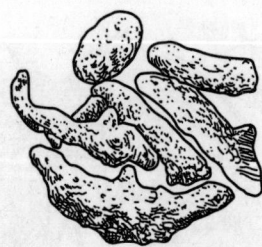

Fig. 5.49. Turmeric. Cured fingers of *Curcuma domestica*.

- General appearance: Primary rhizomes are ovate or pear-shaped and are known as 'bulbs' or 'round turmeric', while the secondary cylindrical lateral rhizomes are known as 'fingers'.
- Size: Fingers or long rhizomes are 4–7 cm long and 1.0–1.5 cm in width.
- Shape: Fingers or long turmeric rhizomes are tapering on both ends. Bulbs are short and thick.
- Outer surface: Longitudinally wrinkled and with transverse rings. Transverse rings are due to the leaf scars.
- Colour: Deep yellow to brown.
- Fracture: Hard, difficult to break.
- Odour: Characteristic, aromatic.
- Taste: Aromatic, pungent and bitter.

Tests

Turmeric, because of curcumins, shows the following reactions. For the tests curcuma powder or evaporated residue of tincture is used.

1. With concentrated sulphuric acid red colour is produced.
2. With solution of sodium or potassium hydroxide red to violet colour is produced.

3. With acetic anhydride and concentrated sulphuric acid it shows violet colour. When this test is seen in ultraviolet light, intense red-coloured fluorescence is seen. This fluorescence test is due to Curcumin III and in Java turmeric only grayish-yellow fluorescence is seen and thus turmeric and Java turmeric can be distinguished.

Uses

It is choleretic and cholagogue. Volatile oil has aromatic and pungent properties (see Part 2).

ANTIMALARIALS

CINCHONA BARK

Countess, Peruvian or Jesuit's bark, Cinchona

Botanical Source

Cinchona is the dried bark of the stem or of the root of *Cinchona calisaya*, *Cinchona ledgeriana*, *Cinchona officinalis* and *Cinchona succirubra* or hybrids of any of the first two species with any of the last two species.

Family

Rubiaceae.

Geographical Source

It is mainly cultivated in Indonesia (Java), Zaire, India, Guatemala and Bolivia.

Characters

Plants are tropical shrubs or trees. Members of the family contain alkaloids of quinoline ring as quinine, isoquinoline ring as emetine and indole ring as yohimbine.

Macroscopy

There are four species and several hybrids of cinchona. The general characters of stem bark and root bark are mentioned here.

1. *General characters of stem bark:* Shape of the bark is curved, quill or double quill. Outer surface is rough, mainly due to longitudinal and transverse cracks, fissures, ridges and protuberances. Cracks and fissures are characteristic for each bark. Greyish patches of moss or lichen are present on the outer surface. Colour of *C. succirubra* is reddish-brown while of other barks is yellowish to brown. Barks are usually up to 30 cm

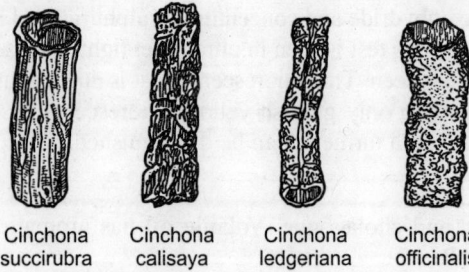

Cinchona   Cinchona   Cinchona   Cinchona
succirubra   calisaya   ledgeriana   officinalis

Fig. 5.50. Barks of *Cinchona* species.

long, 1.5–2 cm in diameter and 2–8 mm thick. Inner surface is striated and its colour may be reddish-brown to yellow according to the variety.

• Fracture is short in outer part and fibrous in inner part.
• Odour is distinct and taste is bitter.

2. *Root bark:* It occurs in channelled pieces. Outer surface is sometimes scaly and inner striated.

Cork: Cork consists of several rows of radially arranged thin-walled cells with reddish-brown contents. Phelloderm is a narrow zone of regular cells.

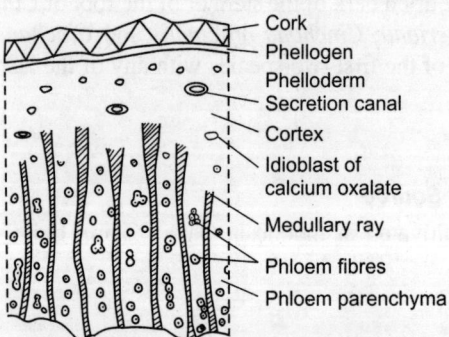

Cork
Phellogen
Phelloderm
Secretion canal
Cortex
Idioblast of calcium oxalate
Medullary ray
Phloem fibres
Phloem parenchyma

Fig. 5.51. T.S. of Cinchona bark.

Cortex: Cortex consists of thin-walled parenchymatous cells. Cells contain amorphous reddish-brown matter, small rounded starch grains and occasionally microcrystals of calcium oxalate. Few idioblasts or secretion cells appearing oval in the transection are present on the inner side.

Phloem: It is wide. It consists of sieve tubes, phloem parenchyma and phloem fibres. Phloem fibres are isolated or in small radial groups. They are spindle-shaped and lignified with striated walls. Medullary rays are 2 to 3-celled wide and radially elongated.

Uses

It is used as antipyretic, analgesic and antimalarial bark (see Part 2).

OXYTOCICS

Oxytocics are drugs which cause contraction of uterus muscle. These agents are used to induce labour. They are also used to treat post-partum haemorrhage.

Methyl ergometrine tablet and methyl ergometrine maleate injection are clinically used in the active management or 3rd stage of labour.

ERGOT

Ergot of Rye, Ergot

Botanical Source

Ergot is the dried sclerotium of the fungus *Claviceps purpurea* Tulasne, arising in the ovary of rye plant *Secale cereale* (Family Gramineae).

Family

Clavipitaceae (Ascomycetes).

Geographical Source

Ergot is cultivated in Czechoslovakia, Germany, Hungary, Switzerland and India.

Morphology

- Size: 1–4 cm long, 2–7 mm wide.
- Shape: Slightly curved, fusiform. sub-cylindrical, tapering at both ends.
- Outer surface: Black to purplish-brown, longitudinally furrowed with occasional transverse cracks.

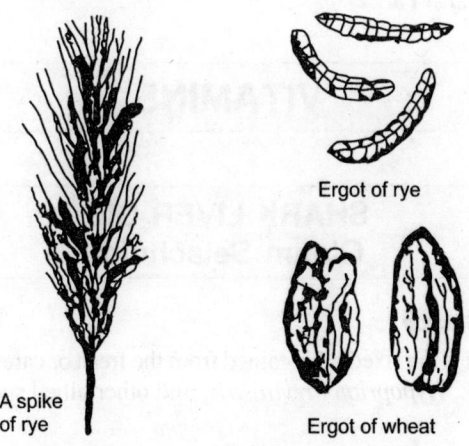

Ergot of rye

A spike of rye

Ergot of wheat

Fig. 5.52. Ergot, *Claviceps purpurea*.

- Fractured surface: It shows a narrow outer layer of purplish-brown rectangular cells often obliterated and a middle layer of black to purple or rose-coloured pseudo-parenchyma, consisting of oval or rounded cells of chitinous cell walls, containing fixed oil and proteins and pale or dark lines radiating from the centre.
- Odour: It is characteristic. It should possess neither rancid nor ammoniacal odour. Ergot powder when treated with sodium hydroxide produces strong smell of trimethylamine.
- Taste: Unpleasant.
- Ergot of good quality has white fracture and has neither ammoniacal nor rancid odour.

Ergot as a drug consists of mostly complete sclerotia with other organic matter limited to just 1% officially.

Chemical Tests

1. Ergot when seen in filtered ultraviolet light shows a red-coloured flourescence. Rye flour is used as food in many European countries and contamination with ergot can be easily detected by this test.
2. **Ergotoxine test:** Extract ergot powder with chloroform and sodium carbonate. Separate the chloroform layer and add to it the reagent consisting of 0.1 gm of *p*-dimethylaminobenzaldehyde, 100 ml of 35% v/v sulphuric acid and 1.5 ml of 5% ferric chloride. A deep blue colour is produced. This reaction is also used for the quantitative estimation of alkaloids by colorimetric method using ergotoxine ethanesulphonate as the standard.

Uses

Ergot has oxytocic action, produces uterine stimulation and hastens the delivery (see also Part 2).

VITAMINS

SHARK LIVER OIL
Oleum Selachoidi

Zoological Source

Shark liver oil is the fixed oil obtained from the fresh or carefully preserved livers of shark, *Hypoprion brevirostris*, and other allied species.

Family

Carcharhinidae.

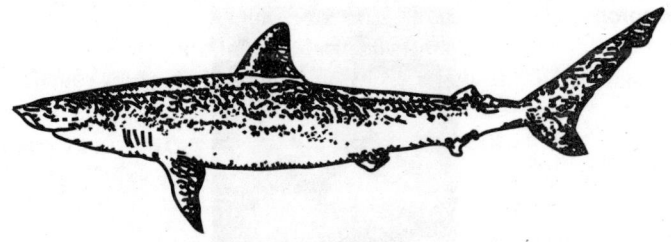

Fig. 5.53. The shark, *Hypoprion brevirostris*.

Geographical Source

Sea coasts of India and other European countries.

Characters

- Shark liver oil is pale yellow to brownish yellow liquid.
- Odour is fishy but not rancid.
- Taste is bland and fishy.
- Shark liver oil is miscible with light petroleum (boiling point 50–60° C), ether and chloroform. It is only slightly soluble in alcohol.

Chemical tests

1. Dissolve 1 drop of shark liver oil in 1 ml of chloroform. On adding sulphuric acid and then shaking, a pale violet colour develops, which in the end becomes brown or blue.
2. Add 5 ml of the oil in a centrifuge tube and add to it 5 ml of benzene. When the solution is centrifuged at 25°C for 25 minutes, no precipitate is produced and the solution remains clear.

Uses

Shark liver oil, admixed with vitamin D, is used as a tonic and nutritive.

AMLA

Embelic myrobalan (Eng.), Amala (Hindi & German); Amlaki (Beng.); Aamlah (Urdu & Persian); Amlaj (Arabic); Nelli (Tamil)

Botanical Source

Amla consists of fresh or dried fruits of *Emblica officinalis* (*Phyllanthus emblica*).

Family

Euphorbiaceae.

Geographical Source

The plant is widely distributed throughout India, Sri Lanka and China.

Morphology

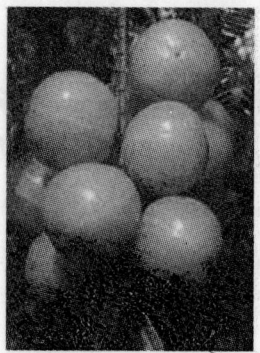

Fig. 5.54. Amla fruit.

- General appearance: Fruit is fleshy, globose, with six pale vertical furrows. It is smooth, shiny with few prominent but minute light coloured specks. A depression left by the removal of peduncle is seen at one end of the fruit, which is a drupe with strong stony endocarp.
- Size: Fruits 1.3–1.6 in diameter.
- Shape: Globose, with 6 pale vertical furrows.
- Colour: Green when fresh unripe, but light yellow when mature; on drying dark brownish to black.
- Fracture: Pericarp hard, not easily removable from the light brownish seed (stone), dried fruit splitting longitudinally.
- Odour: Almost odourless, faintly characteristic.
- Taste: Sour and slightly bitter and sweet with astringent feeling.

Uses

It is considered a rejuvenative tonic in Ayurvedic, Unani and in other alternative medicines. It is a rich source of vitamin C.

ENZYMES

PAPAYA / PAPAIN

Papaw (Eng.), Papaya (Beng, Guj., Hindi); Amba Hindi (Arabic, Persian); Arandkharbuza (Unani); Melonenbaum (German); Pappali (Tamil)

Botanical Source

Papaya fruit and the enzyme papain are obtained from *Carica payapa.*

Family

Caricaceae.

Geographical Source

India, Pakistan, Bangladesh and Sri Lanka.

General (Morphological) Description

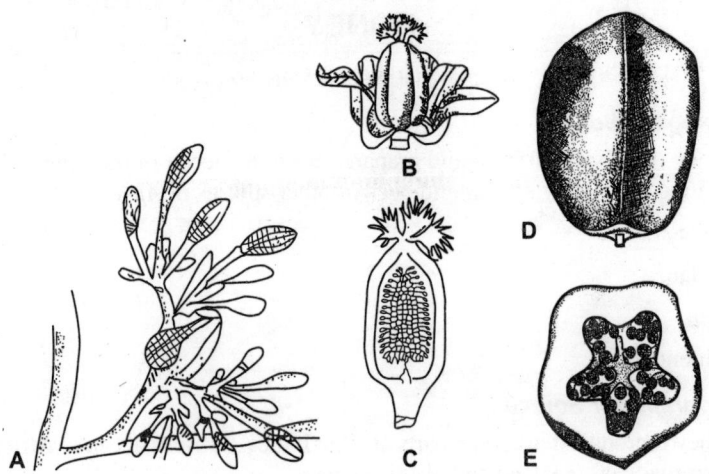

Fig. 5.55. *Carica papaya* (Family Caricaceae). (A) A flower; (B) An inflorescence; (C) A developing fruit (ovary); (D) A mature fruit; (E) Fruit cut in T.S. showing blackish seeds.

- Papaya is a small tree with a straight single stem, growing 5–10 metres tall, with spirally arranged leaves confined to the top of the trunk. The lower part of the trunk is conspicuously scarred showing the remains of earlier leaves and fruits. The leaves are large 40–60 cm in diameter and palmately lobed with 7 lobes.
- The flowers are dioecious.
- The fruit matures into a large 15–40 cm long, 10–25 cm diameter and it is ripe when it feels soft and changes to yellowish colour. The rind of the fruit nearing maturity gives a white, milky juice or latex which contains an albuminoid, a digestive enzyme, papain, also called papayotin. The latex changes its colour to yellowish or somewhat orange on standing (ripening).

Uses

It is an edible fruit. Its powder is used as meat tenderizer and marketed as tablets for indigestion problems and alimentary canal worms' attacks (see also Part 2). It is considered as an anticonstipative. Papain made into paste with water is used to treat bee and wasps stings and mosquito bites.

PHARMACEUTICAL AIDS

HONEY

Madha, Mel, Shehad, Asal (Ar.)

Biological Source

Honey is the saccharine liquid prepared from the nectar of the flowers by the hive-bee *Apis mellifica* and bees of other species of *Apis*.

Family

Apidae.

Order

Hymenoptera.

Geographical Source

Honey is produced in certain parts of West Indies, California, Chile, Africa, Australia, New Zealand and also in India.

Characters

- Honey is viscid, translucent, white to pale yellow or yellow brown-coloured liquid. On keeping its crystals of glucose separate.
- Odour is pleasant and charactristic and taste is sweet. The odour and taste depend on the flowers from which nectar is sucked.
- Specific rotation of honey is +3° to –10°.
- The total ash 0.1–0.8% and weight per ml is 1.35–1.38 g.

Test

Shake 10 ml of honey and 5 ml of ether till they both become miscible. Separate the upper ethereal layer and evaporate it in the porcelain dish. Add to the residue 1 drop of 1% resorcinol hydrochloric acid. In natural honey a transient red colour is obtained, while in artificial invert sugar red colour persists for some time. Sometimes artificial invert sugar is prepared by the enzyme invertase when this test is negative. However, this artificial invert sugar has not got the aromatic taste and smell of the natural honey.

The limits of chloride, sulphate and total ash should be as required in the pharmacopeia.

Uses

Nutritive, demulcent and laxative.

STARCH (AMYLUM)

Botanical Source

Starch consists of polysaccharide granules which on complete hydrolysis yield glucose.

Characters

- Starch occurs as white powder or in irregular angular mass. It is insoluble in cold water. Its specific gravity is 1.60–1.65 and thus being heavier than water it sinks in water. One part of starch forms colloidal solution when heated with 15 parts of water, which when cooled forms translucent jelly.
- With iodine reagent, it gives deep blue colour. The pH of starch depends on its composition or method of preparation.
- Maize starch is neutral or slightly alkaline, rice starch is slightly alkaline, while wheat and potato starches are slightly acidic.
- Starch occurs in simple or compound grains.
- Characters of starch, as seen through microscope, like shape, size, position of hilum, striations and whether they are concentric or eccentric, and in compound starch number of starch grains are characteristic for each starch.
- Viewed under polarized light starch granules show distinct black cross intersecting at the hilum.

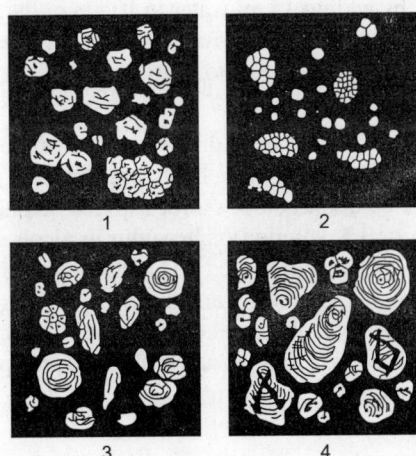

Fig. 5.56. Starches. (1) Wheat, (2) Maize, (3) Rice, and (4) Potato.

Uses

Primarily starch is used as a nutritive. However, it has many other uses (see Part 2).

GUM ACACIA (GUM ARABIC)

Botanical Source
Acacia gum is the dried gummy exudation obtained from stem and branches of *Acacia senegal* and other *Acacia* species.

Family
Leguminosae.

Geographical Source
Sudan, especially Kordofan, Senegal and Senegambia in West Africa and Central Africa.

Characters
Acacia occurs as spherodial or oval tears or pieces of 1–4 cm in diameter. Sometimes it also occurs in angular fragments. It is white, yellow or pale amber and opaque because of numerous minute cracks. It is brittle and breaks easily and fractured surface being transparent and glassy. It has no odour and taste is mucilaginous. It is soluble in water but insoluble in alcohol, though soluble in concentrations below 60%. The solution in water is translucent, viscid and slightly acidic. 10% solution of the gum in water is slightly levorotatory.

Identity Tests
Prepare a solution by adding 15 ml water to 10 gm of the gum by stirring it well. Use this solution for the following tests:

1. To 5 ml of the solution add 0.1 g borax. A stiff translucent mass is formed.
2. Dilute 1 ml of the solution by adding water and add to it few drops of lead subacetate solution. A white bulky precipitate is formed.
3. To 5 ml of the solution add few drops of 1% alcoholic solution of guaicum resin or 1% solution of benzidin in alcohol and hydrogen peroxide. Blue colour is produced due to enzyme oxidase.
4. To 1 ml solution add 4 ml water and dilute hydrochloric acid and boil for few minutes. Hydrolysis takes place and reducing sugars are produced. Add Fehling's solution and heat. A red precipitate of cuprous oxide is produced.

Purity Tests

1. Dilute 1 ml of the solution by adding 10 ml water and keep for few hours. No sediment should be deposited.
2. To 1 ml of the solution add 4 ml of water and few drops of lead acetate solution. No precipitate should be produced. Indian gum, tragacanth gum and other gums produce a precipitate.

3. To 1 ml of solution add 4 ml of water, boil, cool and add 2 drops of N/10 iodine solution. Blue colour shows the presence of starch and brown colour of dextrins.
4. To 1 ml of the solution add 4 ml of water and few drops of 0.1% ferric chloride solution. No blue or black colour should be produced. Blue or black colour indicates the presence of tannins, which may be due to presence of bark or wood in the drug.

Uses

Acacia is demulcent. It is used as an emulsifying and suspnding agent (see Part 2).

[For notes on Indian Acacia and Ghatti Gum see also Part 2.]

TRAGACANTH

Gummi Tragacanthae, Gum Tragacanth, Gum Dragon Anjira (Hindi)

Botanical Source

Tragacanth is the dried gummy exudation obtained from the stem of *Astragalus gummifer* and other *Astragalus* species.

Family

Leguminosae.

Geographical Source

Iran and North Syria supply Persian tragacanth.

Characters

- Gum occurs in flat or curved ribbon-shaped flakes. The flakes are 3 cm long, 1 cm wide and 2 mm thick. Flakes are white, slightly yellow coloured, horny and translucent with transverse or longitudinal ridges. Fracture is short.
- The gum has no odour and practically no taste. With strong iodine solution it shows greenish colour.

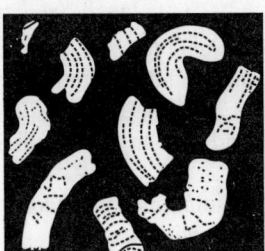

Fig. 5.57. Tragacanth pieces in black background.

- In lower concentrations in water tragacanth gives highly viscous solutions, which are stable to heat and pH.

Uses

In pharmaceutical industry as an emulsifier, thickener and stabilizer. As a herbal remedy it has been used as a purgative and for topical treatment of burns.

AGAR

Agar-agar, Japanese isinglass

Botanical Source

Agar is the dried gelatinous substance obtained by extraction with water, concentration and drying of red algae from various species of *Gelidium*, *Gracilaria* and *Pterocladia*.

Order

Rhodophyceae.

Geographical Source

Japan: *Gelidium amansii* and other *Gelidium* species. Australia: *Gracilaria confervoides*. New Zealand: *Pterocladia lucida* and other allied species.

Characters

- Agar occurs in strips, flakes or coarse powder. Strips are about 60 cm in length and 4 mm wide, translucent, yellowish-white and slightly attached to each other. Odour is slight and taste is mucilaginous.
- Agar is insoluble in cold water, but is soluble in boiling water. On cooling to about 35°C, a firm gel forms that does not melt or liquefy below about 85°C. These setting and melting temperatures are characteristic for agar. Gels formed at agar concentrations greater than 0.5% are rigid, but gelation can take place at concentrations as low as 0.04%.

Tests for Identity

1. Add ruthenium red on powdered drug – *Red colour*.
2. Add 0.5 ml hydrochloric acid to 0.5% aqueous solution and heat on water bath for 30 minutes and divide into two parts:
   (a) Add to the first part 3 ml of 10% caustic soda solution and 2 ml Fehling's solution and heat on water bath – *Reduction takes place due to galactose*.
   (b) Add barium chloride solution to the second part – *White precipitate of barium sulphate is obtained*.
3. Agar is incinerated to ash, dilute hydrochloric acid is added and seen under microscope when skeletons and sponge spicules of diatoms are seen.

As agar does not contain nitrogen so the following tests of gelatin are negative.

1. Heated with soda lime – *No ammonia produced.*
2. Millon's reagent – *No precipitate.*
3. 0.2% solution of agar with tannic acid solution – *No precipitate.*

Uses

Agar is used as a laxative in chronic constipation and as an appetite suppressant. It is used as an excipient for the manufacture of emulsions and fat-free ointment bases. Agar jellies are used for the cultures of micro-organisms; as a solid substrate to contain culture medium for micro-biological work. In the food industry agar is an important gelling material and as a thickener for soups and ice cream.

GELATIN (GELATINUM)

Biological Source

Gelatin is the protein derivative obtained after purifying and evaporating the aqueous extract of skin, bones and tendons of animals. The skin and bones of ox and sheep are used in the preparation.

Family

Bovidae.

Characters

Gelatin occurs in sheets, strips or as granular powder. Gelatin is white or has slight pale yellow colour. It is translucent and has practically no odour and taste. Gelatin is soluble in hot water and 2% solution on cooling forms a jelly. Gelatin is soluble in acetic acid and glycerine but is insoluble in alcohol and ether. It is hard and brittle and breaks with a short fracture.

Tests for identity

1. Heat a small quantity of gelatin in a dry test tube with soda lime. Because of nitrogenous constituent ammonia is evolved.

   Dissolve 0.5 gm gelatin in 100 ml water by heating and use this solution for the following tests:

2. Take few ml of the solution in a test tube and add few drops of 10% tannic acid solution. White to white buff coloured precipitate is produced which does not dissolve on heating.
3. Add Millon's reagent to few ml of the solution. White precipitate is produced which becomes red on heating.
4. Add picric acid solution to the solution of gelatin. Yellow precipitate is produced.

The aforesaid four tests distinguish agar and gelatin. In agar these tests are negative.

Uses

Gelatin is considered a fairly good substitute of blood plasma. It is an important material for pharmaceutical and food industries. Used for the manufacture of capsules and suppositories, and also for coating pills and tablets.

BEESWAX

White and Yellow Beeswax, Cera Alba and Cera Flava,
Shamah Al Nahl (Arabic)

Zoological Source

Beeswax is the purified wax obtained from honeycomb of *Apis mellifica* and other species of *Apis*.

Family

Apidae.

Order

Hymenoptera.

Geographical Source

Jamaica, East and West Africa, India, France and Italy. Also in countries where honey is produced.

Characters

- Wax is white, yellow or yellowish-brown solid having pleasant smell of honey. It breaks with granular fracture. It is insoluble in water, slightly soluble in alcohol, but soluble in chloroform, ether, fixed oil and volatile oils including turpentine oil.
- Specific gravity is 0.958–0.970. Melting point 62–64° C and refractive index at 80°C is 1.4380–1.4420.

Uses

Beeswax is used in ointments as hardening material, in preparations of plaster and polishes.

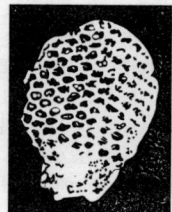

Fig. 5.58. Honey comb.

MISCELLANEOUS DRUGS

LIQUORICE (LICORICE)

Licuorice root, Radix Glycyrrhiza, Sweet root, Mulethi (Hindi),
Jethi Madh (Guj.), Yastimadhu (Sanskrit), Asalassus (Arabic & Persian)

Botanical Source

Licorice consists of peeled and/or unpeeled roots and stolon (and subterranean stems) of the plant *Glycyrrhiza glabra* and other species of *Glycyrrhiza*.

Family

Leguminosae.

Geographical Source

The main supplies of the drug come from Spain, Iran, Iraq, Sicily, Russia, Greece and Asia Minor (Anatolia), Afghanistan, India and Pakistan.

Morphology

- General appearance: Spanish licorice consists of peeled or unpeeled stolons and roots.
- Size: Up to 20 cm in length and 1–2 cm in diameter.
- Shape: Peeled pieces angular, unpeeled straight, unbranched, cylindrical.
- Outer surface: Unpeeled drug is dark reddish-brown, longitudinally wrinkled, stolons bear buds, scale leaves and scars of lateral roots.
- Fracture: Fibrous in bark, splintery in wood.

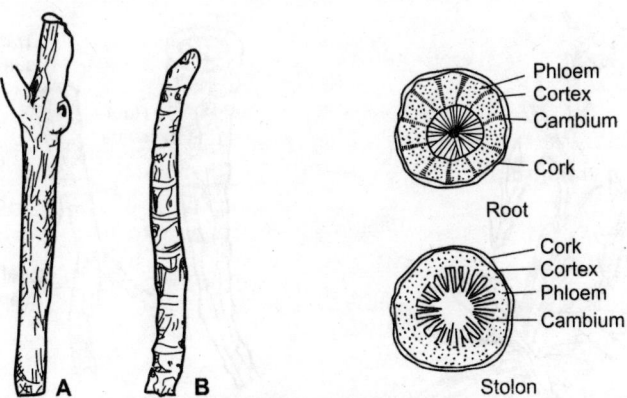

Fig. 5.59. Liquorice, *Glycyrrhiza glabra*. (A) Part of root; (B) Part of stolon; (C) Transverse sections of licorice root and stolon.

- Taste: Sweet, free from bitterness.
- Peeled drug: Outer surface pale yellow, fibrous.
- Smoothed transverse preparation of stolon shows a thin brown cork, narrow phelloderm and radial medullary rays, greyish-yellow phloem with groups of fibres, distinct cambium, yellow xylem with vessels and groups of fibres and central pith.
- Root shows similar appearance but pith is absent and has tetrarch xylem with four primary medullary rays.

Uses

It is expectorant, antispasmodic, anti-ulcer, antiinflammatory and sweetening agent (see Part 2).

PICRORHIZA

Katuki (Sanskrit), Kutki (Hindi), Kadu (Guj.), Katuki (Beng.)

Botanical Source

Picrorhiza consists of dried stolons and rhizomes of *Picrorhiza kurroa.*

Family

Scrophulariaceae.

Geographical Source

The drug is collected in Kashmir and Sikkim.

Morphology

In commerce pieces of rhizomes and stolons 3.8 cm long and 0.3–1 cm in diameter are found. These pieces are more or less cylindrical or slightly

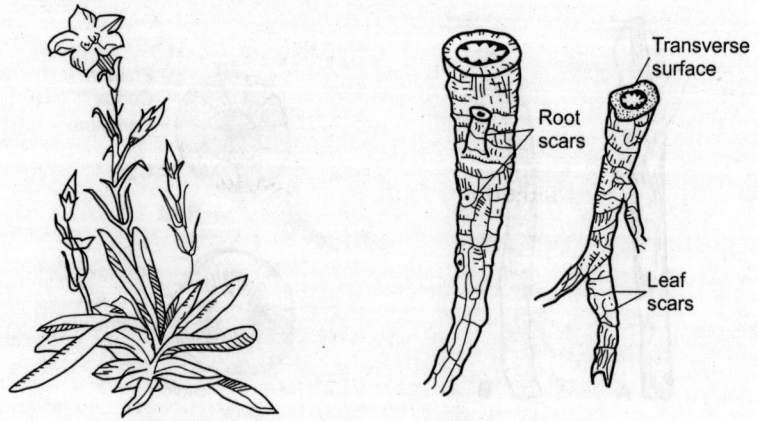

Fig. 5.60. (A) Picrorhiza twig; (B) Picrorhiza roots.

curved with brownish grey cork. Rhizome is covered with remains of black scale leaves and shows root and branch scars and apical bud. The stolons bear scale leaves at distant intervals. Frequently, small protuberances which represent accessory buds are seen both on the rhizomes and stolons. Fracture is short and shows on the inner side a black lacunar surface with whitish xylem ring. Odour is characteristic and taste is very bitter.

Uses

It is a popular bitter tonic, cathartic, stomachic and febrifuge (see Part 2).

DIOSCOREA

Yam, Mexican Yam

Botanical Source

Dioscorea consists of tubers of several species of the genus *Dioscorea*, such as *D. floribunda*, *D. spiculiflora* and *D. villosa*. In India, however, *D. deltoida*, *D. prazeri*, *D. bulbifera* and *D. bellophyla* are found.

Family

Dioscoreaceae.

Geographical Source

D. deltoida is being successfully cultivated in Jammu & Kashmir, Tamil Nadu, Karnataka, Bengal and Maharashtra. *D. floribunda* is also now cultivated in India, while *D. bellophylla* in Pakistan.

Characters

The plant is found growing wild in Western Himalayan region at an altitude of about 3000 metres. It is a climber and possesses tuberous roots, with

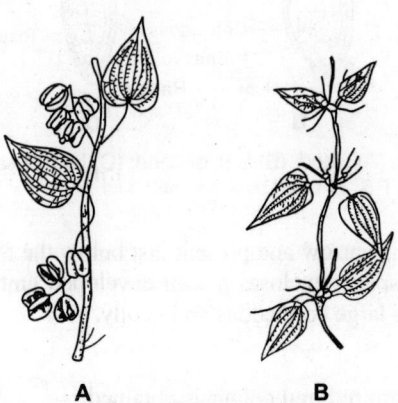

A   **B**

Fig. 5.61. Dioscorea. (A) *Dioscorea deltoida*, a shoot. (B) *Dioscorea belophylla*, a branch with flowers.

tubers which are very large, heavy and brown with adhering soil. It is yet another example of a plant which has highly developed underground part, but a weakly developed shoot, requiring support to hold it above the ground.

Uses

Diosgenin is used for the production of steroidal drugs.

LINSEED

Flax Seed, Semen Lini, Alasi (Hind.), Bizra al Kattan (Arabic)

Botanical Source

Linseed consists of the dried ripe seeds of *Linum usitatissimum* Linn.

Family

Linaceae.

Geographical Source

Argentina, India, Russia, Canada, U.S.A.

Morphology

- Size: 4–6 mm long, 2–3 mm wide and 1.5 mm thick.
- Shape: Elongated ovate, flattened, obliquely pointed at one end.
- Outer surface: In the angle in the depression, hilum is seen and micropyle is adjacent to it. From the hilum the yellowish raphe runs to the chalaza at the flat end of the seed. Testa is glossy, brown to dark and finely pitted.

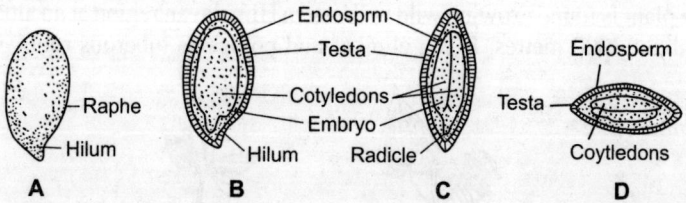

Fig. 5.62. Linseed. (A) Seed; (B) L.S. of seed; (C) L.S. of seed at right angle to the thickness; (D) T.S. of seed.

- Endosperm: It is narrow and present just below the testa and is oily.
- Embryo: Endosperm encloses a well-developed embryo consisting of radicle and two large cotyledons and is oily.

Chemical Tests

1. With ruthenium red, red colour is obtained.
2. It gives cyanogenetic glycoside tests.

Uses

Mucilage has demulcent and soothing action and hence linseed is used in cough and bronchitis. Linseed oil, being a drying oil, is used in paints and varnishes (see Part 2).

SHATAVARI

Shatavar; Shahakul Satavari (Hindi); Satavar (Guj.); Safaid Musli (Unani)

Botanical Source

The drug, Shatavari, consists of the dried tubers or tuberous roots of the plant *Asparagus racemosus*. (The correct botanical identity of the roots of Shatavari continues to be disputed, in spite of the fact that the literature mentions it to be derived from *A. racemosus*.)

Family

Liliaceae.

Geographical Source

The plant grows in the northern part of India, in Himalayan and sub-Himalayan regions.

Characters

- General appearance: The market samples of the drug consist of peeled dried, entire or broken pieces; broken pieces show irregular, uneven transverse surface; external surface shows deep irregular, longitudinal furrows and minute transverse wrinkles. The drug swells considerably on being soaked in water and becomes soft and flaccid.
- Shape: Roots are cylindrical, straight or slightly curved, entire roots taper at both ends.
- Size: 4–12 cm long and 6–12 mm in thickness.
- Fracture: Drug is hard and breaks with uneven fracture. The smooth fractured transverse surface shows a wide bark and a small central narrow wood. Sometimes broken pieces also show a norrow cavity.
- Colour: White to buff, sometimes pale brownish.
- Odour: Odourless.
- Taste: Bland, which becomes slightly bitter after some time.

Uses

As a popular indigenous drug it has uterine blocking activity. For safe delivery, especially in threatened abortion.

PYRETHRUM

Pyrethrum flowers, Insect flowers, Flores Pyrethri

Botanical Source

Pyrethrum consists of dried flower heads of *Chrysanthemum cinerarifolium* and many other species of the genus *Chrysanthemum* e.g. *C. roseus*.

Family

Compositae.

Geographical Source

The plant is a native of Dalmatia (Yugoslavia – Balkans) and is now widely cultivated in Kenya, East Central Africa, Japan, Yugoslavia, Brazil, Ecuador and India.

Characters

The closed flower heads are about 6–9 mm in diameter and open ones 9–11 mm in diameter. They bear a short peduncle which is striated longitudinally. The receptacle is 4–8 mm in diameter. It is flat and without paleae. It is surrounded by an involucre of two to three rows of yellowish or greenish-yellow, lanceolate, hairy bracts with a membranous margin. The receptacle bears numerous yellow tubular florets and a single row of 15–23 white, cream or straw-coloured ligulate florets. The ligulate corollas are 10–20 mm in length and have about 17 veins and 3 apical teeth. The central tooth is often more or less suppressed. Calyx is tubular and membranous.

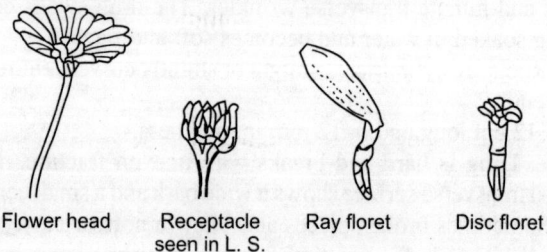

| Flower head | Receptacle seen in L. S. | Ray floret | Disc floret |

Fig. 5.63. Pyrethrum flower.

Ovary is inferior and 5-ribbed with filiform style and bifid stigma. Calyx and gynaecium in tubular florets are same as ligulate florets. Fruit is a 5-ribbed cypsela. Flowers have slightly aromatic odour and bitter acrid taste.

Persian insect flowers have rose colour of ray florets and 10-ribbed fruits.

Uses

Pyrethrum and pyrethrins are used as contact insecticides.

TOBACCO

Tambaku, Tamaku, (Hindi, Beng., Guj., Urdu)

Botanical Source

The drug, Tobacco, consists of the dried leaves of the plant *Nicotiana tabacum*. Of the other species of the genus *Nicotiana*, *N. rustica* also forms the source of tobacco.

Family

Solanaceae.

Geographical Source

The plants grow in many parts of India and are cultivated.

Characters

Nicotiana tabacum is a sturdy annual plant which has stout straight stem bearing a few branches. It grows up to a height of 3 metres. Leaves are large, about 100 cm in length, mostly sessile, ovate, elliptic or lanceolate (Fig. 5.64).

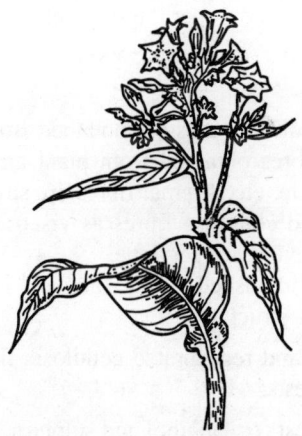

Fig. 5.64. Tobacco, *Nicotiana tabacum* (Family Solanaceae). A branch with leaves and flowers.

Uses

Tobacco is smoked in India in bidis, cigarettes and even as a snuff (see Part 2).

6

Study of Fibres and Surgical Dressings

This chapter 7 of the syllabus deals with the "Study of source, preparation and identification of fibers used in sutures and surgical dressings – cotton, silk, wool and regenerated fibre."

The chapter first gives below the introduction, in general, of fibres, sutures, surgical dressings and regenerated fibres followed by the drugs/materials mentioned above as per the syllabus.

FIBRES

Fibres used in surgical dressings are obtained from plant, animal or are man-made fibres. Fibres obtained from plant are vegetable fibres, e.g. cotton, flax, hemp, jute, etc. Animal fibres are silk and wool. Man-made fibres are regenerated cellulose fibres as viscose and acetate rayon or synthetic fibres like nylon and terylene.

Fibres can be distinguished by the chemical nature of their cell wall and their microscopic structures.

Vegetable fibres and regenerated cellulosic fibres are cellulosic and show the following tests:

1. With Molisch's test (α-naphthol and sulphuric acid) they show violet colour.
2. With chlor-zinc iodine or iodine and sulphuric acid they show blue colour.
3. Vegetable fibres dissolve in cuoxam (copper oxide ammonia) with blue colour.
4. When ignited they do not produce foul smell.

Animal fibres are proteinous in nature and show the following tests:

1. When ignited they burn with unpleasant smell.

2. They are soluble in 5% potassium hydroxide.
3. They are stained permanently with picric acid and show Millon's test.

SUTURES

Both sutures and ligatures are threads or strings specially prepared and sterilised for use in surgery. They are prepared from the same material. The sutures are used for sewing or stitching together tissues like skin, muscle, tendon, etc. by using a needle. A ligature is used to tie and constrict a blood vessel, vein, or artery and no needle is used. Sutures are classified as absorbable and non-absorbable. Absorbable suture is absorbed and digested in the tissues of the body. Absorbable sutures are catgut kangaroo tendons and synthetic absorbable polymers, etc. Non-absorbable sutures are not absorbed and remain in the body, as silk. Others get encapsulated after a long time while some remain as inert implants; silk, cotton, nylon, synthetic polyesters and stainless steel wire belong to this group.

The most essential properties of sutures are:

1. Sterility,
2. Adequate mechanical strength,
3. Non-irritant,
4. Fine gauze, and
5. Time of absorption, if absorbable.

SURGICAL DRESSINGS

A dressing is described as a material applied to protect a wound and favours its healing. A **bandage** is described as a material which holds dressing in place, applies pressure or supports an injured part or checks haemorrhage. 'Surgical dressing' term is utilized to incorporate all structures whether used alone or in conjuction with others to cover a wound.

Functions of dressings

To provide ideal conditions for wound healing by:
(a) Removing wound exudates from the site.
(b) Preventing infection or combating infection.
(c) Giving physical protection to the healing wound.
(d) Giving mechanical support to surrounding tissues.
(e) To protect wound from outside liquids.

Properties of dressings

(a) Should not adhere to the granulating surface.
(b) Should be easy to handle at all stages.
(c) Should be durable.
(d) Should be free from loose threads, ends and fibres.
(e) Should be easily sterilized.

The surgical dressings consist of three parts:

1. Wound facing layer.
2. Absorbent layer.
3. Outer covering.

Wound facing layer: Absorbent fabrics, absorbent gauze, absorbent muslin and absorbent lint mostly of cotton; tenderised fabrics, cellulose fabrics; non-adherent dressing, paraffin gauze dressing; man-made fibre fabrics; metallized dressings, perforated films.

Absorbent layer: Non-woven materials (cotton wool, rayon wool); woven fabrics, gauze absorbent cotton, gauze pads.

Outer layer: Non-extensible bandages – plain bandage, plaster of Paris bandage; Extensible bandage: Non-adhesives – Rubber elastic; Adhesives – Zinc oxide adhesive tapes.

Special dressings: Spray on dressings – Pyroxilin, acrylic polymer. Absorbable haemostats – Human fibrin foam, absorbable gelatin sponge, oxidised cellulose and calcium alginate.

Surgical dressings are prepared from the fibres named earlier and described below.

REGENERATED FIBRES

There are several kinds of regenerated cellulose and are known as rayons or artificial silk. According to the method of preparation they are known as Acetate Rayon, Vicscose Rayon, Nitro Rayon, etc. From the regenerated fibres Viscose Rayon will be described below as an example.

ABSORBENT COTTON

Purified Cotton, Gossypium depuratum

Botanical Source

Absorbent cotton consists of the epidermal trichomes of the seeds of the cultivated species of *Gossypium herbaceum*, *G. hirsutum*, *G. barbadense* and other species of *Gossypium*, freed from adhering impurities, deprived of fat, bleached and sterilized.

Family

Malvaceae. Members of this family contain mucilage and are used as drug (Althae root) and as vegetable (Hibiscus).

Geographical Source

Cotton is a very ancient plant and is cultivated in India and Egypt since 3000 years. At present besides India and Egypt, it is cultivated in the U.S.A., South America and in some parts of Africa.

Collection and Preparation

The plants are shrubs or small trees. The fruit is a 3- to 5-celled capsule (boll) containing numerous seeds. The seeds are covered with hairs. The bolls are collected when ripe, separated from capsule, dried and subjected to a process of ginning whereby seeds are separated. In ginning hairs and seeds are put before the roller in which the space is small which allows only the hairs to pass. In some types of the American ones, gin leaves on the seeds short hairs, known as linters which are removed in the delinter machines. Linters are used for the manufacture of inferior grade of cotton wool. The seeds are used for the preparation of cottonseed oil and oil cake is used as cattle feed. The cotton obtained in this way is raw cotton and contains many impurities as colouring matter and fatty material including wax.

Raw cotton is subjected to process of combing whereby short fibres are separated and used for the preparation of absorbent cotton, while long fibres are spun and woven into cloth.

The short fibres known as comber waste are boiled for 10–15 hours with dilute caustic soda solution under 1–3 atmospheric pressure. This removes wax and much of the colouring matter. It is then washed and treated with solution of chlorinated soda and then with dilute hydrochloric acid. It is then washed with water, dried and recarded into flat sheets. It is packed into packages and usually sterilized.

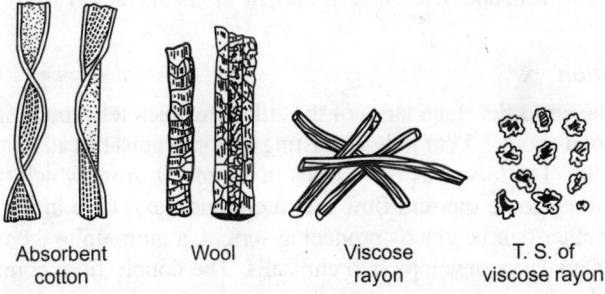

| Absorbent cotton | Wool | Viscose rayon | T. S. of viscose rayon |

Fig. 6.1. Fibres.

Description

Absorbent cotton occurs as white soft, fine filament-like hairs. The hairs are unicellular 2.5–4.5 cm in length and 25–35 μ in diameter. Cotton is odourless and tasteless.

Microscopy

Cotton consists of tubular, filamented, hollow, twisted trichomes. The trichomes are striated and slightly thickened at the edges. The apex is rounded.

Chemical Constituents

Absorbent cotton consists entirely of cellulose.

Storage

Absorbent cotton should be stored in cool place otherwise it becomes non-absorbent by intramolecular rearrangement. It should be wrapped in paper and protected from dust, germs, spores and bacteria. Bacterial attack makes it brittle and dusty and it loses its absorbent power.

Uses

It is used as a filtering medium and in surgical dressings. It absorbs blood, mucus, pus and prevents wound infection by bacteria.

SILK

Biological Source

Silk is the prepared fibre from the cocoons of *Bombyx mori*, the mulberry silk worm and other species of *Bombyx* and *Antheraea* (Order Lepidoptera).

Geographical Source

Fine quality of silk is produced in France and Italy from *Bombyx mori* and other species of *Bombyx* while so called wild silks are produced from *Antheraea mylitta* and *A. assama* (India), *A. yamama* (Japan) and *A. pernyi* (China).

Preparation

Before the chrysalis stage larva of the silkworm secretes around itself an oval cocoon about 2.5 cm long consisting of continuous thread up to 1200 metres long. The larva has two glands in the mouth from which two silk fibroin fibres come out and flow into a common exit tube in the mouth where another pair of glands producing sericin, a gum, unite them. After about 8 days larva develops into chrysalis. The double fibre coming out from the head is spun into a cocoon by movement of the head. If chrysalis was allowed to develop into an insect, silk would be damaged and so cocoons are collected at chrysalis stage and killed by heating at 60–80° C for a few hours or by short exposure of steam. The cocoons are placed in warm water to loosen the gum which causes silk thread to adhere. The ends of thread from 2–15 cocoons are caught up and wound into a single thread which is made up into a hank.

Description

Silk threads are very fine, smooth and solid and are usually yellow in colour. Silk is soft and smooth to the touch and possesses considerable tensile strengh and elasticity. Silk is soluble in curoxam, in 66% sulphuric acid and in concentrated hydrochloric acid. Wool is insoluble in these acids and couxam and can be distinguished.

Chemical Constituents

Silk contains protein fibroin. **Fibroin** does not contain amino acids containing sulphur.

Uses

Silk is used for making ligatures, oiled silk and certain types of sieves.

WOOL

Wool, Animal wool, Sheep's wool

Biological Source

Wool consists of the hairs from the fleece of sheep *Ovis aries*.

Family

Bovidae.

Order

Ungulata.

Geographical Source

Wool is produced in Australia, U.S.A., Argentina, Russia and many other countries including India.

Preparation

As mentioned in the preparation of wool fat, wool fat is removed from wool by washing. Wool is then bleached with sulphur dioxide or hydrogen peroxide and is throughly washed, spread out on wire netting and dried by hot air.

Dcscripton

Wool occurs as loosely felted mass of elastic, lustrous more or less curly hairs, smooth and somewhat slippery to the touch.

Tests

Wool is insoluble in 66% sulphuric acid and in concentrated hydrochloric acid, hot or cold, and in curoxam. Wool, because it contains sulphur containing amino acids, gives black colour with lead acetate and alkali. When seen under microscope wool shows cuticle, cortex and medulla.

Uses

Wool is used as filtering and straining medium and for the manufacture of dresses as flannel and crepe bandages.

VISCOSE RAYON

Botanical Source

Viscose rayon is preferably prepared from the wood cellulose of the wood of common spruce *Picea abies* (*Picea excelsa*) or bleached cotton linters.

Family

Pinanceae.

Preparation

Wood is delignified and wood cellulose is used for the preparation. Wood cellulose is macerated in 15–20% solution of caustic soda for about two hours. It is then squeezed out until it weighs about four times its original weight. The alkaline solution is broken up into small pieces and is allowed to mature for 24 hours in a closed vessel. Carbon disulphide in the proportion of 60 parts to 100 parts of broken cellulose is added. The cellulose swells, become deep orange in colour and gelatinous after 3–4 hours. After ripening for one or two days it forms a viscous fluid of sodium cellulose xanthate, hence the name viscose rayon. The solution is forced through a spinneret into a solution of sulphuric acid and sodium sulphate. The cellulose is regenerated as continuous filament and much of the sulphur is thrown out. The remaining free sulphur is removed with sodium sulphide, and it is bleached, washed and dried till the moisture is 10%.

Description

Viscose rayon fibres are solid and transparent having a diameter of 15–25 μ. They are white and highly lustrous. Seen under microscope the fibre shows grooves along the length. In transverse section the grooves appear as indentations and show an irregular crenate margin.

Tests

Viscose rayon shows tests of cellulose and it is insoluble in 90% formic acid and 90% phenol (distinguishing tests from nylon).

Uses

Viscose rayon is used to make lint, gauze, net and other surgical dressings. It is absorbent similar to absorbent cotton but like cotton it does not lose its absorbency.

APPENDICES

- Classification of Drugs as per the Therapeutic Efficacy (Pharmacological Classification)
- Taxonomic Classification of Drugs
- Chemical Classification of Drugs (Included in ER 1991)
- Medical Glossary

Classification of Drugs
as per the Therapeutic Efficacy
(Pharmacological Classification)

As per the classification mentioned in the syllabus, ER 1991

Common English/ Vernacular Name(s)	Biological Name	Family/N.O.	Main Active Constituent(s)
LAXATIVES			
Aloes/Ghiritkumari, Ghikwar (H), Aliyo (G), Ailwa (U)	*Aloe perryi, A. ferox* and other species of *Aloe*	Liliaceae	Anthraquinones, Glycosides (Aloin: Barbaloin, Iso-barbaloin; Aloe resin)
Rhubarb/Revandchini (H & U)	*Rheum palmatum, R. officinale* and other species of *Rheum*	Polygonaceae	Anthraquinones, as free or reduced derivatives (Rhein, Emodin, Chryso-phenol, etc.)
Senna: Indian senna and Alexandrian senna – leaves and pods	*Cassia angustifolia* and *Cassia acutifolia*	Leguminosae	Sennosides A, B, C & D; other glycosides – Monoanthrones and Dianthrones
Ispaghula/Isapghol (H), Ishabgula (G)	*Plantago ovata*	Plantaginaceae	Mucilage: Pentosan and Aldobionic acid, etc.
Castor oil/ Oleum ricini (L)	*Ricinus communis*	Euphorbiaceae	Glycerides of Ricinoleic acid and Isoricinoleic acids

Common English/ Vernacular Name(s)	Biological Name	Family/N.O.	Main Active Constituent(s)
CARDIOTONICS			
Digitalis, Foxglove leaves, Folia digitalis	*Digitalis purpurea* and *D. lanata*	Scrophulariaceae	Cardiac glycosides: Digitoxin, Gitoxin, Digoxin, etc.
Arjuna bark	*Terminalia arjuna*	Combretaceae	Arjunine, Arjunetin, Arjunolic acid, etc.
CARMINATIVES AND G.I. REGULATORS			
Coriander/Dhania (H), Dhana (G)	*Coriandrum sativum*	Umbelliferae	Volatile oil: Linalool, Geraniol, Borneol, Decenal, etc.
Fennel/Saunf (U), Variyali (G)	*Foeniculum vulgare*	Umbelliferae	Volatile oil: Anethole, Fenchone, etc.
Omum/Ajowan (H & U), Nankhah (P)	*Carum copticum, Trachyspermum ammi, Ptychotis ajowan*	Umbelliferae	Volatile oil: Thymol, Cumene, Terpene, Thymine, etc.
Cardamom, Cardamom seeds/Ilayachi (H & G)	*Elettaria cardamomum* var. *minuscula*	Zingiberaceae	Volatile oil: Cineole, Borneole, Terpene, Alcohols and Esters
Clove, Clove buds or flowers/Lavang (H), Laving (G), Long (U)	*Eugenia caryophyllus*	Myrtaceae	Volatile oil: Eugenol, Acetyl eugenol, Caryophyllenes, etc.
Nutmeg, Myristica/ Jayfal (G), Jaefal (U)	*Myristica fragrans*	Myrtaceae	Volatile oil and fixed oil, Myristicin, Borneole, etc.
Cinnamon/Dalchini (H & U), Taj (G)	*Cinnamomum zeylanicum*	Lauraceae	Volatile oil: Cinnamic aldehyde, Eugenol, etc.
Ginger, Zingiber/ Saunth (H), Soonth (G), Adrak (U)	*Zingiber officinale*	Zingiberaceae	Volatile oil, Gingerol, Gingerone, Zingiberol and Hydrocarbons
Black pepper/ Kali mirch (U), Golmirch	*Piper nigrum*	Piperaceae	Volatile oil, Hydrocarbons, Piperine

Common English/ Vernacular Name(s)	Biological Name	Family/N.O.	Main Active Constituent(s)
Asafoetida, Devil's dung/ Hing (H & G)	*Ferula foetida, F. rubricaulis* and other species of *Ferula*	Umbelliferae	Volatile oil, Resin and Gum, Ferulic acid, Umbellic acid and Umbelliferone

ASTRINGENT

Catechu: Pale/black Gambir/Cutch; Kattha (H & G)	*Uncaria gambier/ Acacia catechu*	Rubiaceae/ Legunimosae	Tannins, Catechins, Phlobatannins, Catechu, Tannic acid, Catechu red

DRUGS ACTING ON NERVOUS SYSTEM

Hyoscyamus (herb), Henbane/Khorasani Ajma (H)	*Hyoscyamus niger*	Solanaceae	Tropane alkaloids: Hyoscyamine, Hyoscine
Belladonna, Deadly nightshade leaves and roots/Sag-Angur Patti (H)	*Atropa belladonna*	Solanaceae	Tropane alkaloids: Atropine, Hyoscyamine, Apoatropine, Hyoscine
Stramonium leaves, Thorn apple leaves/ Jamestown weed	*Datura stramonim* and *Datura tatula*	Solanaceae	Tropane alkaloids: Hyoscyamine and Hyoscine
Withania/Ashwagandha	*Withania somnifera*	Solanaceae	Alkaloids and Steroid lactones
Ephedra, Ma-Huang/ Ephedra (H & U)	*Ephedra sinica* and other species of *Ephedra*	Gnetaceae/ Ephedraceae	Alkaloids: Ephedrine, Pseudoephedrine, Norephedrine
Aconite root, Monkshood/ Vachhnag (G)	*Aconitum nepallus*	Renunculaceae	Alkaloids: Aconine, Benzol aconine, Aconitine
Opium/Afim (H), Afin (G), Afyun (U)	*Papaver somniferum*	Papaveraceae	Opium alkaloids: Morphine, Codeine, Papaverine, Thebaine, etc.
Cannabis, Indian Hemp/ Hashish, Bhang, Ganja, Charas (H, G, U)	*Cannabis sativa*	Cannabinaceae	Resin contains Cannabidiol, Cannabidolic acid, Tetrahydrocannabinol and other constituents

Common English/ Vernacular Name(s)	Biological Name	Family/N.O.	Main Active Constituent(s)
Nux vomica/Kuchla (H), Zer kachuro (G)	*Strychnos nux vomica*	Loganiaceae	Alkaloids: Strychnine, Brucine, Vomicine

ANTI-HYPERTENSIVES

Rauwolfia, Snake root/ Sarpagandha, Chhotachand, Pagla ki Dawa (H & U)	*Rauwolfia serpentina*	Apocyanaceae	Alkaloids: Reserpine, Deserpidine, Serpentine, Rescinnamine, Ajmaline, Ajmalicine, etc.

ANTITUSSIVES

Vasaka leaves, Adhatoda/Adulasa, Sinhmukhi (H & U)	*Adhatoda vasica*	Acanthaceae	Alkaloids: Vasicine, Vasicinone, 6-Hydroxy vacicine and Volatile oil
Balsam Tolu, Tolu Balsam	*Myroxylon balsamum* (*M. toluifera*)	Leguminosae	Resin and Balsamic acids
Holy Basil/Tulsi, Surasa (H & G), Raihan (U & A)	*Ocimum sanctum*	Labiatae	Volatile oil, Eugenol, Methyl eugenol, Caryophyllene, etc.

ANTIRHEUMATICS

Gum Guggul, Indian Bdellium/Gugal, Gugul (S, H & G), Muqil (U)	*Commiphora wighti* (*C. mukul, Balsamo-dendron mukul*)	Burseraceae	Oleo-gum-resin and Steroids (Guggulo-sterols); also Flavonoids and Ellagic acid
Colchicum, Autumn Crocus Corm, Meadow Saffron Corm, Indian Colchicum Corm/ Surinjan (H & U)	*Colchicum autumnale* and *C. luteum*	Liliaceae	Alkaloids: Colchicine & Demicolcine and Colchicoresin

ANTITUMOURS

Catharanthus, Vinca, Madagascar perivinkle/ Baramasi (H & G)	*Catharanthus roseus* (*Vinca rosea*)	Apocyanaceae	Alkaloids: Vinblastine, Vincristine, Catharanthine, Vindoline, etc.

Common English/ Vernacular Name(s)	Biological Name	Family/N.O.	Main Active Constituent(s)
Indian Podophyllum	*Podophyllum hexandrum* (*P. emodi*)	Berberidaceae	Resin: Podophyllotoxin

ANTILEPROTICS

Chalmoogra oil, Hydnocarpus oil, Gynocardia oil	*Hydnocarpus wightiana, H. anthelmintica, H. heterophylla* and *Tarakto-genous kurzii*	Flacourtiaceae/ Bixaceae	Glycerides of fatty acids: Hydnocarpic acid, Chalmoogric acid, Gorlic acid

ANTIDIABETICS

Pterocarpus, Indian Kino Tree, Malabar Kino/ Bija (H), Vijasara, Biyo (G), Bijasara (S & U)	*Pterocarpus marsupium*	Leguminosae (Papilionaceae)	l-Epicatechin, Pterostibene, Essential oil and Fixed oil, Marsupol, Propterol and colouring matter
Gymnema/Gurhmar (H), Meshasringi (S & B), Kharak (A), Khar-e-khasak (P)	*Gymnema sylvestre* (Syn. *Asclepias geminate*)	Asclepiadaceae	Resin, Bitter principle, Gymnemic acid, Quercitol, Lupiol, Stigmasterol, Saponins, etc.

DIURETICS

Caltrop, Puncture vine, Cathead/Gokhru (small and large) (H & U)	*Tribulus terrestris/ Pedalium murex*	Zygophyllaceae	Mucilage, Saponins, Alkaloid, Fatty oil and Resin
Spreading hogweed/ Punarnava (S & Ger.), Godhaparna (H)	*Boerhaavia diffusa*	Nyctaginaceae	Punarvoside

ANTIDYSENTERICS

Ipecacuanha, Ipecac, Rio Ipecac, Johore or Brazilian Ipecac	*Cephaelis ipecacuanha* and *C. acuminata*	Rubiaceae	Alkaloids: Emetine, Cephaeline, Psychotrine, Psychotrine methyl ether

Common English/ Vernacular Name(s)	Biological Name	Family/N.O.	Main Active Constituent(s)
ANTISEPTICS AND DISINFECTANTS			
Benzoin/Loban (H & G)	*Styrax benzoin* and *S. parallelo-neurus*	Styraceae	Balsamic acids: Cinnamic and Benzoic acids and Resins
Myrrh/Bol (H), Hirabol (G)	*Commiphora molmol* and *C. abyssinica*	Burseraceae	Volatile oil, Gum and Resins
Margosa tree/Nim, Neem (H & U), Kohumba (G)	*Azadirachta indica* (Syn. *Melia Azadirachta*)	Meliaceae	Nimbin, Nimbidin, Nimbidiol, Carotenoides, Ascorbic acid
Curcuma, Turmeric/ Haldi (H & U), Zardchob (P)	*Curcuma domestica* (Syn. *C. longa*)	Zingiberaceae	Curcumin, Volatile oil and Resin
ANTIMALARIALS			
Cinchona, Countess bark, Jesuit's bark, Peruvian bark	*Cinchona calisaya* and other species of *Cinchona*	Rubiaceae	Alkaloids: Quinine, Quinidine, Cinchonine, Cinchonidine, etc. and Bitter Glycoside Quinovin
OXYTOCICS			
Ergot, Ergot of Rye	*Claviceps purpurea*	Clavicipitaceae	Alkaloids: Ergometrine, Ergotamine, Ergosine, etc.
VITAMINS			
Shark Liver Oil	*Hypoprion breverostris*	Carcharhinidae	Vitamin A, Glycerides of saturated and unsaturated acids
Embelic Myrobalan/ Amla (H & G), Amlaki (B), Amlah (U & P), Nelli (T), Amlaj (A)	*Emblica officinalis* (Syn. *Phyllanthus emblica*)	Euphorbiaceae	Vitamin C, Tannins: Gallic acid, Ellagici acid and Phyllembelin

Common English/ Vernacular Name(s)	Biological Name	Family/N.O.	Main Active Constituent(s)
ENZYMES			
Papaw, Papain/ Papaya (B, G & H), Pappali (T), Arand-Kharbuza (U)	*Carica papaya*	Caricaceae	Papain (Papayotin) (Papaya's pulp is rich in many other phytochemicals)
Diastase, Amylase	*Hordeum vulgare*	Gramineae	An amylase enzyme
Yeast, Faex medicinalis	*Saccharomyces cerevisiae*	Saccharo-mycetaceae	Vitamin B complex, Proteins and Glycogen
PERFUMES AND FLAVOURING AGENTS			
Peppermint Oil, Corn Mint/ Pudina (B, H, P & U)	*Mentha piperita* (*Mentha arvensis* var. *piperascens*)	Labiatae	Volatile oil: Menthol, Menthofuran, Menthone, Jasmon, etc.
Lemon Oil	*Citrus limonia*, *C. limon*	Rutaceae	Volatile oil: Citral, Citronellal, etc.
Orange Oil	*Citrus aurantium* var. *amara*, *C. sinensis*	Rutaceae	Volatile oil: Decanal, Lemonine
Lemon Grass Oil, East India Lemon Grass Oil, Indian Oil of Verbena	*Cymbopogon flexuosus* and *C. citratus*	*Gramineae*	Volatile oil: Citral
Sandal Wood Oil, White Sandalwood/ Safed Chandan (H)	*Santalum album*	Santalaceae	Volatile oil: Santalol
PHARMACEUTICAL AIDS			
Honey, Mel/Madhu (H), Shehad (U), Asal (A)	*Apis mellifica* and other species of *Apis*	Apidae	Invert Sugar (and Sucrose, Dextrin, Volatile oil)
Starch, Amylum, Wheat Starch, Maize Starch, Rice Starch and Potato Starch	*Triticum sativum*, *Zea mays*, *Oryza sativum* and *Solanum tuberosum*	Grarnineae and Solanaceae	Starch: Amylose and Amylopectin

Common English/ Vernacular Name(s)	Biological Name	Family/N.O.	Main Active Constituent(s)
Acacia, Gum Acacia or Arabic/Babul or Gond Kikar (H)	*Acacia senegal* and other species of *Acacia*	Leguminosae	Gum: Arabin (and Enzyme Oxidase)
Tragacanth Gum, Gum Dragon/Anjira (H)	*Astragalus gummifer* and species of *Astragalus*	Leguminosae	Gum: Bassorin and Tragacanthin
Guar Gum, Guaran/ Guar Gum	*Cyamompsis tetragonolobus*	Leguminosae	Mucilage – Polysaccharides
Pectin, Pectins	Citric fruits: *Citrus aurantium*, *C. limon*	Rutaceae	Pectins: Polymers of glycosidally combined Galacto-uronic acid
Sodium Alginate	*Laminaria* species, *Fucus* species and Brown Sea Weeds	Laminariaceae, Fucaceae, Phaeophyceae	Polysaccharide: Alginic acid
Agar, Agar-agar, Japanese Isinglass	*Gelidium*, *Gracilaria* and *Pterocladia* species	Gelidiaceae (Order Rhodophyceae)	Polysaccharides: Agarose and Agaropectin
Gelatin	Skin, Bones and Tendons of Ox and Sheep	Bovidae	Protein: Glutin
Arachis oil, Peanut oil, Groundnut oil/Fool Sudani Oil (A), Mongphali ka tel (H)	*Arachis hypogea*	Leguminosae	Fixed oil: Glycerides of higher fatty acids and protein with essential amino acids, etc.
Olive oil, Sweet oil, Salad oil/Zaitoon ka Tel (H & U)	*Olea europoea*	Oleaceae	Fixed oil: Glycerides, Fatty acids, Tocopherols, etc.
Beeswax, White or Yellow Beeswax/ Shamah al Nahl (A)	Honeycomb of Bee: *Apis mellifica* and other species of *Apis*	Apidae	Beeswax: Myricin, Cerotic acid, Myricyl and Ceryl alcohols

Common English/ Vernacular Name(s)	Biological Name	Family/N.O.	Main Active Constituent(s)
Lanolin, Wool Fat/ Soof al Kharoof (A)	*Ovis aries*	Bovidae	Wool Fat: Esters of cholesterol and isocholesterol with higher acids
Kaolin, China Clay, Porcelain Clay	Not from biological source	—	Pure Aluminium silicate

MISCELLANEOUS DRUGS

Common English/ Vernacular Name(s)	Biological Name	Family/N.O.	Main Active Constituent(s)
Liquorice, Licorice, Glycyrrhiza, Sweet root/ Mulethi (H), Jeth Madh (G), Asalassus (A & P)	*Glycyrrhiza glabra* and other species of *Glycerriza*	Leguminosae	Glycyrrhizin, Glycyrrhizinic acid, Liquiritin
Garlic/Lasun (H), Lasan (G)	*Allium sativum*	Liliaceae	Alliin
Picrorhiza/Kutki (H), Kadu (G)	*Picrorhiza kurroa*	Scrophulariacea	Picroside I and II and Kutkoside
Dioscorea, Yam, Mexican Yam	*Dioscorea deltioda, D. floribunda* and other species of *Dioscorea*	Dioscoreaceae	Diosgenin, Dioscin
Linseed, Flax Seed/ Alsi (H & U)	*Linum usitatissimum*	Linaceae	Mucilage, Fixed oil, Linamarin
Shatavari, Shakakul, Satavari (H), Satavar (G), Safaid Musli (U)	*Asparagus racemosus*	Liliaceae	Shatavarin I–IV and Starch
Shankhpushpi (H), Vishnukaranti (S), Shankhvalli (M)	*Convolvulus pluricaulis* (Syn. *C. microphyllus*) and *Evolvulus alsinoids*	Convolvulacea	Alkaloid: Shankhpushpine, Volatile oil and Betain and Alkaloid Evolvine
Pyrethrum, Pyrethrum Flowers, Insect Flowers	*Chrysanthemum cinerarifolium, C. roseus*	Compositae	(Oily) Pyrethrines Esters: Pyrethrine I & II, Cinerine I & II, Jasmoline I & II
Tobacco/Tambaku (H, B, G & U)	*Nicotiana tabacum, N. rustica*	Solanaceae	Alkaloids: Nicotine, Nicotyrine, Nomicotine

Common English/ Vernacular Name(s)	Biological Name	Family/N.O.	Main Active Constituent(s)

FIBRES, SUTURES AND SURGICAL DRESSINGS

These are mentioned under a separate chapter. They are included here to complete the classification of all materials.

Common English/ Vernacular Name(s)	Biological Name	Family/N.O.	Main Active Constituent(s)
Absorbent Cotton, Purified Cotton/ Kapas (B, H & S)	*Gossypium herbaceum* and other species of *Gossypium*	Malvaceae	Cellulose (Poly-saccharides of cellobiose units)
Silk	*Bombyx mori* and other species of *Bombyx* and *Antheraea*	Order Lepidoptera	Protein Fibroin
Wool, Animal Wool, Sheep's Wool	*Ovis aries*	Bovidae, Order Ungulata	Protein Keratin
Viscose Rayon	*Picea abies* (*P. excelsa*)	Pinaceae	Cellulose

Abbreviations: A, Arabic; B, Bengali; G, Gujarati; Ger., German; H, Hindi; L, Latin; M, Marathi; P, Persian; S, Sanskrit; T, Tamil; U, Urdu.

Taxonomic Classification of Drugs

Biological Name	Plant Part Used as Drug	Common Name/Phytochemical Class of Compounds
THALLOPHYTA		
ALGAE		
Fucaceae and Laminareacea	Extract	Sodium alginate/Polysaccharide
Gelidiaceae		
Gelidium species	Extract	Agar/Polysaccharide
Gracilaria species	Extract	Agar/Polysaccharide
Pterocladia species	Extract	Agar/Polysaccharide
FUNGI		
Saccharomyces cerevisiae	Yeast – Fungi	Yeast/Protein
Hypocreaceae		
Claviceps purpurea	Sclerotium	Ergot/Alkaloids
GNETACEAE (EPHEDRACEAE)		
Ephedra sinica	Aerial parts	
Ephedra equisetina	Aerial parts	Ephedra herb/Alkaloids
Ephedra gerardiana	Aerial parts	Indian Ephedra herb/Alkaloids
Ephedra nebrodensis	Aerial parts	Indian Ephedra herb/Alkaloids

Biological Name	Plant Part Used as Drug	Common Name/Phytochemical Class of Compounds

ANGIOSPERMAE
MONOCOTYLEDONS

GRAMINEAE

Biological Name	Plant Part Used as Drug	Common Name/Phytochemical Class of Compounds
Cymbopogon spp.	Fresh herb	Lemon grass oil/Volatile oil
Triticum sativum	Seed	Wheat starch/Polysaccharide
Oryza sativa	Seed	Rice starch/Polysaccharide
Zea mays	Seed	Maize starch/Polysaccharide

LILIACEAE

Biological Name	Plant Part Used as Drug	Common Name/Phytochemical Class of Compounds
Colchicum autumnale	Seed and corm	European Colchicum seed and corm/ Alkaloids
Colchicum luteum	Seed and corm	Indian Colchicum seed and corm/ Alkaloids
Aloe species	Dried extract	Aloe/Glycosides
Asparagus racemosus	Roots	Shatavari/Glycosides
Allium sativum	Bulb	Garlic/Volatile oil

ZINGIBERACEAE

Biological Name	Plant Part Used as Drug	Common Name/Phytochemical Class of Compounds
Elettaria cardamomum	Seeds (Fruits)	Cardamom seeds/Volatile oil
Zingiber officinale	Rhizomes	Ginger rhizome/Resins
Curcuma domestica	Rhizomes	Turmeric/Resins

DIOSCORIACEAE

Biological Name	Plant Part Used as Drug	Common Name/Phytochemical Class of Compounds
Dioscorea deltoidea and species	Rhizomes	Dioscorea/Glycosides (Saponins)

DICOTYLEDONS

CANNABINACEAE

Biological Name	Plant Part Used as Drug	Common Name/Phytochemical Class of Compounds
Cannabis sativa	Aerial parts	Cannabis/Resins

POLYGONACEAE

Biological Name	Plant Part Used as Drug	Common Name/Phytochemical Class of Compounds
Rheum palmatum, *R. emodi* and other species of *Rheum*	Rhizomes	Rhubarb – Indian Rhubarb/ Glycosides (Anthraquinones)

Biological Name	Plant Part Used as Drug	Common Name/Phytochemical Class of Compounds
RANNCULACEAE		
Aconitum napellus	Roots	Aconite/Alkaloids
Aconitum chasmanthum	Roots	Aconite/Alkaloids
Aconitum deinorrhizum	Roots	Aconite/Alkaloids
BERBERIDACEAE		
Podophyllum hexandrum	Rhizome (and roots)	Indian Podophyllum/Resins
PAPAVERACEAE		
Papaver somniferum	Capsule's latex	Opium/Alkaloids
LEGUMINOSAE		
Acacia arabica	Gummy exudate	Indian Acacia/Polysaccharide
Acacia senegal	Gummy exudate	Acacia gum/Polysaccharide
Acaica catechu	Dried extract	Catechu/Tannins (Catechins)
Astragalus gummifer	Gummy exudate	Tragacanth gum/Polysaccharide
Myroxylon balsamum	Resin extract	Balsam Tolu/Resin
Glycyrrhiza glabra	Stolons, roots	Glycyrrhiza, Licorice/ Glycosides (Saponins)
Cyamoposis tetragonolobus	Seed endosperm	Guar gum/Polysaccharide
Arachis hypogaea	Seed kernel	Arachis oil, Peanut oil/Fixed oil
PIPERACEA		
Piper nigrum		
ZYGOPHYLLADEAE		
Tribulus terrestris	Fruits	Small Gokhru/ Glycosides (Steroidal Saponins)
LINACEAE		
Linum usitatissimum	Seeds	Linseed/Fixed oil

Biological Name	Plant Part Used as Drug	Common Name/Phytochemical Class of Compounds
EUPHORBIACEAE		
Ricinus communis	Fruits	Castor oil/Fixed oil
Emblica officinalis	Fruits	Amla/Tannins and Vitamin C
RUTACEA		
Citrus arantium var. *amara*	Pericarp (rind)	Bitter orange peel/Volatile oil
Citrus chrysocarpa	Pericarp (rind)	Indian orange peel/Volatile oil
BURSERACEAE		
Commiphora molmol	Stem extract	Myrrh/Resin (Oleo-gum-resin)
MALVACEAE		
Gossypium herbaceum and other species of *Gossypium*	Epidermal trichomes of seed	Cotton/Polysaccharide (Cellulose)
FLACOURTIACEAE		
Hydnocarpus wightiana and other species of *Hydnocarpus*	Seeds	Chaulmoogra oil, Hydnocarpus oil/ Fixed oil
MYRTACEAE		
Eugenia caryophyllus	Unopened flowers	Cloves/Volatile oil
COMBRETACEAE		
Terminalia arjuna	Bark of stem	Arjuna/Tannins and Saponins
MYRISTICACEAE		
Myristica fragrans	Seed – Kernel	Nutmeg seed/Volatile oil
Myristica fragrans	Seed – Arillus	Mace/Volatile oil
UMBELLIFERAE		
Foeniculum vulgare	Fruits	Fennel/Volatile oil
Carum opticum	Fruits	Ajowan/Volatile oil

Biological Name	Plant Part Used as Drug	Common Name/Phytochemical Class of Compounds
Coriandrum sativum	Fruits	Coriander/Volatile oil
Ferula foetida and other species of *Ferula*	Rhizome and root exudate	Asafoetida/Volatile oil, resin and gum

STYRACEAE

Styrax benzoin	Stem exudate	Sumatra benzoin/Balsamic resin
Styrax paralleloneuru	Stem exudate	Sumatra benzoin/Balsamic resin
Styrax tonkinensis	Stem exudate	Siam benzoin/Balsamic resin

LOGANIACEAE

Strychnos nux vomica	Seeds	Nux vomica/Alkaloids

APOCYNACEAE

Rauwolfia serpentina	Roots	Rauwolfia/Alkaloids
Catharanthus roseus	Entire plant	Catharanthus/Alkaloids

NYCTAGINEAE

Boerhavia diffusa	Herb	Punarnava/Alkaloid (Punarnavine)

RUBIACEAE

Cinchona species	Stem and root bark	Cinchona/Alkaloids
Cephaelis ipecacuanha	Root and rhizome	Rio ipecac/Alkaloids
Cephaelis acuminata	Root and rhizome	Cartagena ipecac/Alkaloids
Uncaria gambier	Dried extract of leaves and shoots	Pale Catechu/Tannins – Catechol tannins or Phlobatannins

CONVOLVULACEAE .

Convolvulus pluricaulis	Herb	Shankhpushpi/Alkaloids
Evolvulus alsinoides	Herb	Shankhpushpi/Alkaloids

LABIATAE

Ocimum sanctum	Leaves	Tulsi/Volatile oil
Mentha piperita	Aerial parts	Peppermint or Mentha oil/ Volatile oil

Biological Name	Plant Part Used as Drug	Common Name/Phytochemical Class of Compounds
SOLANACEAE		
Hyoscyamus niger	Herb	Hyoscyamus/Alkaloids
Hyoscyamus muticus	Herb	Egyptian Henbane/Alkaloids
Atropa species	Herb and roots	Belladonna herb and root/Alkaloids
Solanum tuberosum	Potato tubers	Potato starch/Polysaccharide
Withania somnifera	Roots and stem	Withania/Alkaloids and steroids
Nicotiana tabacum	Leaves	Tobacco/Alkaloids
SCROPHULARIACEAE		
Digitalis purpurea	Leaves	Digitalis, Foxglove/Glycosides
Digitalis lanata	Leaves	Digitalis (Lanata)/Glycosides
Picrorhiza kurroa	Stolons and rhizomes	Picrorhiza (Indian Gentian)/ Glycosides (Picrosides)
ACANTHACEAE		
Adhatoda vasica	Leaves	Adhatoda, Vasaka/Alkaloids
PEDALIACEAE		
Pedalium murex	Fruits	Large Gokhru/Alkaloid and resin
PLANTAGINACEAE		
Plantago ovata	Seeds (Husk)	Ispaghula/Carbohydrates (Mucilage)
COMPOSITAE		
Chrysanthemum cinerarifolium	Flowers	Pyrethrum, Insect Flowers/ Pyrethrines
LAURACEAE		
Cinnamomum zeylanicum	Stem bark	Ceylon Cinnamon/Volatile oil
Cinnamom cassia	Stem bark	Cassia/Volatile oil
CARICACEAE		
Carica papaya	Fruits (unripe)	Papaya/Proteolytic enzymes

Biological Name	Plant Part Used as Drug	Common Name/Phytochemical Class of Compounds
OLEACEAE		
Olea europaea	Fruits	Olive oil/Fixed oil
MELIACEAE		
Azadirachta indica Syn. *Melia azadirachta*	Leaves (Twigs)	Neem/Bitter Principles (Nimbidin)
APIDAE		
Apis mellifica	Flowers	Honey, Mel/Carbohydrate
Apis mellifica	Honeycomb	Beeswax/Wax (Myricin)
CARCHARHINIDAE		
Hypoprion brevirostris and other allied species	Livers (of Shark)	Shark liver oil/Vitamins and Fatty acids
BOVIDAE		
Ovis aries	Sheep wool	Lanolin/Wool fat
Various animals (Bovidae Family)	Skin, bones and tendons	Gelatin/Protein (Glutin)

Chemical Classification of Drugs (Included in ER 1991)

1. CARBOHYDRATES AND ORGANIC ACIDS
- **Soluble Saccharides:** Honey
- **Polysaccharides:** Starch, Sodium alginate
- **Mucilage:** Ispaghula seed, Ispaghula husk, Linseed, Agar
- **Gums:** Gum acacia, Gum tragacanth, Indian acacia, Guar gum
- **Cellulose:** Cotton
- **Organic acids:** Tamarind

2. GLYCOSIDES
- **Anthraquinone glycosides:** Senna leaves, Senna pods, Rhubarb, Aloe
- **Cardiac glycosides:** Digitalis leaves
- **Saponin glycosides:** Arjuna bark, Glycyrrhiza, Dioscorea, Shatavari, Gokhru
- **Bitters and bitter glycosides:** Picrorhiza

3. TANNINS
- Pale catechu, Black catechu, Amla (also contains Vit. C)

4. VOLATILE OILS
- Cinnamon bark, Bitter orange peel, Cassia bark, Nutmeg, Mace, Fennel, Ajowain, Coriander, Cardamom, Clove, Ginger, Lemon peel, Tulsi, Garlic, Peppermint oil, Lemon grass oil, Sandalwood oil

5. FIXED OILS, FATS AND WAXES
- Castor oil, Arachis oil, Chaulmoogra oil, Shark liver oil, Lanolin, Beeswax

6. RESINS
- **Balsams:** Balsam of Tolu, Sumatra benzoin, Siam benzoin

- **Gum resins:** Asafoetida, Myrrh
- **Lignans:** Indian podophyllum (included as an anti-cancer drug with Vinca)
- **Miscellaneous resins:** Cannabis, Ginger, Turmeric, Java turmeric

7. PROTEINS
- Gelatin, Yeast

8. ALKALOIDS
- **Pyrrolidine, pyridine and piperidine alkaloids:** Nicotiana, Peppers
- **Tropane alkalolds:** Belladonna herb, Belladonna root, Hyoscyamus herb, Stramonium herb, Datura herb, Indian belladonna, Withania
- **Quinoline alkaloids:** Cinchona bark
- **Isoquinoline alkaloids:** Opium, Ipecac root
- **Indole alkaloids:** Ergot, Nux vomica seeds, Rauwolfia, Catharanthus
- **Quinazoline alkaloids:** Vasaka leaves
- **Alkylamine alkaloids:** Ephedra, Colchicum seed, Colchicum corm, Indian colchicum seed, Indian colchicum corm
- **Unknown structure alkaloids:** Punamava, Shankhpushpi

9. ESTERS
- Pyrethrum

10. VITAMINS
- Shark liver oil, Amla

11. ENZYMES
- Papaya, Diastase, Yeast

12. MINERALS
- Kaolin.

Medical Glossary

Since the drugs included in the syllabus are classified according to the therapeutic efficacy, it is considered more prudent to append a relevent required medical glossary, as given below.

Addison's disease: Deficient secretion of aldosterone and cortisol from the adrenal cortex, causing electrolytic upset, diminution of blood volume, lowered blood pressure, marked anaemia, hypoglycaemia, muscular weakness, gastrointestinal upsets and pigmentation of skin.

Adrenergic: Term applied to sympathetic nerves which liberate adrenaline from their terminations. Opposite to cholinergic.

Allergy: An altered or exaggerated susceptibility to various foreign substances or physical agents which are harmless to the great majority of individuals. It is due to an antigen-antibody reaction, though the antibody formed is not always demonstrable. Hay fever, asthma, urticaria and infantile eczema are allergic conditions.

Anaesthesia: Loss of sensation, general anaesthesia, loss of sensation with loss of consciousness; in local anaesthesia, the nerve conduction is blocked and painful impulses fail to reach the brain.

Analgesic: Insensible to pain; alleviating pain; a drug which relieves pain.

Androgens: Hormones secreted by the testes and adrenal cortex or synthetic substances which control the building up of the protein and the male secondary sex characteristics.

Antagonist: A muscle that relaxes to allow the agonist to perform a movement. When applied to a drug it is one which blocks, nullifies or reverses the effects of another drug.

Anticholinesterase: Enzyme that destroys acetylcholine at the nerve endings. Used for reversing the effects of muscle relaxant drugs.

Anti-inflammatory: Any agent which prevents inflammation.

Antimalarials: Any measure taken to prevent or suppress malaria.

Antimitotic: Any agent which prevents reproduction of cell by mitosis.

Antiphlogistic: Acting against heat, or inflammation.

Antipyretic: Any agent which allays or reduces fever.

Antispasmodic: Any measure used to relieve spasm occurring in muscle.

Antitussive: Any measure which suppresses cough.

Arrhythmia: Any deviation from the normal rhythm, e.g. of the heart.

Arthritis: Inflammation of a joint.

Asthma: Paroxyrnal attack of difficulty in breathing. Bronchial asthma – attack of breathlessness associated with bronchial obstruction or spasm, and characterized by expiratory wheeze. Cardiac asthma – paroxysmal dyspnoea in left ventricular failure.

Astringent: Any agent which contracts organic tissue, thus lessening secretion.

Bronchitis: Inflammation of the bronchi; may be primary or seconday, acute or chronic; the latter can cause right-sided heart failure, especially when associated with gross emphysema.

Bronchodilator: Any agent which dilates the bronchi.

Cancer: A general term which covers many malignant growths in many parts of the body. The growth is purposeless and parasitic, and flourishes at the expense of human host. Characteristics are the tendency to cause local destruction to spread by metastasis, to recover after removal, and to cause toxaemia.

Carcinoma: A malignant tumour of skin of mucous membrane.

Cardiovascular: Pertaining to the heart and blood vessels.

Cathartic: Purgative.

Cholinergic: Applied to parasympathetic nerves which liberate acetyl-choline at their terminations.

Choriocarcinoma: See chorionepithelioma.

Chorionepithelioma: A highly malignant tumour arising from chorionic cells, usually after a hydatiform mole, but may follow abortion or even normal pregnancy, quickly metastasizing especially to the lungs. Cytotoxic drugs have improved the prognosis.

Colitis: Inflammation of the colon. May be acute or chronic, and may be accompanied by ulcerative lesion.

Constipation: An implied chronic condition of infrequent and often difficult evacuation of faeces due to insufficient food or food intake, or to sluggish or disordered action of the bowel musculature of nerve supply, or to habitual failure to empty the rectum. Acute constipation signifies obstruction or paralysis of the gut of sudden onset.

Contraceptive: An agent used to prevent conception.

Convulsions: Involuntary contraction of muscles resulting from abnormal cerebral stimulation from many causes. Occur with or without loss of consciousness.

Cycloplegia: Paralysis of the ciliary muscle of the eye.

Demulcent: A slippery, mucilaginous fluid which allays irritation and soothes inflammation, especially of mucous membranes.

Diaphoretic: An agent which induces perspiration.

Diarrhoea: Deviation from established bowel rhythm characterized by an increase in frequency and fluidity of the stools.

Diuretic: Increasing the flow of urine.

Dysentery: Inflammation of the bowel with evacuation of blood and mucus, accompanied by tenesmus and colic. Amoebic dysentery is caused by protozoon *Entamoeba histolytica*.

Eclampsia: Severe manifestation of toxaemia of pregnancy, associated with fits and coma. Also a sudden convulsive attack.

Emetic: Any agent used to produce vomiting.

Emmenagogue: Medicine intended to restore, or to bring on, the menses.

Expectorant: A drug which promotes or increases the elimination of secretion from respiratory tract by coughing.

Galactorrhoea: Excessive flow of milk. Usually reserved for abnormal or inappropriate secretion of milk.

Glaucoma: A condition where the intraocular pressure is raised. In the acute stage the pain is severe.

Gout: A form of metabolic disorder in which sodium biurate is deposited in the cartilages of the joints, the ears, and elsewhere.

Haemorrhage: The escape of blood from a vessel. Arterial, capillary, venous designate the type of vessels from which it escapes.

Hypertension (Hyperpiesis): Abnormally high tension, by custom alluding to blood pressure and involving systolic and/or diastolic levels. There is no universal agreement on their upper limits of normal, but many cardialogists consider a resting systolic pressure of 160 mmHg and/or a resting diastolic pressure of 100 mmHg to be pathological. The cause may be renal, endocrine, mechanical, or toxic.

Hypnotic: A drug which produces a sleep resembling natural sleep.

Hypotension: Low blood pressure (systolic below 110 mmHg, diastolic below 70 mmHg). May be primary, secondary (e.g. shock, Addison's disease) or postural.

Leukaemia: The leukaemias are now called malignant reticuloses. Blood disease in which the white cells are abnormal in type or number. Classification is according to the kind of leucocyte found and whether the condition is acute or chronic. Acute leukaemia is a rapidly fatal illness, with haemorrhages, ulcerative lesions in the mouth and anaemia.

Lymphosarcoma: A malignant tumour arising from lymphatic tissue.

Myasthenia: Muscular weakness.

Myasthenia gravis: A disorder characterized by marked fatiguability of voluntary muscles, especially those of the eye.

Mydriasis: Abnormal dilation of the pupil of the eye. Drugs which cause mydriasis – mydriatics.

Narcosis: Unconsciousness produced by a drug.

Narcotic: A drug which produces abnormally deep sleep.

Nausea: A feeling of sickness without actual vomiting.

Neoplasm: A new growth; a tumour. Antineoplastic refers to those agents which act against a tumour.

Neurasthenia: A frequently misused term, the precise meaning of which is an uncommon nervous condition consisting of lassitude, inertia, fatigue and loss of initiatives. Restless fidgeting, oversensitivity, undue irritability and often an asthenic physique are also present.

Neuroblastoma: Malignant tumour arising in adrenal medulla from tissues of sympathetic origin. Most cases show a raised urinary catecholamine excretion.

Neuropsychiatry: The combination of neurology and psychiatry. Speciality dealing with organic and functional disease.

Oedema: Abnormal infiltration of tissues with fluid. Cardiac oedema is a dependent oedema of subcutaneous tissues in cardiac failure. Hepatic oedema is caused by osmotic pressure changes in the blood. Pulmonary oedema is a form of waterlogging of the lungs because of left ventricular failure or mitral stenosis. Renal oedema results from disturbed kidney filtration in nephritis.

Ophthalmics: Pertaining to the eye.

Oxytocic: Hastening parturition; an agent promoting uterine contractions.

Parkinsonism: A syndrome of mask-like expression, shuffling gaits, tremor of the limbs and pill-rolling movements of the fingers. Can be drug induced.

Peristalsis: The characteristic movement of the intestines by which the contents are moved along the lumen. It consists of a wave of contraction preceded by the wave of relaxation.

Postpartum: After a birth, after delivery.

Prophylaxis: Prevention or a guarding.

Pyorrhoea: A flow of pus, usually referring to that from teeth sockets. Pyorrhoea alveolaris.

Rheumatoid: Rheumatoid arthritis; a disease of unknown aetiology, characterized by the chronic polyarthritis mainly affecting the smaller peripheral joints, accompanied by general ill-health and resulting eventually in varying degrees of crippling joint, deformities and associated muscle wasting. It is not just a disease of joints. Every system may be involved in some way. Many rheumatologists, therefore, prefer the term "rheumatoid disease". There is some question of it being an autoimmune process. Rheumatoid factors, macro g-globulins found in most people wth severe rheumatoid arthritis. They affect not only joints but lung and nerve tissues and small arteries. It is not yet known whether the organism is the cause of, or the result of, arthritis.

Sclerosis: Term used in pathology to describe abnormal hardening or fibrosis of a tissue – sclerotic. A variably progressive disease of the nervous system, most commonly first affecting young adults, in which patchy, degenerative changes occur in nerve sheath in the brain, spinal cord, and optic nerves, followed by sclerosis. The presenting symptoms can be diverse, ranging from diplopia to weakness or unsteadiness of a limb; disturbances of micturition are common.

Sedative: An agent which lessens functional activity.

Spastic: A condition of muscular rigidity or spasm.

Stomatitis: Inflammation of the mouth.

Sympathetic: A portion of the autonomic nervous system. It is composed of a chain of ganglia on either side of the vertebral column in the thoracolumbar region, and sends fibres to all plain muscle tissue.

Sympathomimetic: Capable of producing changes similar to those produced by stimulation of the sympathetic nerves.

Syndrome: A group of symptoms and/or signs which, occurring together, produce a pattern or symptom complex, typical of a particular disease.

Toxaemia: A generalized poisoning of the body by the products of bacteria or damaged tissues.

Tranquillizers: Do not affect a basic disease; but reduce symptoms so that the patient feels more comfortable and is more accessible to help from psychotherapy.

Ulcer: An open sore on the body surface. Curling's ulcer – a peptic ulcer, associated with extensive burns and scalds. Penetrating ulcer – one which is locally invasive and may erode blood vessels, causing haematemesis or melaena in the case of gastric or duodenal ulcer. Peptic ulcer occurs in the stomach (gastric ulcer); duodenal ulcer occurs in the duodenum. Perforating ulcer – one which erodes through the walls of an organ.

Vasoconstrictor: Any agent which causes a narrowing of the lumen of blood vessels.

Vasodilator: An agent which causes the widening of the lumen of the blood vessels.

Index

A